# Clinical Electrocardiography
## a Simplified Approach

# Clinical Electrocardiography

## a Simplified Approach

### Seventh Edition

**Ary L. Goldberger, MD, FACC**
Professor of Medicine,
Harvard Medical School
Director, Arrhythmia Monitoring Laboratory,
Beth Israel Deaconess Medical Center
Boston, Massachusetts

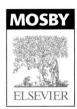

MOSBY

ELSEVIER

1600 John F. Kennedy Boulevard
Suite 1800
Philadelphia, PA 19103-2899

CLINICAL ELECTROCARDIOGRAPHY: A SIMPLIFIED APPROACH     ISBN-13: 978-0-323-04038-9
ISBN-10: 0-323-04038-1

---

**Notice**

Knowledge and best practice in this field are constantly changing. As new research and experience broaden our knowledge, changes in practice, treatment and drug therapy may become necessary or appropriate. Readers are advised to check the most current information provided (i) on procedures featured or (ii) by the manufacturer of each product to be administered, to verify the recommended dose or formula, the method and duration of administration, and contraindications. It is the responsibility of the practitioner, relying on their own experience and knowledge of the patient, to make diagnoses, to determine dosages and the best treatment for each individual patient, and to take all appropriate safety precautions. To the fullest extent of the law, neither the Publisher nor the Author assumes any liability for any injury and/or damage to persons or property arising out or related to any use of the material contained in this book.

The Publisher

---

Previous editions copyrighted 1999, 1994, 1990, 1986, 1981, 1977.

ISBN-13: 978-0-323-04038-9
ISBN-10: 0-323-04038-1

*Acquisitions Editor:* Susan Pioli
*Developmental Editor:* Joan Ryan

Working together to grow
libraries in developing countries

www.elsevier.com | www.bookaid.org | www.sabre.org

ELSEVIER     BOOK AID International     Sabre Foundation

Printed in China

Last digit is the print number:   9   8   7   6   5   4   3   2   1

**FOR**
Ellen, Zach, and Lexy
and for my mother, Blanche Goldberger,
**with love**

# PREFACE

This book is an introduction to electrocardiography. It is written particularly for medical students, house staff, and nurses, and it assumes no previous instruction in ECG reading. The book has been widely used in introductory courses on the subject. Clinicians wishing to review basic electrocardiography have also found it useful.

This new edition is divided into four parts. Part 1 covers the basic principles of electrocardiography, normal ECG patterns, and the major abnormal depolarization (P-QRS) and repolarization (ST-T-U) patterns. Part 2 describes the major abnormalities of heart rhythm and conduction. Part 3 presents an overview and review of the material. Part 4 is primarily a set of unknowns for review and self-assessment. In addition, practice questions are presented at the end of almost all chapters. In reading ECGs, as in learning a new language, fluency is attained only with repetition and review.

The clinical applications of ECG reading have been stressed throughout the book. Each time an abnormal pattern is mentioned, the conditions that might have produced it are discussed. Although the book is not intended to be a manual of therapeutics, general principles of treatment and clinical management are briefly discussed. Separate chapters are devoted to important special topics, including electrolyte and drug effects, cardiac arrest, the limitations and uses of the ECG, and electrical devices, including pacemakers and implantable cardioverter defibrillators (ICDs).

In addition, students are encouraged to approach ECGs in terms of a rational simple differential diagnosis rather than through the tedium of rote memorization. It is comforting for most students to discover that the number of possible arrhythmias that can produce a heart rate of more than 200 beats per minute is limited to just a handful of choices. Only three basic ECG patterns are found with cardiac arrest. Similarly, only a limited number of conditions cause low-voltage patterns, abnormally wide QRS complexes, and so forth.

In approaching any given ECG, "three and a half" essential questions must always be addressed: What does the ECG show and what else could it be? What are the possible causes of this pattern? What, if anything, should be done about it? Most conventional ECG books focus on the first question ("What is it?"), emphasizing pattern recognition. However, waveform analysis is only a first step, for example, in the clinical diagnosis of atrial fibrillation. The following questions must also be considered: What is the differential diagnosis? ("What else could it be?"). Are you sure the ECG actually shows atrial fibrillation, and not another "look-alike pattern," such as multifocal atrial tachycardia, sinus rhythm with atrial premature beats, or even an artifact due to parkinsonian tremor? What could have caused the arrhythmia? Treatment ("What to do?"), of course, depends in part on the answers to these questions.

The continuing aim of this book, therefore, is to present the ECG as it is used in hospital wards, outpatient clinics, emergency departments, and intensive care units, where recognition of normal and abnormal patterns is only the starting point in patient care.

The seventh edition contains updated discussions on multiple topics, including arrhythmias and conduction disturbances, cardiac arrest and sudden death, myocardial ischemia and infarction, drug toxicity, pacemakers, and implantable cardioverter-defibrillators (ICDs). Common pitfalls in ECG interpretation are highlighted. Review questions throughout the text have been revised and updated.

This new edition also includes laminated cards on differential diagnosis for "instant" reference and review.

This edition is dedicated to the memory of my father, Emanuel Goldberger, MD, a pioneer in the development of electrocardiography and the inventor of the $aV_R$, $aV_L$, and $aV_F$ leads. He was coauthor of the first five editions of this textbook.

Finally, I want to thank my students and colleagues for their input and particularly for their challenging questions over the years. I am most grateful to my son, Zach Goldberger, MD, for his many helpful suggestions and comments in the preparation of this new edition.

Ary L. Goldberger, MD

# CONTENTS

# Basic Principles and Patterns

# 1

# Introductory Principles

The *electrocardiogram* (*ECG* or *EKG*) is a graph that records the electrical activity of the heart.

The ECG records these cardiac electrical currents (voltages, potentials) by means of metal *electrodes* placed on the surface of the body.* These metal electrodes are placed on the arms, legs, and chest wall (precordium).

## BASIC CARDIAC ELECTROPHYSIOLOGY

Before the basic ECG patterns are discussed, some elementary aspects of cardiac electrophysiology must be reviewed. Fortunately, only certain simple principles are required for clinical interpretation of ECGs.

The function of the heart is to contract rhythmically and pump blood to the lungs for oxygenation and then to pump this oxygenated blood into the general (systemic) circulation. The signal for cardiac contraction is the spread of electrical currents through the heart muscle. These currents are produced both by *pacemaker*

*As discussed in Chapter 3, the ECG actually records the *differences* in potential between these electrodes.

*cells* and *specialized conducting tissue* within the heart and by the working *heart muscle* itself.

The ECG records only the currents produced by the working heart muscle.

## ELECTRICAL STIMULATION OF THE HEART

In simplest terms, the heart can be thought of as an electrically timed pump. The electrical "wiring" of the heart is outlined in Figure 1-1. Normally, the signal for cardiac electrical stimulation starts in the *sinus node,* also called the *sinoatrial (SA) node.* This node is located in the right atrium near the opening of the superior vena cava. It is a small collection of specialized cells capable of automatically generating an electrical stimulus (signal). From the sinus node, this stimulus spreads first through the right atrium and then into the left atrium. Thus the sinus node functions as the normal *pacemaker* of the heart.

The first phase of cardiac muscle activation is electrical stimulation of the right and left atria. This in turn signals the atria to contract and pump blood simultaneously through the tricuspid and mitral valves into the right and left ventricles. The electrical stimulus then spreads to specialized conduction tissues in the

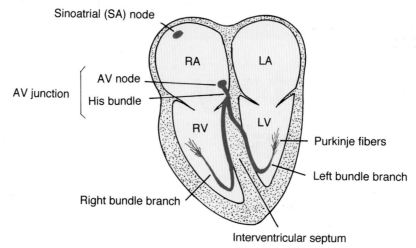

**FIGURE 1-1**   Normally, the cardiac stimulus is generated in the *sinoatrial (SA) node,* which is located in the *right atrium (RA).* The stimulus then spreads through the *RA* and *left atrium (LA).* Next, it spreads through the *atrioventricular (AV)* node and the *bundle of His,* which comprise the *AV junction.* The stimulus then passes into the *left* and *right ventricles (LV and RV)* by way of the *left* and *right bundle branches,* which are continuations of the bundle of His. Finally, the cardiac stimulus spreads to the ventricular muscle cells through the *Purkinje fibers.*

*atrioventricular* (AV) *junction,* which includes the *AV node* and *bundle of His,* and then into the *left* and *right bundle branches,* which transmit the stimulus to the ventricular muscle cells.

The AV junction, which acts as a sort of electrical "bridge" connecting the atria and ventricles, is located at the base of the interatrial septum and extends into the interventricular septum (see Fig. 1-1). The upper (proximal) part of the AV junction is the AV node. (In some texts, the terms *AV node* and *AV junction* are used synonymously.) The lower (distal) part of the AV junction is called the *bundle of His* after the physiologist who described it. The bundle of His then divides into two main branches: the right bundle branch, which distributes the stimulus to the right ventricle, and the left bundle branch,* which distributes the stimulus to the left ventricle (see Fig. 1-1).

---

*The left bundle branch has two major subdivisions called *fascicles.* (These small bundles are discussed in Chapter 7 along with the *hemiblocks.*)

The electrical stimulus spreads simultaneously down the left and right bundle branches into the *ventricular myocardium* (ventricular muscle) by way of specialized conducting cells called *Purkinje fibers.* These fibers are located in the ventricular myocardium.

Under normal circumstances, when the sinus node is pacing the heart (normal sinus rhythm), the AV junction appears to serve primarily as a shuttle, directing the electrical stimulus into the ventricles. Under some circumstances, however, the AV junction can also act as an independent pacemaker of the heart. For example, if the sinus node fails to function properly, the AV junction can act as an *escape* pacemaker. In such cases, an AV junctional rhythm (and *not* sinus rhythm) is present. This produces a distinct ECG pattern (see Chapter 14).

Just as the spread of electrical stimuli through the atria leads to atrial contraction, so the spread of stimuli through the ventricles leads to ventricular contraction, with pumping of blood to the lungs and into the general circulation.*

## CARDIAC CONDUCTIVITY AND AUTOMATICITY

The speed with which electrical impulses are conducted through different parts of the heart varies. For example, conduction is *slowest* through the AV node and *fastest* through the Purkinje fibers. The relatively slow conduction speed through the AV node is of functional importance because it allows the ventricles time to fill with blood before the signal for cardiac contraction arrives.

In addition to *conductivity*, a major electrical feature of the heart is *automaticity*. Automaticity refers to the capacity of certain cardiac cells to function as pacemakers by spontaneously generating electrical impulses that spread throughout the heart. As mentioned earlier, the sinus node normally is the primary pacemaker of the heart because of its inherent automaticity. Under special conditions, however, other cells outside the sinus node (in the atria, AV junction, or ventricles) can also act as independent pacemakers. For example, if the automaticity of the sinus node is depressed, the AV junction can act as a backup (escape) pacemaker.

The term *sick sinus syndrome* is used clinically to describe patients who have severe depression of sinus node function (see Chapter 20). These patients may experience light-headedness or even syncope (fainting) because of excessive *bradycardia* (slow heartbeat). (Sick sinus syn-

drome and other causes of bradycardia are discussed in Part 2 in the section on cardiac arrhythmias.)

In other conditions, the automaticity of pacemakers outside the sinus node may be abnormally increased, and these *ectopic* (non-sinus) pacemakers may compete with the sinus node for control of the heartbeat. A rapid run of ectopic beats results in an abnormal *tachycardia*. (Ectopy is also discussed in detail in Part 2.)

If you understand the normal physiologic stimulation of the heart, you have the basis for understanding the abnormalities of heart rhythm and conduction that produce distinctive ECG patterns. For example, failure of the sinus node to stimulate the heart properly can result in various rhythm disturbances associated with sick sinus syndrome. Blockage of the spread of stimuli through the AV junction can produce various degrees of AV heart block (see Chapter 17). Disease of the bundle branches can produce left or right bundle branch block (see Chapter 7). Finally, any disease process that involves the ventricular muscle itself (e.g., injury of the heart muscle by myocardial infarction) can produce marked changes in the normal ECG patterns.

The first part of this book is devoted to explaining the basis of the normal ECG and then examining the major conditions that cause abnormal depolarization (P and QRS) and repolarization (ST-T and U) patterns. (This alphabet of ECG terms is defined in Chapter 2.) The second part is devoted to describing various abnormal rhythms and AV conduction disturbances (arrhythmias). The third part is a review and extension of material covered in earlier chapters. The fourth part is a collection of "unknowns" for self-assessment. In addition, review questions are included at the end of each chapter. Selected publications are cited in the Bibliography, including freely available online resources.

---

*The initiation of cardiac contraction by electrical stimulation is referred to as *electromechanical coupling*. A key part of this contractile mechanism is the release of calcium ions inside the atrial and ventricular heart muscle cells, which is triggered by the spread of electrical activation.

## REVIEW

An *electrocardiogram* (*ECG* or *EKG*) records the electrical voltages (potentials) produced in the heart. It does this by means of metal *electrodes* (connected to an electrocardiograph) placed on the patient's chest wall and extremities. The potentials recorded on the ECG are produced by the working atrial and ventricular muscle fibers themselves.

Normally, the cardiac stimulus starts in pacemaker cells of the *sinus node,* also called the *sinoatrial (SA) node,* located high in the right atrium near the opening of the superior vena cava. From there the stimulus spreads downward and to the left, through the right and left atria, and reaches the *atrioventricular (AV) node,* located near the top of the interventricular septum (see Fig. 1-1). After a delay, the stimu-

lus spreads through the *AV junction* (*AV node* and *bundle of His*). The bundle of His then subdivides into *right* and *left bundle branches.* The right bundle branch runs down the interventricular septum and into the right ventricle. From there the small *Purkinje fibers* rapidly distribute the stimulus outward into the main muscle mass of the right ventricle. Simultaneously, the left main bundle branch carries the stimulus down the interventricular septum to the muscle mass of the left ventricle, also by way of the Purkinje fibers.

This repetitive sequence of stimulation of the heart is the normal basic process. Disturbances in this process may produce abnormalities of heart rhythm, termed *cardiac arrhythmias.*

## QUESTIONS

1. Label the major parts of the cardiac conduction system shown in this diagram; then trace the spread of the normal cardiac stimulus from the atria to the ventricles.

2. What is an electrocardiogram?

3. *True* or *false.* The ECG directly records only the electrical activity of working heart muscle cells, not that of the pacemaker cells or of the specialized conduction system.

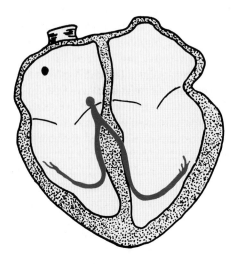

## CHAPTER 2

# Basic ECG Waves

## DEPOLARIZATION AND REPOLARIZATION

In Chapter 1, the general term electrical *stimulation* was applied to the spread of electrical stimuli through the atria and ventricles. The technical term for this cardiac electrical stimulation or activation is *depolarization.* The return of heart muscle cells to their resting state after stimulation (depolarization) is called *repolarization.* These terms are derived from the fact that normal "resting" myocardial cells (atrial and ventricular cells) are polarized; that is, they carry electrical charges on their surface. Figure 2-1*A* shows the resting polarized state of a normal atrial or ventricular heart muscle cell. Notice that the outside of the resting cell is positive and the inside is negative (about –90 mV [millivolts]).*

When a heart muscle cell is stimulated, it depolarizes. As a result, the outside of the cell, in the area where the stimulation has occurred, becomes negative and the inside of the cell becomes positive. This produces a difference in electrical voltage on the outside surface of the cell between the stimulated depolarized area

and the unstimulated polarized area (Fig. 2-1*B*). Consequently, a small electrical current forms and spreads along the length of the cell as stimulation and depolarization occur, until the entire cell is depolarized (Fig. 2-1*C*). The path of depolarization can be represented by an arrow, as shown in Figure 2-1*B*. For individual myocardial cells (fibers), depolarization and repolarization proceed in the same direction. For the entire myocardium, however, depolarization proceeds from the innermost layer (endocardium) to the outermost layer (epicardium), whereas repolarization proceeds in the opposite direction. The mechanism of this difference is not fully understood.

The depolarizing electrical current is recorded by the ECG as a *P wave* (when the atria are stimulated and depolarize) and as a *QRS complex* (when the ventricles are stimulated and depolarize).

After a time, the fully stimulated and depolarized cell begins to return to the resting state. This is known as *repolarization.* A small area on the outside of the cell becomes positive again (Fig. 2-1*D*), and the repolarization spreads along the length of the cell until the entire cell is once again fully repolarized. Ventricular repolarization is recorded by the ECG as the *ST segment, T wave,* and *U wave.* (Atrial repolarization is usually obscured by ventricular potentials.)

The ECG records the electrical activity of a large mass of atrial and ventricular cells, not

---

*Membrane polarization is due to differences in the concentration of ions inside and outside the cell. See the Bibliography for references that present the basic electrophysiology of the *resting membrane potential* and *cellular depolarization* and *repolarization* (the action potential) that underlie the ECG waves recorded on the body surface.

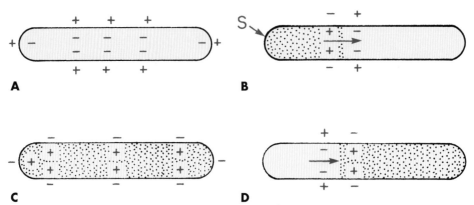

**FIGURE 2-1** Depolarization and repolarization. **A,** The resting heart muscle cell is polarized; that is, it carries an electrical charge, with the outside of the cell positively charged and the inside negatively charged. **B,** When the cell is stimulated (S), it begins to depolarize (*stippled* area). **C,** The fully depolarized cell is positively charged on the inside and negatively charged on the outside. **D,** Repolarization occurs when the stimulated cell returns to the resting state. The direction of depolarization and repolarization is represented by *arrows*. Depolarization (stimulation) of the atria produces the P wave on the ECG, whereas depolarization of the ventricles produces the QRS complex. Repolarization of the ventricles produces the ST-T complex.

that of just a single cell. Because cardiac depolarization and repolarization normally occur in a synchronized fashion, the ECG is able to record these electrical currents as specific waves (P wave, QRS complex, ST segment, T wave, and U wave).

In summary, regardless of whether the ECG is normal or abnormal, it records just two basic events: (1) depolarization, the spread of a stimulus through the heart muscle; and (2) repolarization, the return of the stimulated heart muscle to the resting state.

## BASIC ECG WAVEFORMS: P, QRS, ST, T, AND U WAVES

The spread of stimuli through the atria and ventricles followed by the return of stimulated atrial and ventricular muscle to the resting state produces the electrical currents recorded on the ECG. Furthermore, each phase of cardiac electrical activity produces a specific wave or complex (Fig. 2-2). The basic ECG waves are labeled alphabetically and begin with the P wave:

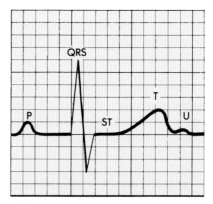

**FIGURE 2-2** The P wave represents atrial depolarization. The PR interval is the time from initial stimulation of the atria to initial stimulation of the ventricles. The QRS represents ventricular depolarization. The ST segment, T wave, and U wave are produced by ventricular repolarization.

- P wave—atrial depolarization (stimulation)

- QRS complex—ventricular depolarization (stimulation)

- ST segment, T wave, and U wave—ventricular repolarization (recovery)

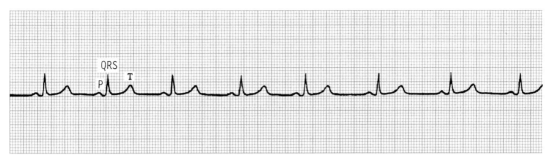

**FIGURE 2-3**  The basic cardiac cycle (P-QRS-T) repeats itself again and again.

The P wave represents the spread of a stimulus through the atria (atrial depolarization). The QRS complex represents stimulus spread through the ventricles (ventricular depolarization). The ST segment and T wave represent the return of stimulated ventricular muscle to the resting state (ventricular repolarization). The U wave is a small deflection sometimes seen just after the T wave. It represents the final phase of ventricular repolarization, although its exact mechanism is not known.

You are probably wondering why no wave or complex represents the return of stimulated atria to their resting state. The answer is that the atrial ST segment (STa) and atrial T wave (Ta) are generally not observed on the normal ECG because of their low amplitudes. (An important exception is described in Chapter 11 in the discussion of acute pericarditis, which often causes PR segment deviation.) Similarly, the routine ECG is not sensitive enough to record any electrical activity during the spread of stimuli through the atrioventricular (AV) junction (AV node and bundle of His). The spread of electrical stimuli through the AV junction occurs between the beginning of the P wave and the beginning of the QRS complex. This interval, known as the *PR interval,* is a measure of the time it takes for a stimulus to spread through the atria and pass through the AV junction.

In summary, the P-QRS-T sequence represents the repetitive cycle of the electrical activity in the heart, beginning with the spread of a stimulus through the atria (P wave) and ending with the return of stimulated ventricular muscle to its resting state (ST-T sequence). As shown in Figure 2-3, this cardiac cycle repeats itself again and again.

## ECG PAPER

The P-QRS-T sequence is recorded on special ECG graph paper that is divided into gridlike boxes (Figs. 2-3 and 2-4). Each of the small boxes is 1 millimeter square (1 mm²). The paper usually moves at a speed of 25 mm/sec. Therefore, horizontally, each unit represents 0.04 second (25 mm/sec × 0.04 sec = 1 mm). Notice that the lines between every five boxes are heavier, so that each 5-mm unit horizontally corresponds to 0.2 second (5 × 0.04 = 0.2). The ECG can therefore be regarded as a moving graph that horizontally corresponds to time, with 0.04- and 0.2-second divisions.

Vertically, the ECG graph measures the voltages, or amplitudes, of the ECG waves or deflections. The exact voltages can be measured because the electrocardiograph is standardized (calibrated) so that a 1-mV signal produces a deflection of 10-mm amplitude (1 mV = 10 mm). In most electrocardiographs, the standardization can also be set at one-half or two-times normal sensitivity.

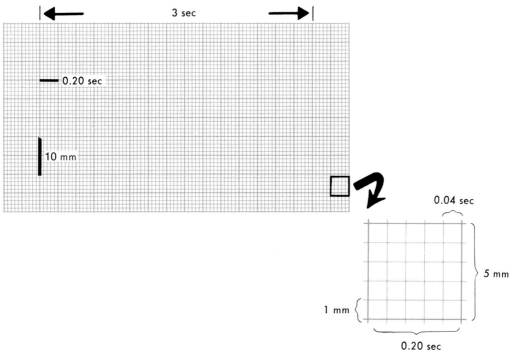

**FIGURE 2-4** The ECG is usually recorded on a graph divided into millimeter squares, with darker lines marking 5-mm squares. Time is measured on the horizontal axis. With a paper speed of 25 mm/sec, each small (1-mm) box side equals 0.04 second and each larger (5-mm) box side equals 0.2 second. The amplitude of any wave is measured in millimeters on the vertical axis.

## BASIC ECG MEASUREMENTS AND SOME NORMAL VALUES

### STANDARDIZATION (CALIBRATION) MARKER

The electrocardiograph must be properly calibrated so that a 1-mV signal produces a 10-mm deflection. The unit may have a special standardization button that produces a 1-mV wave. As shown in Figure 2-5, the standardization mark (St) produced when the machine is correctly calibrated is a square wave 10 mm tall. If the machine is not standardized correctly, the 1-mV signal produces a deflection either more or less than 10 mm and the amplitudes of the P, QRS, and T deflections are larger or smaller than they should be. The standardization

deflection is also important because standardization can be varied in most electrocardiographs (see Fig. 2-5). When very large deflections are present (as occurs, for example, in some patients who have an electronic pacemaker that produces very large spikes or who have high QRS voltage caused by hypertrophy), it may be advisable to take the ECG at one-half standardization to get the entire tracing on the paper. If the ECG complexes are very small, it may be advisable to double the standardization (e.g., to study a small Q wave more thoroughly). Some electronic electrocardiographs do not display the calibration pulse. Instead, they print the paper speed and standardization at the bottom of the ECG paper (25 mm/sec, 10 mm/mV).

**A**          **B**          **C**

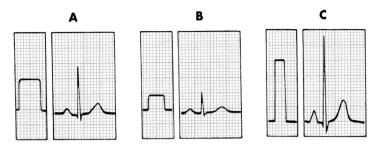

**FIGURE 2-5** Before taking an ECG, the operator must check to see that the machine is properly calibrated, so that the 1-mV standardization mark is 10 mm tall. **A,** Electrocardiograph set at normal standardization. **B,** One half standardization. **C,** Two times normal standardization.

Because the ECG is calibrated, any part of the P, QRS, and T deflections can be described in two ways; that is, both the amplitude (voltage) and the width (duration) of deflection can be measured. Thus it is possible to measure the amplitude and width of the P wave, the amplitude and width of the QRS complex, the amplitude of the ST segment deviation (if present), and the amplitude of the T wave. For clinical purposes, if the standardization is set at 1 mV = 10 mm, the height of a wave is usually recorded in millimeters, not millivolts. In Figure 2-3, for example, the P wave is 1 mm in amplitude, the QRS complex is 8 mm, and the T wave is about 3.5 mm.

A wave or deflection is also described as positive or negative. By convention, an *upward* deflection or wave is called *positive*. A *downward* deflection or wave is called *negative*. A deflection or wave that rests on the baseline is said to be *isoelectric*. A deflection that is partly positive and partly negative is call *biphasic*. For example, in Figure 2-6, the P wave is positive, the QRS complex is biphasic (initially positive, then negative), the ST segment is isoelectric (flat on the baseline), and the T wave is negative.

This chapter examines P, QRS, ST, T, and U waves in a general way. The measurements of heart rate, PR interval, QRS width, and QT interval are considered in detail, along with their normal values.

## P WAVE

The P wave, which represents atrial depolarization, is a small positive (or negative) deflection

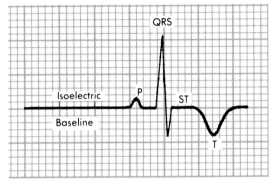

**FIGURE 2-6** The P wave is positive (upward), and the T wave is negative (downward). The QRS complex is biphasic (partly positive, partly negative), and the ST segment is isoelectric (neither positive nor negative).

before the QRS complex. (The normal values for P wave amplitude and width are described in Chapter 6.)

## PR INTERVAL

The PR interval is measured from the beginning of the P wave to the beginning of the QRS complex (Fig. 2-7). The PR interval may vary slightly in different leads, and the shortest PR interval should be noted. The PR interval represents the time it takes for the stimulus to spread through the atria and pass through the AV junction. (This physiologic delay allows the ventricles to fill fully with blood before ventricular depolarization occurs.) In adults the normal PR interval is between 0.12 and 0.2 second (three to five small box sides). When conduction through the AV junction is

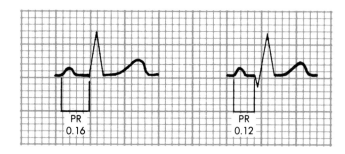

**FIGURE 2-7** Measurement of the PR interval (see text).

impaired, the PR interval may become prolonged. Prolongation of the PR interval above 0.2 second is called *first-degree heart block* (see Chapter 17).

## QRS COMPLEX

One of the most confusing aspects of electrocardiography for the beginning student is the nomenclature of the QRS complex. As noted previously, the QRS complex represents the spread of a stimulus through the ventricles. However, not every QRS complex contains a Q wave, an R wave, and an S wave—hence the confusion. The bothersome but unavoidable nomenclature becomes understandable if you remember several basic features of the QRS complex (see Fig. 2-8): When the initial deflection of the QRS complex is negative (below the baseline), it is called a *Q wave*; the first positive deflection in the QRS complex is called an *R wave*; a negative deflection following the R wave is called an *S wave*. Thus the following QRS complex contains a Q wave, an R wave, and an S wave:

In contrast, the following complex does not contain three waves:

If, as shown, the entire QRS complex is positive, it is simply called an *R wave*. If the entire complex is negative, however, it is termed a *QS wave* (not just a Q wave, as might be expected).

Occasionally, the QRS complex contains more than two or three deflections. In such cases, the extra waves are called *R'* (R prime) *waves* if they are positive and *S'* (S prime) *waves* if they are negative.

Figure 2-8 shows the various possible QRS complexes and the nomenclature of the respective waves. Notice that capital letters (QRS) are used to designate waves of relatively large amplitude and small letters (qrs) label relatively small waves.

The QRS nomenclature is confusing at first, but it allows you to describe any QRS complex over the phone and to evoke in the mind of the trained listener an exact mental picture of the complex named. For example, in describing an ECG you might say that lead $V_1$ showed an rS complex ("small r, capital S"):

You might also describe a QS ("capital Q, capital S") in lead $aV_F$:

**How to Name the QRS Complex**

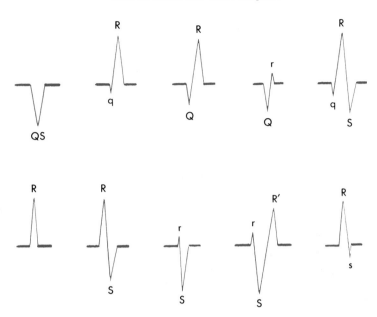

**FIGURE 2-8**  QRS nomenclature (see text).

## QRS WIDTH (INTERVAL)

The QRS width, or interval, represents the time required for a stimulus to spread through the ventricles (ventricular depolarization) and is normally 0.1 second or less (Fig. 2-9). If the spread of a stimulus through the ventricles is slowed, for example, by a block in one of the bundle branches, the QRS width is prolonged. (The full differential diagnosis of a wide QRS complex is discussed in Chapters 12 and 24.)

## ST SEGMENT

The ST segment is that portion of the ECG cycle from the end of the QRS complex to the beginning of the T wave (Fig. 2-10). It represents the beginning of ventricular repolarization. The normal ST segment is usually *isoelectric* (i.e., flat on the baseline, neither positive nor negative), but it may be slightly elevated or depressed normally (usually by less than 1 mm). Some pathologic conditions such as myocardial infarction (MI) produce characteristic abnormal devia-

**QRS Interval**

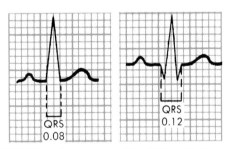

**FIGURE 2-9**  Measurement of the QRS width (interval) (see text).

tions of the ST segment. The very beginning of the ST segment (actually the junction between the end of the QRS complex and the beginning of the ST segment) is sometimes called the *J point*. Figure 2-10 shows the J point and the normal shapes of the ST segment. Figure 2-11 compares a normal isoelectric ST segment with abnormal ST segment elevation and depression.

## J Point, ST Segment, and T Wave

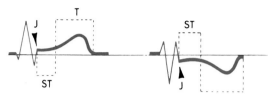

FIGURE 2-10    Characteristics of the normal ST segment and T wave. The junction (J) is the beginning of the ST segment.

### ST Segments

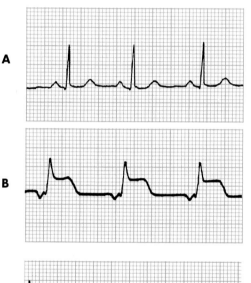

FIGURE 2-11    ST segments. **A,** Normal. **B,** Abnormal elevation. **C,** Abnormal depression.

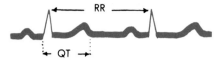

FIGURE 2-12    Measurement of the QT interval. The RR interval is the interval between two consecutive QRS complexes (see text).

When the T wave is positive, it normally rises slowly and then abruptly returns to the base-line.* When it is negative, it descends slowly and abruptly rises to the baseline. The *asymmetry* of the normal T wave contrasts with the symmetry of T waves in certain abnormal conditions such as myocardial infarction (see Chapters 8 and 9) and a high serum potassium level (see Chapter 10).

### QT INTERVAL

The QT interval is measured from the beginning of the QRS complex to the end of the T wave (Fig. 2-12). It primarily represents the return of stimulated ventricles to their resting state (ventricular repolarization). The normal values for the QT interval depend on the heart rate. As the heart rate increases (the RR interval shortens),[†] the QT normally shortens; as the heart rate decreases (the RR interval lengthens), the QT interval lengthens.

The QT should be measured in the ECG lead (see Chapter 3) that shows the longest intervals. You can measure several intervals in that lead and use the average value. When the QT interval is long, it is often difficult to measure because the end of the T wave may merge imperceptibly with the U wave. As a result, you may be measuring the QU interval rather than the QT interval.

### T WAVE

The T wave represents part of ventricular repolarization. A normal T wave has an asymmetric shape; that is, its peak is closer to the end of the wave than to the beginning (see Fig. 2-10).

---

*The exact point at which the ST segment ends and the T wave begins is arbitrary and sometimes impossible to define precisely.
†The interval between successive QRS complexes is termed the *RR interval.*

| TABLE 2-1 | QT Interval | |
|---|---|---|
| **Upper Limits of Normal (Estimated)** | | |
| Measured RR interval (sec) | Heart rate (per min) | QT interval upper normal limits (sec) |
| 1.50 | 40 | 0.50 |
| 1.20 | 50 | 0.48 |
| 1.00 | 60 | 0.43 |
| 0.86 | 70 | 0.40 |
| 0.80 | 75 | 0.39 |
| 0.75 | 80 | 0.37 |
| 0.67 | 90 | 0.35 |
| 0.60 | 100 | 0.34 |
| 0.50 | 120 | 0.31 |
| 0.40 | 150 | 0.27 |

Table 2-1 shows approximate upper normal limits for the QT interval with different heart rates. Unfortunately, there is no simple rule for determining the normal limits of the QT interval. As a result of this problem, another index of the QT was devised. It is the *rate-corrected* QT or $QT_c$. The rate-corrected QT can be obtained by dividing the actual QT by the square root of the RR interval (both measured in seconds):

$$QT_c = \frac{QT}{\sqrt{RR}}$$

Normally, the $QT_c$ is less than or equal to about 0.44 second.*

*As a general rule:* At heart rates of 80/min or less, a measured QT interval of more than half the RR interval is always prolonged. It is also important to note, however, that at heart rates below 80/min, the QT may be less than half the RR and still be significantly prolonged, and at heart rates above 80/min, a QT more than half the RR is not necessarily prolonged (see Table 2-1).

*A number of other formulas have been proposed for calculating a rate-corrected QT interval. None is ideal or universally accepted. Some authors give the upper limits of the $QT_c$ as 0.43 sec in men and 0.45 sec in women.

A number of factors can abnormally prolong the QT interval (Fig. 2-13). For example, this interval can be prolonged by certain drugs used to treat cardiac arrhythmias (e.g., amiodarone, disopyramide, dofetilide, ibutilide, procainamide, quinidine, and sotalol), as well as a large number of other types of agents (tricyclic antidepressants, phenothiazines, pentamidine, and so forth). Specific electrolyte disturbances (low potassium, magnesium, or calcium levels) are important causes of QT prolongation. Hypothermia also prolongs the QT interval by slowing the repolarization of myocardial cells. The QT interval may be prolonged with myocardial ischemia and infarction (especially during the evolving phase) and with subarachnoid hemorrhage. QT prolongation may predispose patients to potentially lethal ventricular arrhythmias. (See the discussion of torsades de pointes in Chapter 16.) The differential diagnosis of a long QT is summarized in Chapter 24.

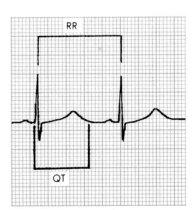

**FIGURE 2-13** Abnormal QT interval prolongation in a patient taking quinidine. The QT interval (0.6 sec) is markedly prolonged for the heart rate (65 beats/min) (see Table 2-1). The rate-corrected QT interval (normally 0.44 sec or less) is also prolonged (0.63 sec).* Prolonged ventricular repolarization may predispose patients to develop torsades de pointes, a life-threatening ventricular arrhythmia (see Chapter 16).

*In Fig. 2-13, find the $QT_c$.

$$QT_c = \frac{QT}{\sqrt{RR}} = \frac{0.60}{\sqrt{0.92}} = 0.63$$

The QT interval may be shortened by digitalis in therapeutic doses or by hypercalcemia, for example. Because the lower limits of normal for the QT interval have not been well defined, only the upper limits are given in Table 2-1.

### U WAVE

The U wave is a small, rounded deflection sometimes seen after the T wave (see Fig. 2-2). As noted previously, its exact significance is not known. Functionally, U waves represent the last phase of ventricular repolarization. Prominent U waves are characteristic of hypokalemia (see Chapter 10). Very prominent U waves may also be seen in other settings, for example, in patients taking drugs such as sotalol or one of the phenothiazines or sometimes after patients have had a cerebrovascular accident. The appearance of very prominent U waves in such settings, with or without actual QT prolongation, may also predispose patients to ventricular arrhythmias (see Chapter 16).

Normally, the direction of the U wave is the same as that of the T wave. Negative U waves sometimes appear with positive T waves. This abnormal finding has been noted in left ventricular hypertrophy and myocardial ischemia.

## CALCULATION OF HEART RATE

Two simple methods can be used to measure the heart rate (number of heartbeats per minute) from the ECG: box counting method and QRS counting method.

### BOX COUNTING METHOD

The easier way, when the heart rate is regular, is to count the number of large (0.2-sec) boxes between two successive QRS complexes and divide a constant (300) by this. (The number of large time boxes is divided into 300 because $300 \times 0.2 = 60$ and the heart rate is calculated in beats per minute or 60 seconds.)

For example, in Figure 2-14, the heart rate is 75 beats/min, since four large time boxes are counted between successive R waves ($300 \div 4 =$

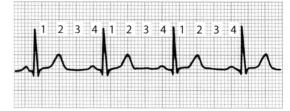

**FIGURE 2-14** Heart rate (beats per minute) can be measured by counting the number of large (0.2-sec) time boxes between two successive QRS complexes and dividing 300 by this number. In this example, the heart rate is calculated as $300 \div 4 = 75$ beats/min.

75). Similarly, if two large time boxes are counted between successive R waves, the heart rate is 150 beats/min. With five intervening large time boxes, the heart rate is 60 beats/min.

When the heart rate is fast or must be measured very accurately from the ECG, you can modify the approach as follows: Count the number of small (0.04-sec) boxes between successive R waves and divide a constant (1500) by this number. In Figure 2-14, 20 small time boxes are counted between QRS complexes. Therefore the heart rate is $1500 \div 20 = 75$ beats/min. (The constant 1500 is used because $1500 \times 0.04 = 60$ and the heart rate is being calculated in beats per 60 seconds.)

### QRS COUNTING METHOD

If the heart rate is irregular, the first method will not be accurate because the intervals between QRS complexes vary from beat to beat. In such cases you can determine an average rate simply by counting the number of QRS complexes in some convenient time interval (e.g., every 6 seconds or every 10 seconds) and multiplying this number by the appropriate factor to obtain the rate in beats per 60 seconds.

- Counting the number of QRS complexes in 6-second intervals (and then multiplying this number by 10; Fig. 2-15) can be easily done in most acute settings because the top of the ECG paper used in bedside cardiac monitors

**FIGURE 2-15** Measurement of heart rate (beats per minute) by counting the number of QRS complexes in a 6-second interval and multiplying this number by 10. In this example, 10 QRS complexes occur in 6 seconds. Therefore the heart rate is $10 \times 10 = 100$ beats/min. The *arrows* point to 3-second markers.

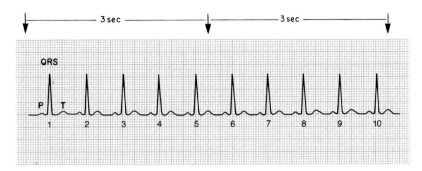

and telemetry units is generally scored with vertical marks every 3 seconds* (see Fig. 2-14).

- For conventional, full 12-lead ECG recordings, the rhythm strip at the bottom of the chart generally displays 10 consecutive seconds of data, so the number of QRS complexes in this entire interval can be multiplied by 10 to obtain the heart rate.

By definition, a heart rate exceeding 100 beats/min is termed *tachycardia*, and a heart rate slower than 60 beats/min is called *bradycardia*. (In Greek, *tachys* means "swift," whereas *bradys* means "slow.") Thus during exercise you probably develop a sinus tachycardia, but during sleep or relaxation your pulse rate may drop into the 50s or even lower, indicating a sinus bradycardia.

## THE ECG AS A COMBINATION OF ATRIAL AND VENTRICULAR WAVEFORMS

The ECG actually consists of two separate but normally related parts: an atrial ECG, represented by the P wave; and a ventricular ECG, represented by the QRS-T sequence. With com-

pletely normal rhythm, when the sinus node is pacing the heart, the P wave (atrial stimulation or depolarization) always precedes the QRS complex (ventricular stimulation or depolarization) because the atria are electrically stimulated first. Therefore the P-QRS-T cycle is usually considered as a unit. In some abnormal conditions, however, the atria and the ventricles can be stimulated by separate pacemakers. For example, suppose that the AV junction is diseased and stimuli cannot pass from the atria to the ventricles. In this situation, a new (subsidiary) pacemaker located below the level of the block in the AV junction may take over the task of pacing the ventricles while the sinus node continues to pace the atria. In this case, stimulation of the atria is independent of stimulation of the ventricles, and the P waves and QRS complexes have no relation to each other. This type of arrhythmia is called *complete heart block* and is described in detail in Chapter 17. (Figure 17-5 shows an example of this abnormal condition in which the atrial and ventricular ECGs are independent of each other.)

## THE ECG IN PERSPECTIVE

Up to this point, this chapter has considered only the basic components of the ECG. Several general items need to be emphasized before actual ECG patterns are discussed.

1. The ECG is a recording of cardiac *electrical* activity. It does not directly measure the

---

*If 3-second marks are not present, you can simply count the number of QRS cycles in any 15-cm interval and multiply this number by 10. On the ECG graph, 1 sec = 25 mm = 2.5 cm; therefore, 15 cm = 6 seconds of data.

*mechanical* function of the heart (i.e., how well the heart is contracting and performing as a pump). Thus a patient with acute pulmonary edema may have a normal ECG. Conversely, a patient with a grossly abnormal ECG may have normal cardiac function.

2. The ECG does not directly depict abnormalities in cardiac structure such as ventricular septal defects and abnormalities of the heart valves. It only records the electrical changes produced by structural defects. In some patients, however, the clinician can infer a specific structural diagnosis such as mitral stenosis, pulmonary embolism, or myocardial infarction from the ECG because typical electrical abnormalities may develop in such patients.

3. The ECG does not record *all* the heart's electrical activity. The electrodes placed on the surface of the body record only the currents that are transmitted to the area of electrode placement. Therefore there are actually "silent" electrical areas of the heart. For example, the ECG is not sensitive enough to record depolarization of pacemaker cells in

the sinus node occurring just before the P wave. As noted earlier, the conventional electrocardiograph does not generally record repolarization of the atria. (For an important exception, see the discussion of pericarditis in Chapter 11.) In addition, the conventional ECG does not detect the spread of stimuli through the AV junction. The electrical activity of the AV junction can be recorded using a special apparatus and a special electrode placed in the heart *(His bundle electrogram)*. Further, the ECG records the summation of electrical potentials produced by innumerable cardiac muscle cells. Therefore the presence of a normal ECG does not necessarily mean that all these heart muscle cells are being depolarized and repolarized in a normal way.

For these reasons, the ECG must be regarded as any other laboratory test, with proper consideration for both its uses and its limitations (see Chapter 23).

The 12 ECG leads are described in Chapter 3. Normal and abnormal ECG patterns are discussed in subsequent chapters.

## REVIEW

The ECG, whether normal or abnormal, records two basic physiologic processes: *depolarization* and *repolarization:*

1. Depolarization (the spread of stimulus through the heart muscle) produces the P wave from the atria and the QRS complex from the ventricles.

2. Repolarization (the return of stimulated muscle to the resting state) produces the atrial ST segment and T wave (which are ordinarily not seen on the ECG) and the ventricular ST segment, T wave, and U wave.

ECGs are recorded on special paper that is divided into gridlike boxes. Each small box is

$1 \text{ mm}^2$. Each millimeter horizontally represents 0.04 second. Each 0.2 second is denoted by a heavier vertical line. ECG deflections are usually standardized so that a 1-mV signal produces a 10-mm deflection. Therefore each millimeter vertically represents 0.1 mV. Each 5-mm interval is denoted by a heavier horizontal line.

Four basic intervals are measured on the ECG:

1. The *heart rate*, measured in beats/min can be quickly calculated in two ways:
   Method 1 (box counting): Count the number of large (0.2-sec) time boxes between two successive R waves, and divide the constant 300 by this number (see Fig. 2-14).

If you want a more accurate measurement of the rate, divide the constant 1500 by the number of small (0.04-sec) time boxes between two successive R waves.

Method 2 (QRS counting): Count the number of QRS complexes that occur every 6 or 10 seconds, and multiply this number by 10 or 6, respectively.

2. The *PR interval* is measured from the beginning of the P wave to the beginning of the QRS complex. The normal PR interval is from 0.12 to 0.2 second.

3. The *QRS interval* is normally 0.1 second or less in width.

4. The *QT interval* is measured from the beginning of the QRS complex to the end of the T wave. It varies with the heart rate, becoming shorter as the heart rate increases.

These four intervals can be considered the "vital signs" of the ECG because they give essential information about the electrical stability (or instability) of the heart.

## QUESTIONS

1. Calculate the heart rate in each of the following examples.

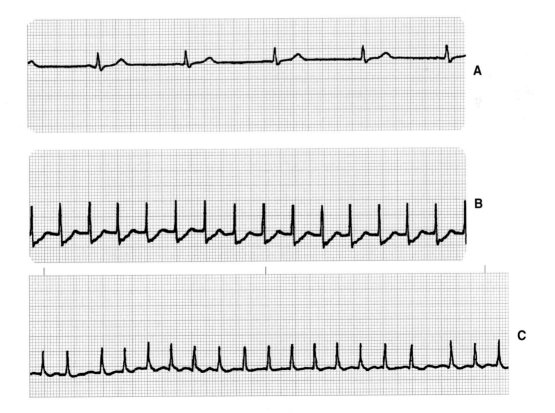

2. Name the major abnormality in each example.

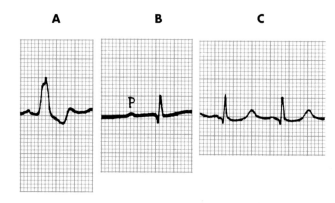

3. Slowing of conduction in the atrioventricular (AV) node is most likely to do which of the following?
   a. Prolong the PR interval
   b. Prolong the QRS interval
   c. Prolong the QT interval
   d. All of the above

4. A block in the left bundle branch is most likely to do which of the following?
   a. Prolong the PR interval
   b. Prolong the QRS interval
   c. Prolong the QT interval
   d. All of the above

5. Name the component waves of the QRS complexes shown below.

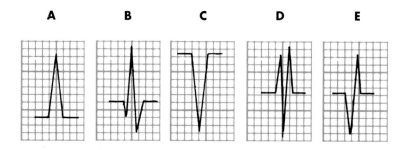

6. Name four factors that may prolong the QT interval.

7. Which of the following events is never observed on a clinical 12-lead ECG?
   a. Atrial depolarization
   b. Atrial repolarization
   c. His bundle depolarization
   d. Ventricular depolarization
   e. Ventricular repolarization

## CHAPTER 3

# ECG Leads

As discussed in Chapter 1, the heart produces electrical currents similar to those of the familiar dry cell battery. The strength or voltage of these currents and the way they are distributed throughout the body over time can be measured by a suitable recording instrument such as an electrocardiograph.

The body acts as a conductor of electricity. Therefore recording electrodes placed some distance from the heart, such as on the arms, legs, or chest wall, are able to detect the voltages of the cardiac currents conducted to these locations. The usual way of recording these voltages from the heart is with the 12 standard ECG leads. The leads actually show the differences in voltage (potential) between electrodes placed on the surface of the body.

Taking an ECG is like recording an event such as a baseball game with a video camera. Multiple camera angles are necessary to capture the event completely. One view is not enough. Similarly, multiple ECG leads must be recorded to describe the dynamic electrical activity of the heart adequately. Figure 3-1 shows the ECG patterns that are obtained when electrodes are placed at various points on the chest. Notice that each lead presents a different pattern.

Figure 3-2 is an ECG illustrating the 12 leads. The leads can be subdivided into two groups: the six *limb (extremity)* leads (shown in the left two columns) and the six *chest (precordial)* leads (shown in the right two columns).

The six limb leads—I, II, III, $aV_R$, $aV_L$, and $aV_F$—record voltage differences by means of electrodes placed on the extremities. They can be further divided into two subgroups based on their historical development: three standard *"bipolar"* limb leads (I, II, and III), and three augmented *"unipolar"* limb leads ($aV_R$, $aV_L$, and $aV_F$).

The six chest leads—$V_1$, $V_2$, $V_3$, $V_4$, $V_5$, and $V_6$—record voltage differences by means of electrodes placed at various positions on the chest wall.

The 12 ECG leads can also be viewed as 12 "channels." In contrast to television channels (which can be tuned to different events), however, the 12 ECG channels (leads) are all tuned to the *same* event (the P-QRS-T cycle), with each lead viewing the event from a different angle.

## LIMB (EXTREMITY) LEADS

### STANDARD LIMB LEADS: I, II, AND III

The limb (extremity) leads are recorded first. In connecting a patient to an electrocardiograph, first place metal electrodes on the arms and legs. The right leg electrode functions solely as an electrical ground, so you need concern yourself with it no further. As shown in Figure 3-3, the arm electrodes are attached just above the wrist and the leg electrodes are attached above the ankles.

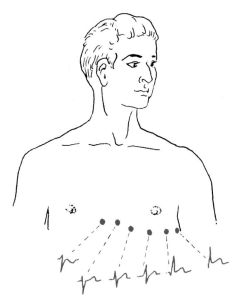

FIGURE 3-1    Multiple chest leads give a three-dimensional view of cardiac electrical activity.

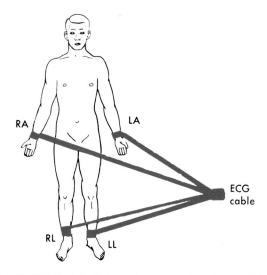

FIGURE 3-3    Metal electrodes are used to take an ECG. The right leg (RL) electrode functions solely as a ground to prevent alternating-current interference. LA, left arm; LL, left leg; RA, right arm.

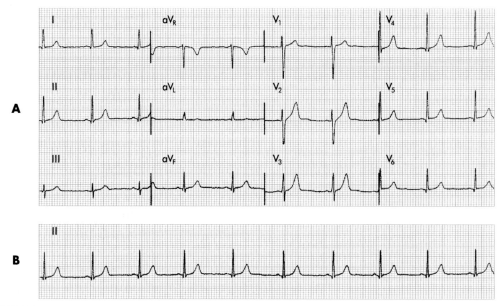

FIGURE 3-2    A, Sample ECG showing the 12 standard leads. B, A lead II rhythm strip recorded simultaneously. What is the approximate heart rate? (Answer: about 80 beats/min)

The electrical voltages of the heart are conducted through the torso to the extremities. Therefore an electrode placed on the right wrist detects electrical voltages equivalent to those recorded below the right shoulder. Similarly, the voltages detected at the left wrist or anywhere else on the left arm are equivalent to those recorded below the left shoulder. Finally, voltages detected by the left leg electrode are comparable to those at the left thigh or near the groin. In clinical practice, the electrodes are attached to the wrists and ankles simply for convenience.*

As mentioned, the limb leads consist of standard "bipolar" (I, II, and III) and augmented (aV$_R$, aV$_L$, and aV$_F$) leads. The bipolar leads were so named historically because they record the differences in electrical voltage between two extremities.

Lead I, for example, records the difference in voltage between the left arm (LA) and right arm (RA) electrodes:

$$\text{Lead I} = \text{LA} - \text{RA}$$

Lead II records the difference between the left leg (LL) and right arm (RA) electrodes:

$$\text{Lead II} = \text{LL} - \text{RA}$$

Lead III records the difference between the left leg (LL) and left arm (LA) electrodes:

$$\text{Lead III} = \text{LL} - \text{LA}$$

Consider what happens when you turn on the electrocardiograph to lead I. The LA electrode detects the electrical voltages of the heart that are transmitted to the left arm. The RA electrode detects the voltages transmitted to the right arm. Inside the electrocardiograph, the RA voltages are subtracted from the LA voltages, and the difference appears at lead I. When lead

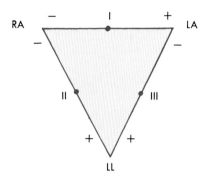

**Einthoven's Triangle**

**FIGURE 3-4** Orientation of leads I, II, and III. Lead I records the difference in electrical potentials between the left arm and right arm. Lead II records it between the left leg and right arm. Lead III records it between the left leg and left arm.

II is recorded, a similar situation occurs between the voltages of LL and RA. When lead III is recorded, the same situation occurs between the voltages of LL and LA.

Leads I, II, and III can be represented schematically in terms of a triangle, called *Einthoven's triangle* after the Dutch physiologist who invented the electrocardiograph in the early 1900s. At first the ECG consisted only of recordings from leads I, II, and III. Einthoven's triangle (Fig. 3-4) shows the spatial orientation of the three standard limb leads (I, II, and III). As you can see, lead I points horizontally. Its left pole (LA) is positive and its right pole (RA) is negative. Therefore lead I = LA − RA. Lead II points diagonally downward. Its lower pole (LL) is positive and its upper pole (RA) is negative. Therefore lead II = LL − RA. Lead III also points diagonally downward. Its lower pole (LL) is positive and its upper pole (LA) is negative. Therefore lead III = LL − LA.

Einthoven, of course, could have hooked the leads up differently. Yet because of the way he arranged them, the bipolar leads are related by the following simple equation:

$$\text{Lead I} + \text{Lead III} = \text{Lead II}$$

---

*Obviously, if you are taking an ECG on an amputee or someone with a cast, you have to place the electrodes below or near the shoulders or groin, depending on the circumstance.

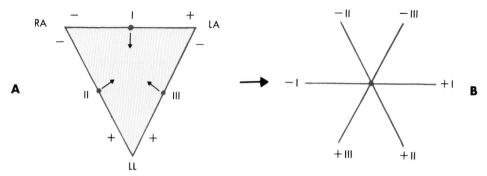

**FIGURE 3-5** **A,** Einthoven's triangle. **B,** The triangle is converted to a triaxial diagram by shifting leads I, II, and III so that they intersect at a common point.

In other words, add the voltage in lead I to that in lead III and you get the voltage in lead II.* You can test this equation by looking at Figure 3-2. Add the voltage of the R wave in lead I (+9 mm) to the voltage of the R wave in lead III (+4 mm) and you get +13 mm, the voltage of the R wave in lead II. You can do the same with the voltages of the P waves and T waves.

It is a good practice to scan leads I, II, and III rapidly when you first look at a mounted ECG. If the R wave in lead II does not seem to be the sum of the R waves in leads I and II, this may be a clue that the leads have been recorded incorrectly or mounted improperly.

*Einthoven's equation* is simply the result of the way the bipolar leads are recorded; that is, the LA is positive in lead I and negative in lead III and thus cancels out when the two leads are added:

$$I = L\cancel{A} - RA$$
$$II = LL - L\cancel{A}$$
$$I + III = LL - RA = II$$

---

*This rule is only approximate. It is exact when the three standard limb leads are recorded simultaneously, using a three-channel electrocardiograph, because the peaks of the R waves in the three leads do *not* occur simultaneously. The exact rule is as follows: The voltage at the peak of the R wave (or at any point) in lead II equals the sum of the voltages in leads I and III at points occurring simultaneously.

Thus, in electrocardiography, one plus three equals two.

In summary, leads I, II, and III are the standard (bipolar) limb leads, which, historically, were the first invented. These leads record the differences in electrical voltage between selected extremities.

In Figure 3-5, Einthoven's triangle has been redrawn so that leads I, II, and III intersect at a common central point. This was done simply by sliding lead I downward, lead II rightward, and lead III leftward. The result is the *triaxial* diagram in Figure 3-5B. This diagram, a useful way of representing the three bipolar leads, is employed in Chapter 5.

## AUGMENTED LIMB (EXTREMITY) LEADS: $aV_R$, $aV_L$, AND $aV_F$

Nine leads have been added to the original three "bipolar" extremity leads. In the 1930s, Dr. Frank N. Wilson and his colleagues at the University of Michigan invented the "unipolar" limb leads and also introduced the six "unipolar" chest leads, $V_1$ through $V_6$. A short time later, Dr. Emanuel Goldberger invented the three augmented unipolar limb leads: $aV_R$, $aV_L$, and $aV_F$. The abbreviation *a* refers to *augmented;* *V* to *voltage;* *R, L,* and *F* to *right arm, left arm,* and *left foot* (leg), respectively. Today 12 leads are routinely employed, consisting of the six limb leads (I, II, III, $aV_R$, $aV_L$, and $aV_F$) and the six precordial leads ($V_1$ to $V_6$).

A so-called unipolar lead records the electrical voltages at one location relative to an electrode with close to zero potential rather than relative to the voltages at another single extremity, as in the case of the bipolar limb leads.* The zero potential is obtained inside the electrocardiograph by joining the three extremity leads to a central terminal. Because the sum of the voltages of RA, LA, and LL equals zero, the central terminal has a zero voltage. The $aV_L$ and $aV_F$ leads are derived in a slightly different way because the voltages recorded by the electrocardiograph have been augmented 50% over the actual voltages detected at each extremity. This augmentation is also done electronically inside the electrocardiograph.†

Just as Einthoven's triangle represents the spatial orientation of the three standard limb leads, the diagram in Figure 3-6 represents the spatial orientation of the three augmented limb leads. Notice that each of these "unipolar" leads can also be represented by a line (axis) with a positive and negative pole. Because the diagram has three axes, it is also called a *triaxial* diagram.

As would be expected, the positive pole of lead $aV_R$, the right arm lead, points upward and to the patient's right arm. The positive pole of lead $aV_L$ points upward and to the patient's left arm. The positive pole of lead $aV_F$ points downward toward the patient's left foot.

Furthermore, just as leads I, II, and III are related by Einthoven's equation, so leads $aV_R$, $aV_L$, and $aV_F$ are related:

$$aV_R + aV_L + aV_F = 0$$

In other words, when the three augmented limb leads are recorded, their voltages should total zero. Thus the sum of the P wave voltages is zero, the sum of the QRS voltages is zero, and the sum of the T wave voltages is zero. Using Figure 3-2, test this equation by adding the QRS voltages in the three unipolar limb leads ($aV_R$, $aV_L$, and $aV_F$).

It is also a good practice to scan leads $aV_R$, $aV_L$, and $aV_F$ rapidly when you first look at a mounted ECG. If the sum of the waves in these three leads does not equal zero, the leads may have been recorded incorrectly or mounted improperly.

The 12 ECG leads have two major features, which have already been described. They have both a specific *orientation* and a specific *polarity*.

Thus the axis of lead I is oriented horizontally, and the axis of lead $aV_R$ points diagonally downward. The orientation of the standard (bipolar) leads is shown in Einthoven's triangle (see Fig. 3-5), and the orientation of the augmented (unipolar) limb leads is diagrammed in Figure 3-6.

The second major feature of the ECG leads, their polarity, can be represented by a line (axis) with a positive and a negative pole. (The

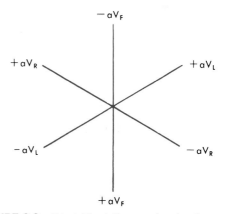

**FIGURE 3-6** Triaxial lead diagram showing the relationship of the three augmented ("unipolar") leads ($aV_R$, $aV_L$, and $aV_F$). Notice that each lead is represented by an axis with a positive and negative pole. The term *unipolar* was used to mean that the leads record the voltage in one location relative to about zero potential, instead of relative to the voltage in one other extremity.

---

*Although so-called unipolar leads (like bipolar leads) are represented by axes with positive and negative poles, the historical term *unipolar* does not refer to these poles; rather it refers to the fact that unipolar leads record the voltage in one location relative to an electrode with close to zero potential.

†Augmentation was developed to make the complexes more readable.

polarity and spatial orientation of the leads are discussed further in Chapters 4 and 5 when the normal ECG patterns seen in each lead are considered and the concept of electrical axis is explored.)

Do not be confused by the difference in meaning between ECG electrodes and ECG leads. An *electrode* is simply the metal plate used to detect the electrical currents of the heart in any location. An ECG *lead* shows the differences in voltage detected by electrodes. For example, lead I presents the differences in voltage detected by the left and right arm electrodes. Therefore a lead is a means of recording the differences in cardiac voltages obtained by different electrodes.

## RELATIONSHIP BETWEEN LIMB (EXTREMITY) LEADS

Einthoven's triangle in Figure 3-4 shows the relationship of the three standard limb leads (I, II, and III). Similarly, the triaxial diagram in Figure 3-7 shows the relationship of the three augmented limb leads (aV$_r$, aV$_l$, and aV$_F$). For convenience, these two diagrams can be combined so that the axes of all six limb leads intersect at a common point. The result is the *hexaxial* lead diagram shown in Figure 3-7. The hexaxial

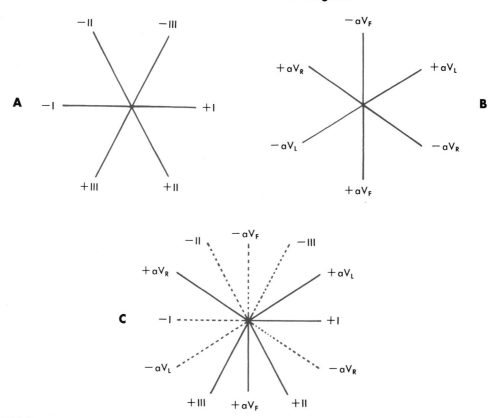

**Derivation of Hexaxial Lead Diagram**

FIGURE 3-7    **A,** Triaxial diagram of the so-called bipolar leads (I, II, and III). **B,** Triaxial diagram of the augmented limb leads (aV$_R$, aV$_L$, and aV$_F$). **C,** The two triaxial diagrams can be combined into a hexaxial diagram that shows the relationship of all six limb leads. The negative pole of each lead is now indicated by a *dashed line.*

diagram shows the spatial orientation of the six extremity leads (I, II, III, $aV_R$, $aV_L$, and $aV_F$).

The exact relationships among the three augmented extremity leads and the three standard extremity leads can also be described mathematically. For present purposes, however, the following simple guidelines allow you to get an overall impression of the similarities between these two sets of leads.

As you might expect by looking at the hexaxial diagram, the pattern in lead $aV_L$ usually resembles that in lead I. The positive poles of lead $aV_R$ and lead II, on the other hand, point in opposite directions. Therefore the P-QRS-T pattern recorded by lead $aV_R$ is generally the reverse of that recorded by lead II. For example, when lead II shows a qR pattern

lead $aV_R$ usually shows an rS pattern

Finally, the pattern shown by lead $aV_F$ usually but not always resembles that shown by lead III.

## CHEST (PRECORDIAL) LEADS

The chest leads ($V_1$ to $V_6$) show the electrical currents of the heart as detected by electrodes placed at different positions on the chest wall. The precordial leads used today are also considered "unipolar" leads in that they measure the voltage in any one location relative to about zero potential (Box 3-1). These chest leads are recorded simply by means of electrodes at six designated locations on the chest wall* (Fig. 3-8). Two points are worth mentioning here:

*Sometimes, in special circumstances (e.g., a patient with suspected right ventricular infarction or congenital heart disease), additional leads are placed on the right side of the chest. For example, lead $V_{3R}$ is equivalent to lead $V_3$, but the electrode is placed to the right of the sternum.

---

| BOX 3-1 | Conventional Placement of ECG Chest Leads |
|---|---|

Lead $V_1$ is recorded with the electrode in the fourth intercostal space just to the right of the sternum.

Lead $V_2$ is recorded with the electrode in the fourth intercostal space just to the left of the sternum.

Lead $V_3$ is recorded on a line midway between leads $V_2$ and $V_4$.

Lead $V_4$ is recorded in the midclavicular line in the fifth interspace.

Lead $V_5$ is recorded in the anterior axillary line at the same level as lead $V_4$.

Lead $V_6$ is recorded in the midaxillary line at the same level as lead $V_4$.

---

1. The fourth intercostal space can be located by placing your finger at the top of the sternum and moving it slowly downward. After you move your finger down about $1\frac{1}{2}$ inches, you can feel a slight horizontal ridge. This is called the *angle of Louis*, which is located where the manubrium joins the body of the sternum (see Fig. 3-8). The second intercostal space is just below and lateral to this point. Move down two more spaces. You are now in the fourth interspace and ready to place lead $V_4$.

2. Chest lead placement in females is complicated by breast tissue, which may result in misplacement of the chest leads. In taking ECGs on women, you must remember to place the electrode *under* the breast for leads $V_3$ to $V_6$. If, as often happens, the electrode is placed *on* the breast, electrical voltages from higher interspaces are recorded. Also, never use the nipples to locate the position of any of the chest lead electrodes, even in men, because nipple location varies greatly.

The chest leads, like the six limb leads, can be represented diagrammatically (Fig. 3-9). Like the other leads, each chest lead has a positive and negative pole. The positive pole of

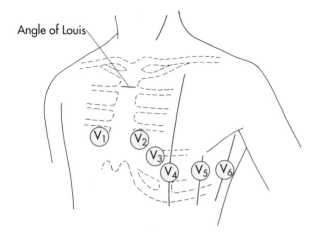

Angle of Louis

**FIGURE 3-8**   Locations of the electrodes for the chest (precordial) leads.

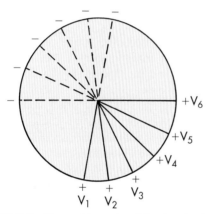

**FIGURE 3-9**   The positive poles of the chest leads point anteriorly, and the negative poles (*dashed lines*) point posteriorly.

each chest lead points anteriorly, toward the front of the chest. The negative pole of each chest lead points posteriorly, toward the back (see the dashed lines in Fig. 3-9).

## THE 12-LEAD ECG: FRONTAL AND HORIZONTAL PLANE LEADS

You may now be wondering why 12 leads are used in clinical electrocardiography. Why not 10 or 22 leads? The reason for exactly 12 leads is partly historical, a matter of the way the ECG has evolved over the years since Einthoven's original 3 limb leads. There is nothing sacred about the electrocardiographer's dozen. In some situations, for example, additional leads are recorded by placing the chest electrode at different positions on the chest wall. Multiple leads are used for good reasons. The heart, after all, is a three-dimensional structure, and its electrical currents spread out in all directions across the body. Recall that the ECG leads were described as being like video cameras by which the electrical activity of the heart can be viewed from different locations. To a certain extent, the more points that are recorded, the more accurate the representation of the heart's electrical activity.

The importance of multiple leads is illustrated in the diagnosis of myocardial infarction (MI). An MI typically affects one localized portion of either the anterior or inferior portion of the left ventricle. The ECG changes produced by an anterior MI are usually best shown by the chest leads, which are close to and face the injured anterior surface of the heart. The changes seen with an inferior MI usually appear only in leads such as II, III, and aVF, which face the injured inferior surface of the heart (see Chapters 8 and 9). The 12 leads therefore provide a three-dimensional view of the electrical activity of the heart.

## Frontal Plane Leads

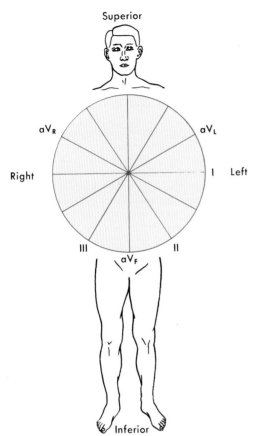

**FIGURE 3-10** Spatial relationships of the six limb leads, which record electrical voltages transmitted onto the frontal plane of the body.

## Horizontal Plane Leads

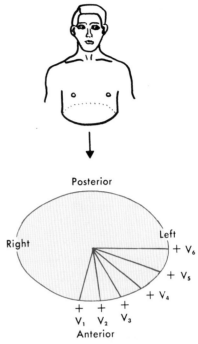

**FIGURE 3-11** Spatial relationships of the six chest leads, which record electrical voltages transmitted onto the horizontal plane.

Specifically, the six limb leads (I, II, III, $aV_R$, $aV_L$, $aV_F$) record electrical voltages transmitted onto the *frontal* plane of the body (Fig. 3-10). (In contrast, the six precordial leads record voltages transmitted onto the *horizontal* plane.) The frontal plane can be illustrated by the image of facing a large window: The window is parallel to the frontal plane of your body. Similarly, heart voltages directed upward and downward and to the right and left are recorded by the frontal plane leads.

The six chest leads ($V_1$ through $V_6$) record heart voltages transmitted onto the *horizontal* plane of the body (Fig. 3-11). The horizontal plane cuts your body into an upper and a lower half. Similarly, the chest leads record heart voltages directed anteriorly (front) and posteriorly (back), and to the right and left.

The 12 ECG leads are therefore divided into two sets: the 6 extremity leads (3 unipolar and 3 bipolar), which record voltages on the frontal plane of the body; and the 6 chest (precordial) leads, which record voltages on the horizontal plane. Together these 12 leads provide a three-dimensional picture of atrial and ventricular depolarization and repolarization. This multilead display is analogous to having 12 video cameras continuously recording cardiac electrical activity from different angles.

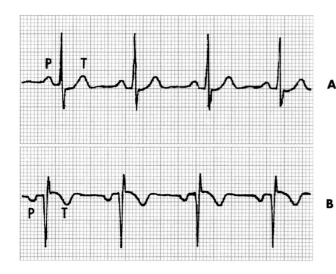

A

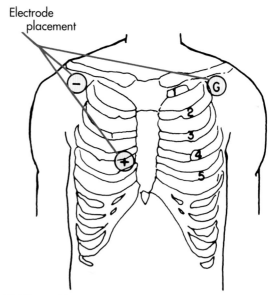

B **FIGURE 3-12** Rhythm strips from a cardiac monitor taken moments apart but showing exactly opposite patterns. This is because the polarity of the electrodes was reversed in the lower strip **(B)**.

## CARDIAC MONITORS AND MONITOR LEADS

### BEDSIDE CARDIAC MONITORS

Up to now, this chapter has considered only the standard 12-lead ECG. It is not always necessary or feasible to record a full 12-lead ECG, however. For example, many patients require continuous monitoring for a prolonged period. In such cases, special cardiac monitors are used to give a continuous beat-to-beat record of cardiac activity from one monitor lead. Such ECG monitors are ubiquitous in intensive care units, operating rooms, and postoperative care units, as well as in a variety of other inpatient settings.

Figure 3-12 is a rhythm strip recorded from a monitor lead obtained by means of three disk electrodes on the chest wall. As shown in Figure 3-13, one electrode (the positive one) is usually pasted in the $V_1$ position. The other two are placed near the right and left shoulders. One serves as the negative electrode and the other as the ground.

When the location of the electrodes on the chest wall is varied, the resultant ECG patterns also vary. In addition, if the polarity of the

**FIGURE 3-13** Monitor lead. A chest electrode (+) is placed at the lead $V_1$ position (between the fourth and fifth ribs on the right side of the sternum). The negative (−) electrode is placed near the right shoulder. A ground electrode (G) is placed near the left shoulder. This lead is therefore a modified $V_1$. Another configuration is to place the negative electrode near the left shoulder and the ground electrode near the right shoulder.

electrodes changes (e.g., the negative electrode is connected to the $V_1$ position and the positive electrode to the right shoulder), the ECG shows a completely opposite pattern (see Fig. 3-12).

## AMBULATORY ECG TECHNOLOGY: HOLTER MONITORS AND LOOP (PATIENT-ACTIVATED EVENT) RECORDERS

The cardiac monitors just described are useful for patients confined to a bed or chair. Sometimes, however, the ECG needs to be recorded in ambulatory patients over longer periods. A special portable system, designed in 1961 by N. J. Holter, records the continuous ECG of patients as they go about their daily activities.

The Holter monitors currently in use consist of electrodes placed on the chest wall that are connected to a special portable analog or digital ECG recorder. The patient can then be monitored over a long period (typically 24 hours). Two ECG leads are usually recorded. The ECG data are played back, and the P-QRS-T complexes are displayed on a special screen for analysis and annotation. Printouts of any portion of the ECG can be obtained for further study and permanent records.

Portable external *loop* or *patient-activated ECG monitors* are also available to record ECGs in individuals with more intermittent symptoms. These "event recorders" are designed with replaceable electrodes so that patients can be monitored for prolonged periods (typically up to 2 weeks) as they go about their usual activities. The ECG is continuously recorded and then automatically erased unless the patient presses an event button. When patients experience a symptom (e.g., light-headedness, palpitations, chest discomfort), they can push a button so that a portion of the ECG obtained during the symptom is stored. The saved ECG includes a continuous rhythm strip just before the button was pressed (e.g., 45 sec), as well as a recording after the event mark (e.g., 15 sec). The stored ECGs can be transmitted by phone to an analysis station for immediate diagnosis.

Event recorders can also be used to monitor the ECG for asymptomatic drug effects and potentially important toxicities (e.g., excessive prolongation of the QT interval with drugs such as sotalol, quinidine, or dofetilide) or to detect other potentially *proarrhythmic effects* (see Chapter 19) of drugs.

## REVIEW

The electrical currents produced during atrial and ventricular depolarization and repolarization are detected by electrodes placed on the extremities and chest wall; 12 leads are usually recorded:

1. The six *limb (extremity)* leads record voltages from the heart that are directed onto the frontal plane of the body. (This plane divides the body into front and back halves.) The extremity leads include three standard ("bipolar") limb leads (I, II, and III) and three augmented ("unipolar") limb leads ($aV_R$, $aV_L$, and $aV_F$).
   a. A standard *"bipolar"* lead records the difference between voltages from the heart

detected at two extremities. The standard limb leads can be represented by Einthoven's triangle (see Fig. 3-4). They are related by the equation:

$$II = I + III.$$

A *"unipolar"* lead records voltages at one point relative to an electrode with close to zero potential. The unipolar limb leads can also be represented by a triaxial diagram (see Fig. 3-6). They are related by the equation:

$$aV_R + aV_L + aV_F = 0.$$

b. The three standard limb leads and the three augmented limb leads can be mapped on the same diagram so that the axes of all six leads intersect at a common point, producing the *hexaxial lead diagram*.

c. As a general rule, the P-QRS-T pattern in lead I resembles that in lead aV$_L$. Leads aV$_R$ and II usually show reverse patterns. Lead aV$_F$ usually resembles lead III.

2. The six *chest (precordial)* leads (V$_1$ to V$_6$) record voltages from the heart as directed onto the horizontal plane of the body (dividing the body into an upper and a lower half).

They are taken with electrodes in specific anatomic locations (see Fig. 3-8).

In addition to the 12 conventional leads, ECGs can be taken in special ways. Monitor leads, in which electrodes are placed on the chest, are generally used in cardiac and intensive care units (CCUs and ICUs). Continuous ECGs are often recorded with the Holter apparatus for a period of 24 or more hours in ambulatory patients who are suspected of having a transient or an unpredictable arrhythmia. Very sporadic symptoms can be correlated with ECG rhythm changes by using patient-activated event recorders for periods of up to 2 weeks or so.

## QUESTIONS

1. Leads I and II are shown below. Draw the P-QRS-T pattern in lead III.

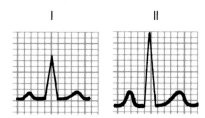

2. Leads I, II, and III are shown below. What is wrong with them?

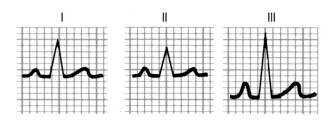

3. Draw the hexaxial lead diagram that shows the six frontal plane (limb) leads.

4. Why does the P-QRS-T pattern in lead aV$_R$ usually show a reverse of the pattern seen in lead II?

## CHAPTER 4

# The Normal ECG

The previous chapters reviewed the cycle of atrial and ventricular depolarization and repolarization detected by the ECG as well as the 12-lead system used to record this electrical activity. This chapter describes the P-QRS-T patterns seen normally in each of the 12 leads. Fortunately, you do not have to memorize 12 or more separate patterns. Rather, if you understand a few basic ECG principles and the sequence of atrial and ventricular depolarization, you can predict the normal ECG patterns in each lead.

As the sample ECG in Figure 3-2 shows, each of the 12 leads appears to be different. In some leads, for example, the P waves are positive (upward); in others, they are negative (downward). In some leads, the QRS complexes are represented by an rS wave; in other leads, they are represented by RS or qR waves. Finally, the T waves are positive in some leads and negative in others. What determines this variety in the appearance of ECG complexes in the different leads, and how does the repetitive cycle of cardiac electrical activity produce such different patterns in these leads?

## THREE BASIC "LAWS" OF ELECTROCARDIOGRAPHY

To answer the preceding questions, you need to understand three basic ECG "laws" (Fig. 4-1):

1. A *positive (upward) deflection* appears in any lead if the wave of depolarization spreads toward the positive pole of that lead. Thus if the path of atrial stimulation is directed downward and to the patient's left, toward the positive pole of lead II, a positive (upward) P wave is seen in lead II (Figs. 4-2 and 4-3). Similarly, if the ventricular stimulation path is directed to the left, a positive deflection (R wave) is seen in lead I (see Fig. 4-1A).

2. A *negative (downward) deflection* appears in any lead if the wave of depolarization spreads toward the negative pole of that lead (or away from the positive pole). Thus if the atrial stimulation path spreads downward and to the left, a negative P wave is seen in lead $aV_R$ (see Figs. 4-2 and 4-3). If the ventricular stimulation path is directed entirely away from the positive pole of any lead, a negative QRS complex (QS deflection) is seen (see Fig. 4-1B).

3. If the mean depolarization path is directed at right angles (perpendicular) to any lead, a small *biphasic deflection* (consisting of positive and negative deflections of equal size) is usually seen. If the atrial stimulation path spreads at right angles to any lead, a biphasic P wave is seen in that lead. If the ventricular stimulation path spreads at right

## Three Basic Laws of Electrocardiography

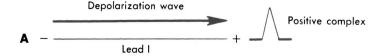

Depolarization wave

Positive complex

**A** Lead I

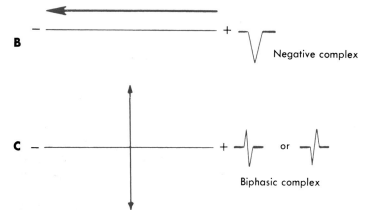

**B** Negative complex

**C** Biphasic complex

or

**FIGURE 4-1** **A,** A positive complex is seen in any lead if the wave of depolarization spreads toward the positive pole of that lead. **B,** A negative complex is seen if the depolarization wave spreads toward the negative pole (away from the positive pole) of the lead. **C,** A biphasic (partly positive, partly negative) complex is seen if the mean direction of the wave is at right angles (perpendicular) to the lead. These three basic laws apply to both the P wave (atrial depolarization) and the QRS complex (ventricular depolarization).

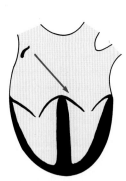

**FIGURE 4-2** With normal sinus rhythm, the atrial depolarization wave *(arrow)* spreads from the right atrium downward toward the atrioventricular (AV) junction and left leg.

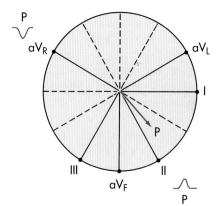

**FIGURE 4-3** With sinus rhythm, the normal P wave is negative (downward) in lead aV$_R$ and positive (upward) in lead II. Recall that with normal atrial depolarization the arrow points down toward the patient's left (see Fig. 4-2), away from the positive pole of lead aV$_R$ and toward the positive pole of lead II.

angles to any lead, the QRS complex is biphasic (see Fig. 4-1C). A biphasic QRS complex may consist of either an RS pattern or a QR pattern.

In summary, when the mean depolarization wave spreads toward the positive pole of any lead, it produces a positive (upward) deflection. When it spreads toward the negative pole (away from the positive pole) of any lead, it produces a negative (downward) deflection. When it spreads at right angles to any lead axis, it produces a biphasic deflection.

Mention of repolarization—the return of stimulated muscle to the resting state—has deliberately been omitted. The subject is touched on later in this chapter in the discussion of the normal T wave.

Keeping the three ECG laws in mind, all you need to know is the direction in which depolarization spreads through the heart at any time. Using this information, you can predict what the P waves and the QRS complexes look like in any lead.

## NORMAL P WAVE

The P wave, which represents atrial depolarization, is the first waveform seen in any cycle. Atrial depolarization is initiated by the sinus node in the right atrium (see Fig. 1-1). The atrial depolarization path therefore spreads from right to left and downward toward the atrioventricular (AV) junction. The spread of atrial depolarization can be represented by an arrow* that points downward and to the patient's left (see Fig. 4-2).

Figure 3-7C, which shows the spatial relationship of the six frontal plane (limb) leads, is

redrawn in Figure 4-3. Notice that the positive pole of lead a$V_r$ points upward in the direction of the right shoulder. The normal path of atrial depolarization spreads downward toward the left leg (away from the positive pole of lead a$V_r$). Therefore, with normal sinus rhythm, lead a$V_r$ always shows a negative P wave. Conversely, lead II is oriented with its positive pole pointing downward in the direction of the left leg (see Fig. 4-3). Therefore, the normal atrial depolarization path is directed toward the positive pole of that lead. When normal sinus rhythm is present, lead II always records a positive (upward) P wave.

In summary, when normal sinus rhythm is present, the P wave is always negative in lead a$V_r$ and positive in lead II.

Using the same principles of analysis, can you predict what the P wave looks like in leads II and a$V_r$ when the heart is being paced not by the sinus node but by the AV junction (AV junctional rhythm)? When the AV junction (or an *ectopic* pacemaker in the lower part of either atrium) is pacing the heart, atrial depolarization must spread up the atria in a *retrograde* direction, which is just the opposite of what happens with normal sinus rhythm. Therefore, an arrow representing the spread of atrial depolarization with AV junctional rhythm points upward and to the right (Fig. 4-4), just the opposite of what occurs with normal sinus rhythm. The spread of atrial depolarization upward and to the right results in a positive P wave in lead a$V_R$, since the stimulus is spreading toward the positive pole of that lead (Fig. 4-5). Conversely, lead II shows a negative P wave.

AV junctional rhythms are considered in detail in Part Two. The topic is introduced in this chapter simply to show how the polarity of the P waves in lead a$V_r$ and lead II depends on the direction of atrial depolarization and how the patterns can be predicted using simple basic principles.

At this point, you need not be concerned with the polarity of P waves in the other 10 leads. You can usually obtain all the clinical

---

*Because the arrows used to represent cardiac electrical potentials have both specific direction and specific magnitude, they are *vectors*. The details of *vectorcardiography* lie outside the scope of this book, although vectorial principles are used throughout the discussions.

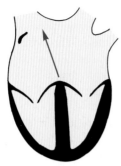

**FIGURE 4-4** When the atrioventricular (AV) junction (or an ectopic pacemaker in the low atrial area) acts as the cardiac pacemaker (junctional or low atrial rhythm), the atria are depolarized in a retrograde (backward) fashion. In this situation, an *arrow* representing atrial depolarization points upward toward the right atrium. The opposite of the pattern is seen with sinus rhythm.

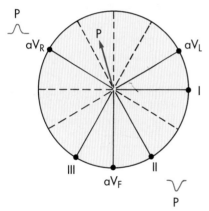

**FIGURE 4-5** With atrioventricular (AV) junctional rhythm (or low atrial ectopic rhythm), the P waves (if seen) are upward (positive) in lead $aV_R$ and downward (negative) in lead II.

information you need to determine whether the sinus node is pacing the atria by simply looking at the P waves in leads II and $aV_R$. The size and shape of these waves in other leads may be important in determining whether left or right atrial enlargement is present (see Chapter 6).

## NORMAL QRS COMPLEX

The principles used to predict P waves can also be applied in deducing the shape of the QRS waveform in the various leads. The QRS, which represents ventricular depolarization, is somewhat more complex than the P wave, but the same basic ECG rules apply to both.

To predict what the QRS looks like in the different leads, you must first know the direction of ventricular depolarization. Although the spread of atrial depolarization can be represented by a single arrow, the spread of ventricular depolarization consists of two major sequential phases:

1. The first phase of ventricular depolarization is of relatively brief duration (shorter than 0.04 sec) and small amplitude. It results from spread of the stimulus through the interventricular septum. The septum is the first part of the ventricles to be stimulated. Furthermore, the left side of the septum is stimulated first (by a branch of the left bundle of His). Thus depolarization spreads from the left ventricle to the right across the septum. Phase one of ventricular depolarization (septal stimulation) can therefore be represented by a small arrow pointing from the left septal wall to the right (Fig. 4-6A).

2. The second phase of ventricular depolarization involves simultaneous stimulation of the main mass of both the left and right ventricles from the inside (endocardium) to the outside (epicardium) of the heart muscle. In the normal heart, the left ventricle is electrically predominant. In other words, it electrically overbalances the right ventricle. Therefore, an arrow representing phase two of ventricular stimulation points toward the left ventricle (Fig. 4-6B).

In summary, the ventricular depolarization process can be divided into two main phases: stimulation of the interventricular septum (represented by a short arrow pointing through the septum into the right ventricle), and simultaneous left and right ventricular stimulation (represented by a larger arrow pointing through the left ventricle and toward the left chest).

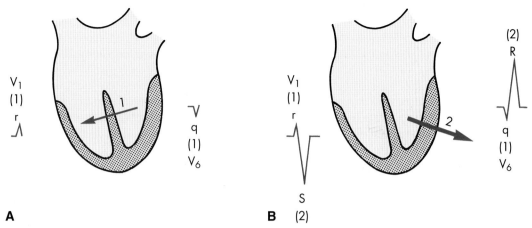

**FIGURE 4-6**  **A,** The first phase of ventricular depolarization proceeds from the left wall of the septum to the right. An *arrow* representing this phase points through the septum from the left to the right side. **B,** The second phase involves depolarization of the main bulk of the ventricles. The *arrow* points through the left ventricle because this ventricle is normally electrically predominant. The two phases produce an rS complex in the right chest lead ($V_1$) and a qR complex in the left chest lead ($V_6$).

Now that the ventricular stimulation sequence has been outlined, you can begin to predict the types of QRS patterns this sequence produces in the different leads. For the moment, the discussion is limited to QRS patterns normally seen in the chest leads (the horizontal plane leads).

## CHEST LEADS

As discussed in Chapter 3, lead $V_1$ shows voltages detected by an electrode placed on the right side of the sternum (fourth intercostal space). Lead $V_6$, a left chest lead, shows voltages detected in the left midaxillary line (see Fig. 3-8). What does the QRS complex look like in these leads (see Fig. 4-6)? Ventricular stimulation occurs in two phases:

1. The first phase of ventricular stimulation, septal stimulation, is represented by an arrow pointing to the right, reflecting the left-to-right spread of the depolarization stimulus through the septum (see Fig. 4-6A). This small arrow points toward the positive pole of lead $V_1$. Therefore the spread of stim-ulation to the right during the first phase produces a small positive deflection (r wave) in lead $V_1$. What does lead $V_6$ show? The left-to-right spread of septal stimulation produces a small negative deflection (q wave) in lead $V_6$. Thus the same electrical event (septal stimulation) produces a small positive deflection (or r wave) in lead $V_1$ and a small negative deflection (q wave) in a left precordial lead, like lead $V_6$. (This situation is analogous to the one described for the P wave, which is normally positive in lead II but always negative in lead $aV_r$.)

2. The second phase of ventricular stimulation is represented by an arrow pointing in the direction of the left ventricle (see Fig. 4-6B). This arrow points away from the positive pole of lead $V_1$ and toward the negative pole of lead $V_6$. Therefore, the spread of stimulation to the left during the second phase results in a negative deflection in the right precordial leads and a positive deflection in the left precordial leads. Lead $V_1$ shows a deep negative (S) wave, and lead $V_6$ displays a tall positive (R) wave.

In summary, with normal QRS patterns, lead $V_1$ shows an rS type of complex. The small initial r wave represents the left-to-right spread of septal stimulation. This wave is sometimes referred to as the *septal r wave* because it reflects septal stimulation. The negative (S) wave reflects the spread of ventricular stimulation forces during phase two, away from the right and toward the dominant left ventricle. Conversely, viewed from an electrode in the $V_6$ position, septal and ventricular stimulation produce a qR pattern. The q wave is a *septal q wave*, reflecting the left-to-right spread of the stimulus through the septum away from lead $V_6$. The positive (R) wave reflects the leftward spread of ventricular stimulation voltages through the left ventricle.

Once again, to reemphasize, the same electrical event, whether depolarization of the atria or ventricles, produces very different looking waveforms in different leads because the spatial orientation of the leads is different.

What happens *between* leads $V_1$ and $V_6$? The answer is that as you move across the chest (in the direction of the electrically predominant left ventricle), the R wave tends to become relatively larger and the S wave becomes relatively smaller. This increase in height of the R wave, which usually reaches a maximum around lead $V_4$ or $V_5$, is called *normal R wave progression*. Figure 4-7 shows examples of normal R wave progression.

At some point, generally around the $V_3$ or $V_4$ position, the ratio of the R wave to the S wave becomes 1. This point, where the amplitude of the R wave equals that of the S wave, is called the *transition zone* (see Fig. 4-7). In the ECGs of some normal people, the transition may be seen as early as lead $V_2$. This is called *early transition*. In other cases, the transition zone may not appear until leads $V_5$ and $V_6$. This is called *delayed transition*.

Examine the set of normal chest leads in Figure 4-8. Notice the rS complex in lead $V_1$ and the qR complex in lead $V_6$. The R wave tends to become gradually larger as you move toward the left chest leads. The transition zone, where the R wave and S wave are about equal, is in lead $V_4$. In normal chest leads, the R wave voltage does not have to become literally larger as you go from leads $V_1$ and $V_6$. The overall trend should show a relative increase, however. In Figure 4-8, for example, notice that the complexes in leads $V_2$ and $V_3$ are about the same and that the R wave in lead $V_5$ is taller than the R wave in lead $V_6$.

In summary, the normal chest lead ECG shows an rS-type complex in lead $V_1$ with a steady increase in the relative size of the R wave toward the left chest and a decrease in S wave amplitude. Leads $V_5$ and $V_6$ generally show a qR-type complex.*

The concept of *normal R wave progression* is key in distinguishing normal and abnormal ECG patterns. For example, imagine the effect that an anterior wall myocardial infarction (MI) would have on normal R wave progression. Anterior wall infarction results in the death of myocardial cells and the loss of normal positive (R wave) voltages. Therefore, one major ECG sign of an anterior wall infarction is the loss of normal R wave progression in the chest leads (see Chapters 8 and 9).

An understanding of normal R wave progression in the chest leads also provides a basis for recognizing other basic ECG abnormalities. For example, consider the effect of left or right ventricular hypertrophy (enlarged muscle mass) on the chest lead patterns. As mentioned previously, the left ventricle is normally electrically predominant and left ventricular depolarization produces deep (negative) S waves in the

---

*Normal chest lead patterns may show slight variation from the patterns discussed thus far. For example, in some normal ECGs, lead $V_1$ shows a QS pattern, not an rS pattern. In other normal chest lead patterns, the septal q wave in the left chest leads may not be seen; thus leads $V_5$ and $V_6$ show an R wave and not a qR complex. On still other normal ECGs, leads $V_5$ and $V_6$ may show a narrow qRs complex as a normal variant (see Fig. 3-2, lead $V_4$) and lead $V_1$ may show a narrow rSr'.

## Normal R Wave Progression

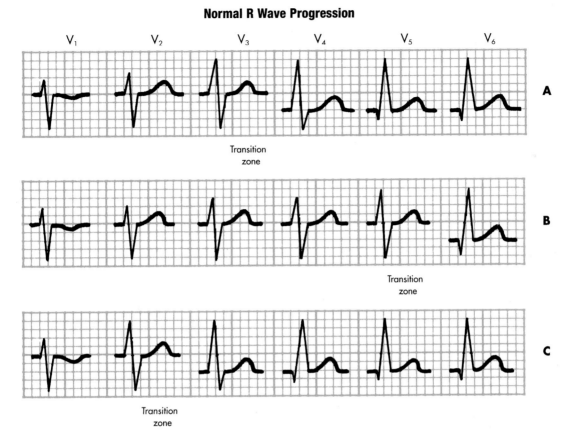

**FIGURE 4-7**  R waves in the chest leads normally become relatively taller from lead $V_1$ to the left chest leads. **A,** Notice the transition in lead $V_3$. **B,** Somewhat delayed R wave progression, with the transition in lead $V_5$. **C,** Early transition in lead $V_2$.

### Normal Chest Lead ECG

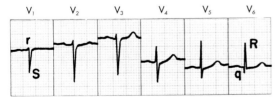

**FIGURE 4-8**  The transition is in lead $V_4$. In lead $V_1$, notice the normal septal r wave as part of an rS complex. In lead $V_6$, the normal septal q is part of a qR complex.

right chest leads with tall (positive) R waves in the left chest leads. With left ventricular hypertrophy, these left ventricular voltages are further increased, resulting in very tall R waves in the left chest leads and very deep S waves in the right chest leads. On the other hand, right ventricular hypertrophy shifts the balance of electrical forces to the right, producing tall positive waves (R waves) in the right chest leads (see Chapter 6).

## LIMB (EXTREMITY) LEADS

Of the six limb leads (I, II, III, $aV_R$, $aV_L$, and $aV_F$), lead $aV_r$ is the easiest to visualize. The

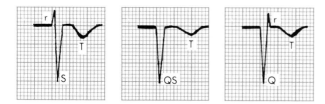

**FIGURE 4-9** Lead aV$_R$ normally shows one of three basic negative patterns: an rS complex, a QS complex, or a Qr complex. The T wave also is normally negative.

positive pole of lead aV$_R$ is oriented upward and toward the right shoulder. The ventricular stimulation forces are oriented primarily toward the left ventricle. Therefore lead aV$_R$ normally shows a predominantly negative QRS complex. Lead aV$_R$ may display any of the QRS-T complexes shown in Figure 4-9. In all cases, the QRS is predominantly negative. The T wave in lead aV$_R$ is also normally negative.

The QRS patterns in the other five limb leads are somewhat more complicated. The reason is that the QRS patterns in the limb leads show considerable normal variation. For example, the limb leads in the ECGs of some normal people may show qR-type complexes in leads I and aV$_L$ and rS-type complexes in leads III and aV$_F$ (Fig. 4-10). The ECGs of other people may show just the opposite picture, with qR complexes in leads II, III, and aV$_F$ and RS complexes in lead aV$_l$ and sometimes lead I (Fig. 4-11).

What accounts for this marked normal variability in the QRS patterns shown in the limb leads? The patterns that are seen depend on the electrical position of the heart. The term *electrical position* is virtually synonymous with *mean QRS axis*, which is described in greater detail in Chapter 5.

In simplest terms the electrical position of the heart may be described as either *horizontal* or *vertical:*

■ When the heart is electrically horizontal *(horizontal QRS axis)*, ventricular depolarization is directed mainly horizontally and to the left in the frontal plane. As the frontal plane diagram in Figure 3-10 shows, the positive poles of leads I and aV$_L$ are oriented horizontally and to the left. Therefore, when the heart is electrically horizontal, the QRS voltages are directed toward leads I and aV$_L$. Consequently, a tall R wave (usually as part of a qR complex) is seen in these leads.

■ When the heart is electrically vertical *(vertical QRS axis)*, ventricular depolarization is directed mainly downward. In the frontal

## Normal Horizontal QRS Axis

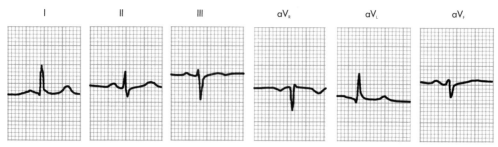

**FIGURE 4-10** With a horizontal QRS position (axis), leads I and aV$_L$ show qR complexes, lead II shows an RS complex, and leads III and aV$_F$ show rS complexes.

## Normal Vertical QRS Axis

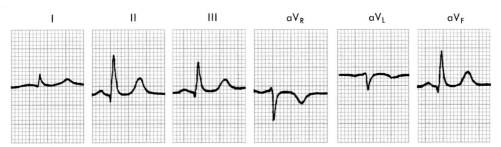

**FIGURE 4-11** With a vertical QRS position (axis), leads II, III, and aV$_F$ show qR complexes, but lead aV$_L$ (and sometimes lead I) shows an RS complex. This is the reverse of the pattern that occurs with a normal horizontal axis.

plane diagram (see Fig. 3-10), the positive poles of leads II, III, and aV$_F$ are oriented downward. Therefore, when the heart is electrically vertical, the QRS voltages are directed toward leads II, III, and aV$_F$. This produces a tall R wave (usually as part of a qR complex) in these leads.

The concepts of electrically horizontal and electrically vertical heart positions can be expressed in another way. When the heart is electrically horizontal, leads I and aV$_l$ show qR complexes similar to the qR complexes seen normally in the left chest leads (V$_5$ and V$_6$). Leads II, III, and aV$_F$ show rS or RS complexes similar to those normally seen in the right chest leads. Therefore, when the heart is electrically horizontal, the patterns in leads I and aV$_l$ resemble those in leads V$_5$ and V$_6$ whereas the patterns in leads II, III, and aV$_F$ resemble those in the right chest leads. Conversely, when the heart is electrically vertical, just the opposite patterns are seen in the limb leads. With a vertical heart, leads II, III, and aV$_F$ show qR complexes similar to those seen in the left chest leads, and leads I and aV$_L$ show rS-type complexes resembling those in the right chest leads.

Dividing the electrical position of the heart into vertical and horizontal variants is obviously an oversimplification. In Figure 4-12, for example, leads I, II, aV$_L$, and aV$_F$ all show positive QRS complexes. Therefore, this tracing has features of *both* the vertical and the horizontal variants. (Sometimes this pattern is referred to as an "intermediate" heart position.)

For present purposes, however, you can regard the QRS patterns in the limb leads as

## Normal Intermediate QRS Axis

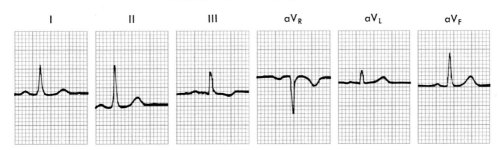

**FIGURE 4-12** Limb leads sometimes show patterns that are hybrids of vertical and horizontal variants, with R waves in leads I, II, III, aV$_L$, and aV$_F$. This represents an intermediate QRS axis and is also a normal variant.

basically variants of either the horizontal or the vertical QRS patterns described.

In summary, the limb leads in normal ECGs can show a variable QRS pattern. Lead $aV_R$ normally always records a predominantly negative QRS complex (Qr, QS, or rS). The QRS patterns in the other limb leads vary depending on the electrical position (QRS axis) of the heart. With an electrically vertical axis, leads II, III, and $aV_F$ show qR-type complexes. With an electrically horizontal axis, leads I and $aV_L$ show qR complexes. Therefore, it is not possible to define a single normal ECG pattern; rather, there is a normal variability. Students and clinicians must familiarize themselves with the normal variants in both the chest leads and the limb leads.

## NORMAL ST SEGMENT

As noted in Chapter 2, the normal ST segment, representing the early phase of ventricular repolarization, is usually isoelectric (flat on the baseline). Slight deviations (generally less than 1 mm) may be seen normally. As described in Chapter 9, the ECGs of certain healthy people show more marked ST segment elevations as a normal variant (early repolarization pattern). Finally, examine the ST segments in the right chest leads ($V_1$ and $V_2$) of Figure 3-2. Notice that they are short and the T waves appear to take off almost from the J point (junction of the QRS complex and ST segment). This pattern of an early takeoff of the T wave in the right chest leads is not an uncommon finding in healthy individuals.

## NORMAL T WAVE

Ventricular repolarization—the return of stimulated muscle to the resting state—produces the ST segment, T wave, and U wave. Deciding whether the T wave in any lead is normal is generally straightforward. As a rule, the T wave follows the direction of the main QRS deflection. Thus when the main QRS deflection is positive (upright), the T wave is normally positive.

Some more specific rules about the direction of the normal T wave can be formulated. The normal T wave is always negative in lead $aV_R$ but positive in lead II. Left-sided chest leads such as $V_4$ to $V_6$ normally always show a positive T wave.

The T wave in the other leads may be variable. In the right chest leads ($V_1$ and $V_2$), the T wave may be normally negative, isoelectric, or positive, but it is almost always positive from lead $V_3$ to $V_6$.* Furthermore, if the T wave is positive in any chest lead, it must remain positive in all chest leads to the left of that lead. Otherwise, it is abnormal. For example, if the T wave is negative in leads $V_1$ and $V_2$ and becomes positive in lead $V_3$, it should normally remain positive in leads $V_4$ to $V_6$.

The polarity of the T wave in the limb leads also depends on the electrical axis of the heart. With a horizontal axis, the main QRS deflection is positive in leads I and $aV_L$ and the T wave is also positive in these leads. With an electrically vertical axis, the QRS is positive in leads II, III, and $aV_F$ and the T wave is also positive in these leads. On some normal ECGs with a vertical axis, however, the T wave may be negative in lead III.

---

*In children and in some normal adults, a downward T wave may extend as far left as lead $V_3$ or $V_4$ in leads with an rS- or RS-type complex. This is known as the *juvenile T wave pattern*.

## REVIEW

The three basic "laws" of electrocardiography are as follows:

1. A *positive (upward) deflection* is seen in any lead if depolarization spreads toward the positive pole of that lead.

2. A *negative (downward) deflection* is seen if depolarization spreads toward the negative pole (or away from the positive pole) of any lead.

3. If the mean depolarization path is directed at right angles *(perpendicular)* to any lead, a small *biphasic (RS or QR) deflection* is seen.

Atrial depolarization starts in sinus node and spreads downward and to the patient's left, toward the positive pole of lead II and away from the positive pole of lead $aV_R$. Therefore, with normal sinus rhythm the P wave is always positive in lead II and negative in lead $aV_R$.

Ventricular depolarization consists of two sequential phases:

1. The first phase is stimulation of the ventricular septum from left to right. This produces a small (septal) r wave in the right chest leads and a small (septal) q wave in the left chest leads.

2. During the second major phase of ventricular depolarization, the stimulus spreads simultaneously outward through the right and left ventricles. Because the mass of the normal left ventricle overbalances the mass of the right ventricle, the spread of depolarization through the left ventricle predominates on the normal ECG. This spread of a stimulus through the left ventricle produces a tall R wave in the left chest leads (e.g., $V_5$ and $V_6$) in association with a small initial q wave. In the right chest leads ($V_1$ and $V_2$), the stimulus produces a deep S wave associated with a small initial r wave.

Chest leads between these extreme positions show a relative increase in R wave amplitude and a decrease in S wave amplitude.

In the limb (extremity) leads, the shape of the QRS complex varies with the electrical position (axis) of the heart:

1. When the heart is electrically horizontal, leads I and $aV_L$ show a qR pattern.

2. When the heart is electrically vertical, leads II, III, and $aV_F$ show a qR pattern.

The normal T wave generally follows the direction of the main deflection of the QRS complex in any lead. In the chest leads, the T wave may normally be negative in leads $V_1$ and $V_2$. In most adults the T wave becomes positive by lead $V_2$ and remains positive in the left chest leads. In the limb leads, the T wave is always positive in lead II and negative in lead $aV_R$. When the heart is electrically horizontal, the QRS complex and T wave are positive in leads I and $aV_L$. When the heart is electrically vertical, the QRS complex and T wave are positive in leads II, III, and $aV_F$.

# QUESTIONS

1. Examine the 12-lead ECG and lead II rhythm strip shown below. Then answers these questions:

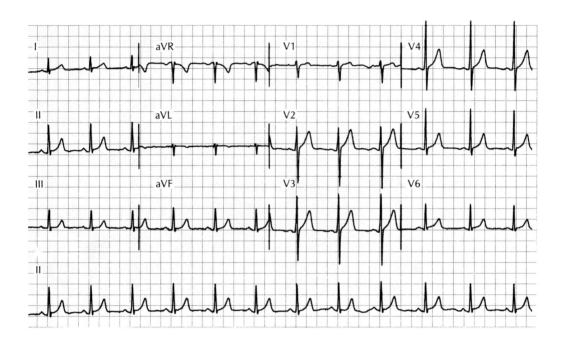

   a. Is normal sinus rhythm present?
   b. In the limb leads, is the QRS axis electrically vertical or electrically horizontal?
   c. In the chest leads, where is the transition zone?
   d. Is the PR interval normal?
   e. Is the QRS interval normal?
   f. Are the T waves in the chest leads normal?

2. On the following ECG, is sinus rhythm present?

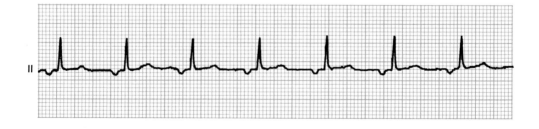

# Electrical Axis and Axis Deviation

**N**ormal ECG patterns in the chest and limb (extremity) leads were discussed in Chapter 4. The general terms *horizontal heart* (or *horizontal QRS axis*) and *vertical heart* (or *vertical QRS axis*) were used to describe the normal variations in QRS patterns seen in the extremity leads. In this chapter the concept of electrical axis is refined, and methods are presented for estimating the QRS axis quickly and simply.

## MEAN QRS AXIS: DEFINITION

The depolarization stimulus spreads through the ventricles in different directions from instant to instant. For example, it may be directed toward lead I at one moment and toward lead III the next. The mean direction of the QRS complex, or *mean QRS electrical axis*, can also be described. If you could draw an arrow to represent the overall, or mean, direction in which the QRS complex is pointed in the frontal plane of the body, you would be drawing the electrical axis of the QRS complex. The term *mean QRS axis* therefore describes the general direction in the frontal plane toward which the QRS complex is predominantly pointed.

Since the QRS axis is being defined in the frontal plane, the QRS is being described only in reference to the six limb leads (the six frontal plane leads). Therefore the scale of reference used to measure the mean QRS axis is the diagram of the frontal plane leads (described in Chapter 3 and depicted again in Fig. 5-1). Einthoven's triangle can easily be converted into a triaxial lead diagram by having the axes of the three standard limb leads (I, II, and III) intersect at a central point (Fig. 5-1*A*). Similarly the axes of the three augmented limb leads (aV$_R$, aV$_L$, and aV$_F$) also form a triaxial lead diagram (Fig. 5-1*B*). These two triaxial lead diagrams can be combined to produce a hexaxial lead diagram (Fig. 5-1*C*). You will be using this diagram to determine the mean QRS axis and describe axis deviation.

As noted in Chapter 3, each lead has a positive and negative pole (see Fig. 5-1*C*). As a wave of depolarization spreads toward the positive pole, an upward (positive) deflection occurs. As a wave spreads toward the negative pole, a downward (negative) deflection is inscribed.

Finally, a scale is needed to determine or calculate the mean QRS axis. By convention, the positive pole of lead I is said to be at 0°. All points below the lead I axis are positive, and all points above that axis are negative (Fig. 5-2). Thus toward the positive pole of lead aV$_L$ (−30°), the scale becomes negative. Downward toward the positive poles of leads II, III, and

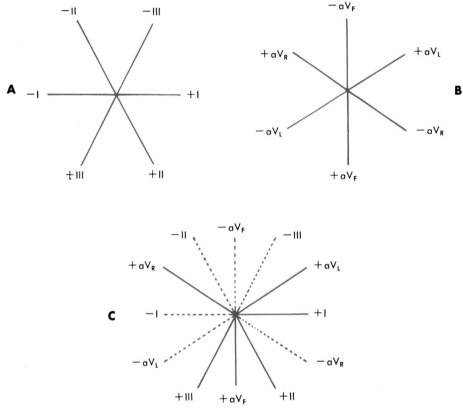

**FIGURE 5-1   A,** Relationship of leads I, II, and III. **B,** Relationship of leads aV$_R$, aV$_L$, and aV$_F$. **C,** These diagrams have been combined to form a hexaxial lead diagram. Notice that each lead has a positive and negative pole. The negative poles are designated by *dashed lines.*

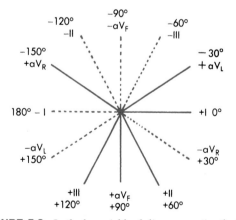

**FIGURE 5-2**   In the hexaxial lead diagram, notice that each lead has an angular designation, with the positive pole of lead I at 0°. All leads above lead I have negative angular values, and the leads below it have positive values.

aV$_F$, the scale becomes more positive (lead II at +60°, lead aV$_F$ at +90°, and lead III at +120°).

The completed hexaxial diagram used to measure the QRS axis is shown in Figure 5-2. By convention again, an electrical axis that points toward lead aV$_L$ is termed *leftward* or *horizontal.* An axis that points toward leads II, III, and aV$_F$ is *rightward* or *vertical.*

## MEAN QRS AXIS: CALCULATION

In calculating the mean QRS axis, you are answering this question: In what general direction or toward which lead axis is the QRS complex predominantly oriented? In Figure 5-3, for example, notice the tall R waves in leads II, III, and aV$_F$. These waves indicate that the

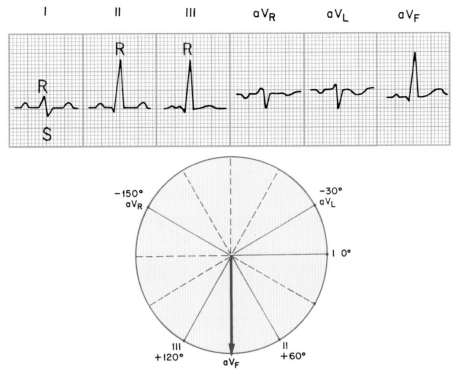

**FIGURE 5-3** Mean QRS axis of +90° (see text).

heart is electrically vertical *(vertical electrical axis)*. Furthermore, the R waves are equally tall in leads II and III.* Therefore, by simple inspection, the mean electrical QRS axis can be seen to be directed between the positive poles of leads II and III and toward the *positive pole* of lead $aV_F$ (+90°).

As a general rule, the mean QRS axis points midway between any two leads that show tall R waves of equal height.

In Figure 5-3, the mean electrical axis could have been calculated a second way. Recall from Chapter 3 that if a wave of depolarization is oriented at right angles to any lead axis, a biphasic complex (RS or QR) is recorded in that lead. Reasoning in a reverse manner, if you find a

biphasic complex in any of the extremity leads, the mean QRS axis must be directed at 90° to that lead. Now look at Figure 5-3 again. Do you see any biphasic QRS complexes? Obviously, lead I is biphasic and shows an RS pattern. Therefore the mean electrical axis must be directed at right angles to lead I. Since lead I on the hexaxial lead scale is at 0°, the mean electrical axis must be at right angles to 0° or at either –90° or +90°. If the axis were –90°, the depolarization forces would be oriented away from the positive pole of lead $aV_F$ and that lead would show a negative complex. In Figure 5-3, lead $aV_F$ shows a positive complex (tall R wave); therefore the axis must be +90°.

Figure 5-4 presents another example. By inspection, the mean QRS axis is obviously horizontal, since leads I and $aV_L$ are positive and leads II, III, and $aV_F$ are predominantly negative. The precise electrical axis can be calculated

---

*In Figure 5-3, three leads (II, III, and $aV_F$) have R waves of equal height. In this situation, the electrical axis points toward the middle lead (i.e., toward lead $aV_F$ or at +90°).

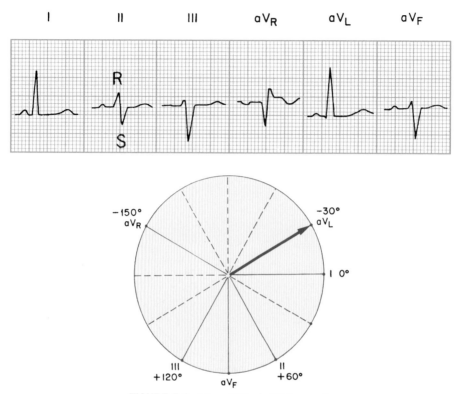

**FIGURE 5-4** Mean QRS of –30° (see text).

by looking at lead II, which shows a biphasic RS complex. Therefore the axis must be at right angles to lead II. Because lead II is at +60° on the hexaxial scale (see Fig. 5-2), the axis must be either –30° or +150°. If it were +150°, leads II, III, and aV$_F$ would be positive. Clearly, the axis is –30°.

Another example is given in Figure 5-5. The QRS complex is positive in leads II, III, and aV$_F$. Therefore the axis is relatively vertical. Because the R waves are of equal magnitude in leads I and III, the mean QRS axis must be oriented between these two leads, or at +60°.

Alternatively, in Figure 5-5, the QRS axis can be calculated by looking at lead aV$_L$, which shows a biphasic RS-type complex. The axis must be at right angles to lead aV$_L$ (–30°); that is, it must be oriented at either –120° or +60°. Obviously, the axis is at +60°. The electrical axis

must be oriented toward lead II, which shows a tall R wave.

A second general rule can now be given: The mean QRS axis is oriented at right angles to any lead showing a biphasic complex. In this situation, the mean QRS axis points in the direction of leads showing tall R waves.

Still another example is provided in Figure 5-6. The electrical axis is seen to be oriented away from leads II, III, and aV$_F$ and toward leads aV$_R$ and aV$_L$, which show positive complexes. Because the R waves are of equal magnitude in leads aV$_R$ and aV$_L$, the axis must be oriented precisely between these leads, or at –90°. Alternatively, look at lead I, which shows a biphasic RS complex. In this case the axis must be directed at right angles to lead I (0°); that is, it must be either –90° or +90°. Because the axis is oriented away from the positive pole of lead aV$_F$

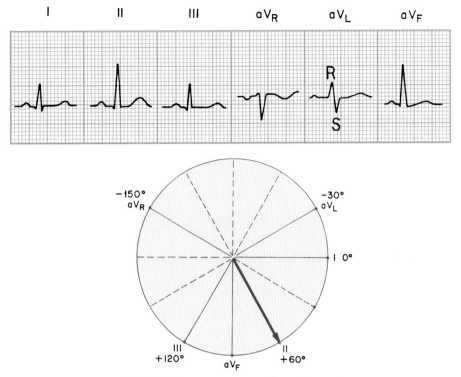

**FIGURE 5-5**   Mean QRS axis of +60° (see text).

and toward the negative pole of that lead, it must be –90°.

Again, look at Figure 5-7. Because lead $aV_R$ shows a biphasic RS-type complex, the electrical axis must be at right angles to the axis of that lead. The axis of $aV_R$ is at –150°; therefore the electrical axis in this case must be either –60° or +120°. Clearly, it is –60° because lead $aV_L$ is positive and lead III shows a negative complex.*

These basic examples should establish the ground rules for calculating the mean QRS axis.

Such calculations are generally only an estimate or a near approximation, however. An error of 10° or 15° is not clinically significant. Thus it is perfectly acceptable to calculate the axis from leads in which the QRS complex is nearly biphasic or from two leads in which the R (or S) waves are of approximately equal amplitude.*

---

*In Figure 5-7, the QRS axis can also be calculated by looking at lead I, which shows an R wave of equal amplitude with the S wave in lead II. The mean QRS axis must be oriented between the positive pole of lead I (0°) and the negative pole of lead II (–120°). Therefore the axis must be at –60°.

---

*For example, when the R (or S) waves in two leads have similar but not identical voltages, the mean QRS axis does not lie exactly between these two leads. Instead, it points more toward the lead with the larger amplitude. Similarly, if a lead shows a biphasic (RS or QR) deflection with the R and S (or Q and R) waves *not* of identical amplitude, the mean QRS axis does *not* point exactly perpendicular to that lead. If the R wave is larger than the S (or Q) wave, the axis points slightly less than 90° away from the lead. If the R wave is smaller than the S (or Q) wave, the axis points slightly more than 90° away from that lead.

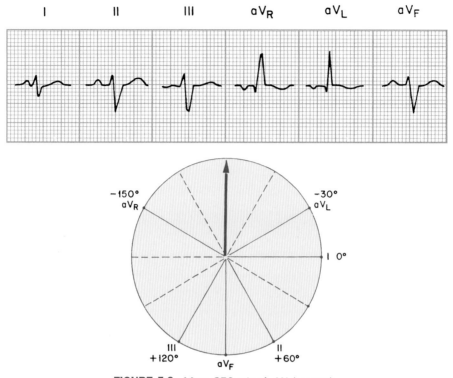

**FIGURE 5-6** Mean QRS axis of –90° (see text).

In summary, the mean QRS axis can be determined on the basis of one or both of the following rules:

- The mean QRS axis points midway between the axes of two extremity leads that show tall R waves of equal amplitude.

- The mean QRS axis points at 90° (right angles) to any extremity lead that shows a biphasic (QR or RS) complex and in the direction of leads that show relatively tall R waves.

## AXIS DEVIATION

The mean QRS axis is a basic measurement that should be made on every ECG. In the ECGs of most normal people, this axis lies between –30° and +100°. An axis of –30° or more negative is described as *left axis deviation (LAD)*, and one

that is +100° or more positive is termed *right axis deviation (RAD)*. In other words, LAD is an abnormal extension of the mean QRS axis found in persons with an electrically horizontal heart, and RAD is an abnormal extension of the mean QRS axis in persons with an electrically vertical heart.

The mean QRS axis is determined by the anatomic position of the heart and the direction in which the stimulus spreads through the ventricles (i.e., the direction of ventricular depolarization):

1. The influence of *cardiac anatomic position* on the electrical axis can be illustrated by the effects of respiration. When a person breathes in, the diaphragm descends and the heart becomes more vertical in the chest cavity. This change generally shifts the QRS electrical axis vertically (to the right).

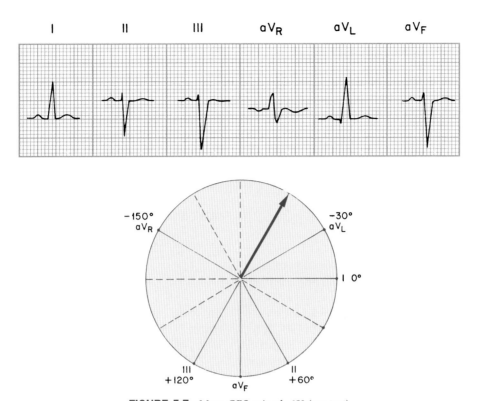

**FIGURE 5-7** Mean QRS axis of –60° (see text).

(Patients with emphysema and chronically hyperinflated lungs usually have anatomically vertical hearts and electrically vertical QRS axes.) Conversely, when the person breathes out, the diaphragm ascends and the heart assumes a more horizontal position in the chest. This generally shifts the QRS electrical axis horizontally (to the left).

2. The influence of the *direction of ventricular depolarization* can be illustrated by left anterior hemiblock, in which the spread of stimuli through the more superior and leftward portions of the left ventricle is delayed and the mean QRS axis shifts to the left (see Chapter 7). By contrast, with right ventricular hypertrophy (RVH), the QRS axis shifts to the right.

Recognition of RAD and LAD is quite simple:

1. RAD exists if the QRS axis is found to be +100° or more positive. Recall that when leads II and III show tall R waves of equal height, the QRS axis must be +90°. As an approximate rule, if leads II and III show tall R waves and the R wave in lead III exceeds the R wave in lead II, RAD is present. In addition, lead I shows an RS pattern with the S wave deeper than the R wave is tall (Figs. 5-8 and 5-9).

2. LAD exists if the QRS axis is found to be –30° or more negative. In the ECG shown in Figure 5-4, the QRS axis is exactly –30°. Notice that lead II shows a biphasic (RS)

**Right Axis Deviation**

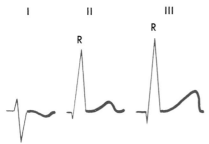

**FIGURE 5-8**   Right axis deviation (mean QRS axis more positive than +100) can be determined by inspecting leads I, II, and III. Notice that the R wave is taller in lead III than in lead II.

complex. Remember that the location of lead II is aligned at +60° (see Fig. 5-2) and a biphasic complex indicates that the electrical axis must be at right angles to that lead (at either –30° or +150°). Thus with an axis of –30°, lead II shows an RS complex with the R and S waves of equal amplitude. If the electrical axis is more negative than –30° (LAD), lead II shows an RS complex with the S wave deeper than the R wave is tall (Figs. 5-10 and 5-11).

The rules for recognizing QRS axis deviation can be summarized as follows:

■ RAD is present if the R wave in lead III is taller than the R wave in lead II. Notice that with RAD, lead I shows an RS-type complex

**Left Axis Deviation**

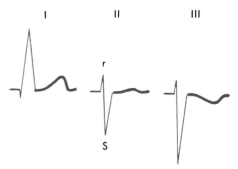

**FIGURE 5-10**   Left axis deviation (mean QRS axis more negative than –30°) can be determined by simple inspection of leads I, II, and III. Notice that lead II shows an rS complex (with the S wave of greater amplitude than the r wave).

in which the S wave is deeper than the R wave is tall (see Figs. 5-8 and 5-9).

■ LAD is present if lead I shows a tall R wave, lead III shows a deep S wave, and lead II shows either a biphasic RS complex (with the amplitude of the S wave exceeding the height of the r wave) (see Figs. 5-10 and 5-11) or a QS complex. Leads I and aV$_L$ both show R waves.

In Chapter 4, the terms *electrically vertical* and *electrically horizontal* heart positions (mean QRS axes) were introduced. This chapter has added the terms *left axis deviation* and *right axis devia-*

**Right Axis Deviation**

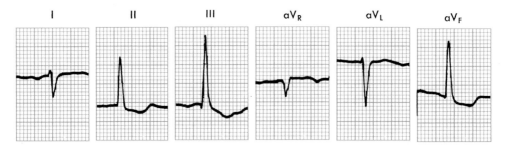

**FIGURE 5-9**   Notice the R waves in leads II and III, with the R wave in lead III being larger than the one in lead II, from a patient with right axis deviation.

## Left Axis Deviation

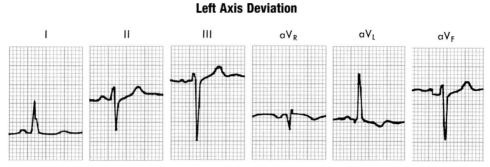

**FIGURE 5-11**  Notice the rS complex in lead II, from a patient with left axis deviation.

*tion.* What is the difference between these terms? Electrically vertical and electrically horizontal heart positions are qualitative. With an electrically vertical mean QRS axis, leads II, III, and $aV_F$ show tall R waves. With an electrically horizontal mean QRS axis, leads I and $aV_L$ show tall R waves. With an electrically vertical heart, the actual mean QRS axis may be normal (e.g., +80°) or abnormally rightward (e.g., +120°). Similarly, with an electrically horizontal heart, the actual axis may be normal (0°) or abnormally leftward (−50°).

RAD therefore is simply an extreme form of a vertical mean QRS axis, and LAD is an extreme form of a horizontal mean QRS axis. Saying that a patient has an electrically vertical or horizontal mean QRS axis does not, in fact, tell whether actual axis deviation is present.

### AXIS DEVIATION: INSTANT RECOGNITION

For beginning students, precise calculation of the QRS axis is not as important as answering the following key questions: Is the QRS axis normal, or is LAD or RAD present? The answer can be obtained simply by inspecting the QRS complex from leads I and II (Fig. 5-12).

If the area under the QRS complex in both leads is positive, the axis must be normal. If the QRS complex is predominantly positive in lead I and negative in lead II, LAD is present. If the QRS complex is predominantly negative in lead I and positive in lead II, RAD (or at least borderline RAD) is present. (Very rarely, the QRS

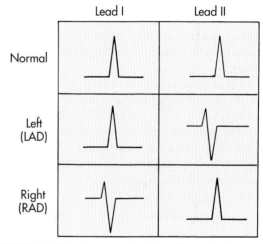

**FIGURE 5-12**  Simple method for telling whether the QRS axis is normal using leads I and II. LAD, left axis deviation; RAD, right axis deviation.

will be predominantly negative in both leads I and II. In such unusual cases, extreme right or left axis deviation will be present.)

### CLINICAL SIGNIFICANCE

Axis deviation may be encountered in a variety of settings. RAD, with a mean QRS axis +100° or more, is sometimes seen in the ECGs of normal hearts. RVH is an important cause of RAD, however (see Chapter 6). Another cause is myocardial infarction of the lateral wall of the left ventricle. In this setting, loss of the normal leftward depolarization forces may lead "by default" to a rightward axis (see Fig. 8-11). Left posterior fascicular block is a much rarer cause of RAD (see Chapter 7). The ECGs of patients with chronic lung disease (emphysema or chronic bronchitis) often show RAD. Finally, a sudden shift in the mean QRS axis to the right (not necessarily causing actual RAD) may occur with acute pulmonary embolism (see Chapters 11 and 24).

LAD, with a mean QRS axis of –30° or more, is also seen in several settings. Patients with left ventricular hypertrophy (LVH) sometimes but not always have LAD (see Chapter 6). Left anterior hemiblock is a fairly common cause of marked deviation (more negative than –45°). LAD may be seen in association with left bundle branch block (see Chapter 7). It may also occur in the absence of apparent cardiac disease.

RAD or LAD is not necessarily a sign of significant underlying heart disease, however. Nevertheless, its recognition (Figs. 5-12 and 5-13) often provides supportive evidence for LVH or RVH, ventricular conduction disturbance (left anterior or posterior fascicular block), or another disorder (see Chapter 24).

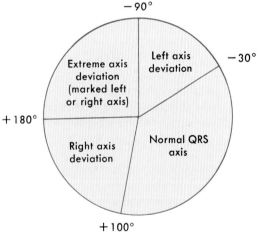

**FIGURE 5-13** Normal QRS axis and axis deviation. Most ECGs show either a normal axis or left or right axis deviation. Occasionally, the QRS axis is between –90° and 180°. Such an extreme shift may be caused by marked left or right axis deviation.

Finally, the limits for LAD and RAD (–30° to +100°) used in this book are necessarily arbitrary. Some authors use different criteria (e.g., 0° to +90°). These apparent discrepancies reflect the important fact that no absolute parameters have been established in clinical electrocardiography—only general criteria can be applied. The same problems will be encountered in the discussion of LVH and RVH (see Chapter 6) because different voltage criteria have been described by various authors.

On rare occasions, all six limb leads show biphasic (QR or RS) complexes, which makes it impossible to calculate the mean frontal plane QRS axis. In such cases, the term *indeterminate axis* is used (Fig. 5-14). An indeterminate QRS axis may occur as a normal variant, or it may be seen in a variety of pathologic settings.

## MEAN ELECTRICAL AXIS OF THE P WAVE AND T WAVE

To this point, this chapter has considered only the mean electrical axis of the QRS complex in the frontal plane. The same principles can be applied to the mean electrical axes of the P wave and T wave in the frontal plane.

For example, when sinus rhythm is present, the normal P wave is always negative in lead $aV_R$ and positive in lead II. Normally, therefore, the P wave is generally directed toward the positive pole of lead II (see Fig. 4-3), which makes the normal mean P wave axis about +60°. On the other hand, if the atrioventricular (AV) junction (and not the sinus node) is pacing the heart, the atria are stimulated in a retrograde way. When AV junctional rhythm is present, atrial depolarization spreads upward, toward lead $aV_R$ and away from lead II (see Fig. 4-5). In this situation, lead $aV_R$ may show a positive P wave and lead II a negative P wave, and the mean P wave axis may be about –150°.

The same principles can be used in calculating the mean electrical axis of the T wave in the frontal plane. As a rule, the mean T wave axis

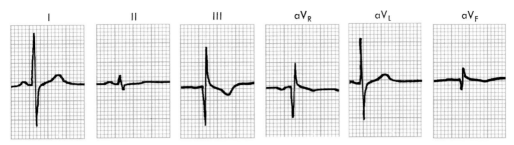

**FIGURE 5-14**   Indeterminate axis. Notice the biphasic complexes (RS or QR) in all six frontal plane leads.

and the mean QRS axis normally point in the same general (but not identical) direction. In other words, when the electrical position of the heart is horizontal, T waves normally are positive in leads I and aV$_L$, in association with tall R waves in those leads. When the electrical position is vertical, T waves are normally positive in leads II, III, and aV$_F$, in association with

tall R waves in those leads. (The T wave is often normally negative in lead III, however, regardless of the electrical position of the heart.)

In summary, the concept of mean electrical axis can be applied to the QRS complex, P wave, or T wave. The mean electrical axis describes the general or overall direction of depolarization or repolarization in the frontal plane.

# REVIEW

The term *mean QRS axis* describes the general direction in which the QRS axis is pointed in the frontal plane of the body. Therefore the mean QRS axis is measured in reference to the six limb (frontal plane) leads. These leads can be arranged in the form of a hexaxial (six axes) diagram (see Fig. 5-1*C*).

The approximate mean QRS axis can be determined by using one of the following rules:

1. The axis will be pointed midway between the positive poles of any two leads that show R waves of equal height.

2. The axis will be pointed at right angles (perpendicular) to any lead that shows a biphasic complex and toward other leads that show tall R waves.

The normal mean QRS axis lies between –30° and +100°. An axis more negative than –30° is defined as *left axis deviation (LAD).* An axis more

positive than +100° is defined as *right axis deviation (RAD).* LAD is an extreme form of a horizontal electrical axis. RAD is an extreme form of a vertical electrical axis:

1. LAD can be readily recognized if *lead II* shows an RS complex in which the S wave is deeper than the R wave is tall. In addition, *lead I* shows a tall R wave and *lead III* shows a deep S wave. LAD is seen in the ECGs of patients with left ventricular hypertrophy, left anterior fascicular block (hemiblock), and certain other pathologic conditions. Sometimes it is seen in the ECGs of healthy people.

2. RAD is present if the R wave in *lead III* is taller than the R wave in *lead II.* In addition, *lead I* shows an rS complex. RAD can be seen in several conditions, including right ventricular hypertrophy, lateral wall myocardial infarction, chronic lung disease, and left

posterior fascicular block (hemiblock) (see Chapter 24). In addition, RAD is sometimes seen in the ECGs of normal people.

More rarely, the QRS complex is biphasic in all six limb leads. This makes the mean electrical axis *indeterminate*.

The mean electrical axis of the P wave and T wave can be estimated in the same manner as the mean QRS axis. With normal sinus rhythm, the normal P wave is about +60° (positive P wave in lead II). Normally, the T wave axis in the frontal plane is similar to the QRS axis. Therefore the T waves are normally positive in leads with a predominantly positive QRS complex.

# QUESTIONS

1. Based on the six limb leads (I, II, III, aV$_R$, aV$_L$, and aV$_F$) shown below, what is the approximate mean QRS axis?

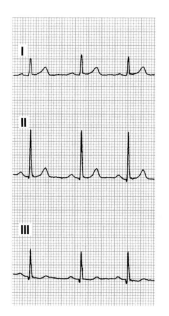
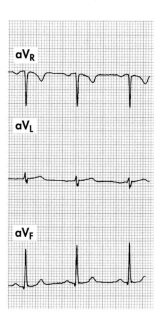

2. Tracings *A*, *B*, and *C* are, in mixed order, leads I, II, and III from an ECG with a mean QRS axis of −30°. Based on this information, can you sort out which lead is which?

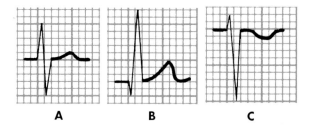

    **A**         **B**         **C**

3. Which of the following conditions does not cause right axis deviation?
    a. Reversal of left and right arm electrodes
    b. Severe chronic obstructive pulmonary disease
    c. Lateral wall myocardial infarction
    d. Acute pulmonary embolism
    e. Left anterior fascicular block (hemiblock)

## CHAPTER 6

# Atrial and Ventricular Enlargement

The basics of the normal ECG were described in the first five chapters. From this point, attention is focused primarily on abnormal ECG patterns. This chapter discusses the effects of enlargement of the four cardiac chambers on the ECG.

*Cardiac enlargement* refers to either *dilation* of a heart chamber or *hypertrophy* of the heart muscle:

1. In dilation of a chamber, the heart muscle is *stretched* and the chamber becomes enlarged. For example, with congestive heart failure (CHF) caused by acute aortic valve regurgitation, the left ventricle dilates.

2. In cardiac hypertrophy, the heart muscle fibers actually *increase in size,* with resultant enlargement of the chamber. For example, aortic stenosis, which obstructs the outflow of blood from the left ventricle, leads to hypertrophy of the left ventricular muscle. Other situations (described later in this chapter) can result in hypertrophy of the atria and right ventricle.

When cardiac hypertrophy occurs, the total number of heart muscle fibers does not increase; rather, each individual fiber becomes larger. One predictable ECG effect of cardiac hypertrophy is an increase in the voltage or duration of the P wave or QRS complex. Not uncommonly, hypertrophy and dilation occur together.

Both dilation and hypertrophy usually result from some type of chronic *pressure* or *volume load* on the heart muscle. The following sections discuss the ECG patterns seen with enlargement of each of the four cardiac chambers, beginning with the right atrium.

## RIGHT ATRIAL ABNORMALITY

Overload of the right atrium (either dilation or actual hypertrophy) may increase the voltage of the P wave. To recognize a large P wave, you must know the dimensions of the normal P wave.

When the P wave is positive, its amplitude is measured in millimeters from the upper level of the baseline, where the P wave begins, to the peak of the wave. A negative P wave is measured from the lower level of the baseline to the lowest point of the P wave. (Measurement of the height and width of the P wave is shown in Figure 6-1.)

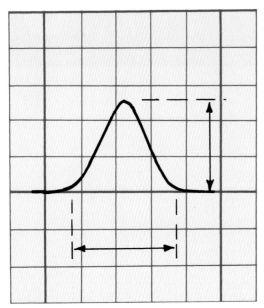

**FIGURE 6-1** The normal P wave is usually no more than 2.5 mm in height and less than 0.12 sec in width.

## Right Atrial Abnormality (Overload)

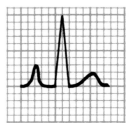

**FIGURE 6-2** Tall narrow P waves may indicate right atrial abnormality or overload (formerly referred to as *P pulmonale* pattern).

Normally, the P wave in every lead is less than or equal to 2.5 mm (0.25 mV) in amplitude and less than 0.12 second (three small boxes) in width. A P wave exceeding either of these dimensions in any lead is abnormal.

Overload of the right atrium may produce an abnormally tall P wave (greater than 2.5 mm). Because pure right atrial abnormality (RAA) generally does not increase the total duration of atrial depolarization, however, the width of the P wave is normal (less than 0.12 sec). The abnormal P wave in RAA is sometimes referred to as *P pulmonale* because the atrial enlargement that it signifies often occurs with severe pulmonary disease (Fig. 6-2). An example of RAA is presented in Figure 6-3.

The tall narrow P waves characteristic of RAA can usually be seen best in leads II, III, aV_F, and sometimes V_1. The ECG diagnosis of P pulmonale can be made by finding a P wave exceeding 2.5 mm in any of these leads. *Echocardiographic* evidence suggests, however, that the finding of a tall peaked P wave does not consistently correlate with RAA. On the other hand, patients may have actual right atrial overload and not tall P waves. In other words, tall

## Right Atrial Abnormality

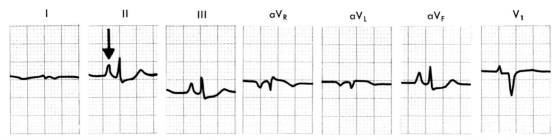

**FIGURE 6-3** Tall P waves (*arrow*) are seen in leads II, III, aV_F, and V_1 from the ECG of a patient with chronic lung disease. This is sometimes called the *P pulmonale* pattern.

peaked P waves are of limited sensitivity and specificity in the diagnosis of right atrial enlargement (see Chapter 23).

RAA is seen in a variety of clinical settings. It is usually associated with right ventricular enlargement. Two of the most common clinical causes of RAA are pulmonary disease and congenital heart disease. The pulmonary disease may be either acute (bronchial asthma, pulmonary embolism) or chronic (emphysema, bronchitis). Congenital heart lesions that produce RAA include pulmonic valve stenosis, atrial septal defects, Ebstein's anomaly (a malformation of the tricuspid valve), and tetralogy of Fallot.

## LEFT ATRIAL ABNORMALITY

Enlargement of the left atrium by dilation or actual hypertrophy also produces predictable changes in the P wave. Normally, the left atrium depolarizes after the right atrium. Thus left atrial enlargement should prolong the total duration of atrial depolarization, indicated by an abnormally wide P wave. Left atrial enlargement (LAE) characteristically produces a wide P wave with duration of 0.12 second or more (at least three small boxes). With enlargement of the left atrium, the amplitude (height) of the P wave may be either normal or increased.

Some patients, particularly those with coronary artery disease, may have broad P waves without detectable enlargement of the left atrium. The abnormal P waves probably represent an atrial conduction delay in a normal-sized chamber. Therefore, rather than the term *left atrial enlargement,* the more general term *left atrial abnormality (LAA)* is being used increasingly to describe these abnormally broad P waves.

Figure 6-4 illustrates the characteristic P wave changes seen in LAA. As shown, the P wave sometimes has a distinctive humped or notched appearance (Fig. 6-4*A*). The second hump corresponds to the delayed depolarization of the left atrium. These humped P waves are usually best seen in one or more of the limb leads (Fig. 6-5). The older term *P mitrale* is sometimes still used to describe wide P waves seen with LAA because these waves were first described in patients with rheumatic mitral valve disease.

In patients with LAA, lead $V_1$ sometimes shows a distinctive biphasic P wave (Fig. 6-6; see Fig. 6-4*B*). This wave has a small initial positive deflection and a prominent, wide negative deflection. The negative component is longer than 0.04 second in duration or 1 mm or more in depth. The prominent negative deflection corresponds to the delayed stimulation of the enlarged left atrium. Remember that anatomically the left atrium is situated posteriorly, up against the esophagus, whereas the right atrium lies anteriorly, against the sternum. The initial positive deflection of the P wave in lead $V_1$ therefore indicates right atrial depolarization,

**Left Atrial Abnormality**

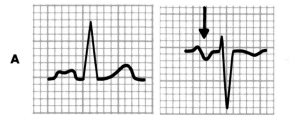

**FIGURE 6-4** Left atrial abnormality/enlargement may produce the following: **A,** wide, sometimes notched P waves in one or more limb leads (formerly referred to as *P mitrale* pattern); and/or **B,** wide biphasic P waves in lead $V_1$.

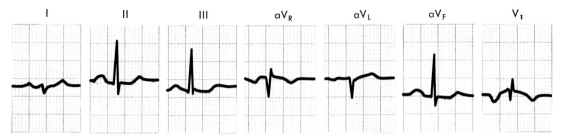

**FIGURE 6-5** Broad, humped P waves from the ECG of a patient with left atrial enlargement (abnormality).

## Atrial Enlargement (Abnormality)

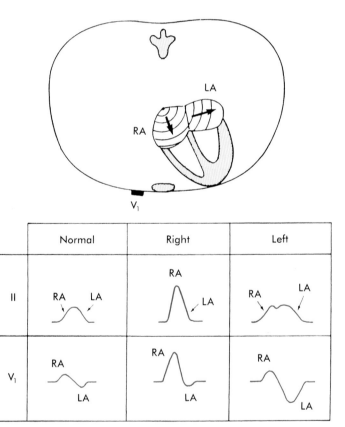

**FIGURE 6-6** Overload of the right atrium (RA) may cause tall peaked P waves in the limb or chest leads. An abnormality of the left atrium (LA) may cause broad, often notched P waves in the limb leads and a biphasic P wave in lead $V_1$ with a prominent negative component representing delayed depolarization of the left atrium. (Modified from Park MK, Guntheroth WG: *How to Read Pediatric ECGs*, 3rd ed. St. Louis, Mosby, 1992.)

whereas the deep negative deflection is a result of left atrial depolarization voltages directed posteriorly (away from the positive pole of lead V$_1$).

In some cases of LAA, you may see both the broad, often humped P waves in leads I and II and the biphasic P wave in lead V$_1$. In other cases, only broad, notched P waves are seen. Sometimes a biphasic P wave in lead V$_1$ is the only ECG evidence of LAA.

Clinically, LAA may occur in a variety of settings, including the following:

■ Valvular heart disease, particularly aortic stenosis, aortic regurgitation, mitral regurgitation, and mitral stenosis*

■ Hypertensive heart disease, which causes left ventricular enlargement and eventually LAA

■ Cardiomyopathies

■ Coronary artery disease

The patterns of LAA and RAA are summarized schematically in Figure 6-6. Patients with enlargement of both atria *(biatrial enlargement or abnormality)* may show a combination of patterns (e.g., tall and wide P waves).

## RIGHT VENTRICULAR HYPERTROPHY

Although atrial enlargement (dilation or hypertrophy) may produce prominent changes in the P wave, the QRS complex is modified primarily by ventricular *hypertrophy.* The resultant ECG effects indicate actual hypertrophy of the ventricular muscle and not simply ventricular dilation.

---

*With mitral stenosis, valvular obstruction to the emptying of the left atrium into the left ventricle eventually results in a backup of pressure through the pulmonary vessels to the right ventricle. Therefore, with advanced mitral stenosis, the ECG may show a combination of LAA (or atrial fibrillation) and signs of right ventricular hypertrophy (RVH), as depicted in Figure 23-1.

You can predict the ECG changes produced by both right ventricular hypertrophy (RVH) and left ventricular hypertrophy (LVH) based on what you already know about normal QRS patterns. Normally, the left and right ventricles depolarize simultaneously, and the left ventricle is electrically predominant because it has greater mass (see Chapter 4). As a result, leads placed over the right side of the chest (e.g., V$_1$) record rS-type complexes.

In these rS-type complexes, the deep negative S wave indicates the spread of depolarization voltages away from the right and toward the left side. Conversely, leads placed over the left chest (e.g., V$_5$, V$_6$) record a qR-type complex:

In this complex, the tall positive R wave indicates the predominant depolarization voltages that point to the left and are generated by the left ventricle.

If sufficient hypertrophy of the right ventricle occurs, the normal electrical predominance of the left ventricle can be overcome. In this situation, what type of QRS complex might you expect to see in the right chest leads? With RVH, the right chest leads show tall R waves, indicating the spread of positive voltages from the hypertrophied right ventricle toward the right (Fig. 6-7). Figures 6-8 and 6-9 show actual examples of RVH. Instead of the rS complex normally seen in lead V$_1$, a tall positive (R) wave indicates marked hypertrophy of the right ventricle.

How tall does an R wave in lead V$_1$ have to be to make a diagnosis of RVH? In adults, the normal R wave in lead V$_1$ is generally smaller than the S wave in that lead. An R wave exceeding the S wave in lead V$_1$ is suggestive but not

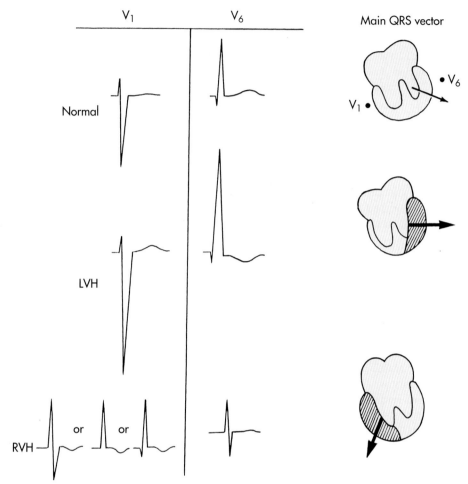

**FIGURE 6-7** The QRS patterns with left ventricular hypertrophy (LVH) and right ventricular hypertrophy (RVH) can be anticipated based on the abnormal physiology. Notice that left ventricular hypertrophy exaggerates the normal pattern, causing deeper right precordial S waves and taller left precordial R waves. By contrast, right ventricular hypertrophy shifts the QRS vector to the right, causing increased right precordial R waves.

diagnostic of RVH. Sometimes a small q wave precedes the tall R wave in lead $V_1$ (see Fig. 6-8).

Along with tall right chest R waves, RVH often produces two additional ECG signs: right axis deviation (RAD) and T wave inversions in right to mid-precordial leads.

RVH affects both depolarization (QRS complex) and repolarization (ST-T complex). For reasons not fully understood, hypertrophy of the heart muscle alters the normal sequence of repolarization. With RVH, the characteristic repolarization change is the appearance of inverted T waves in the right and middle chest leads (see Figs. 6-8 and 6-9). These right chest T wave inversions were formerly referred to as a *right ventricular "strain" pattern.* A preferable term is *T wave inversions associated with right ventricular overload.*

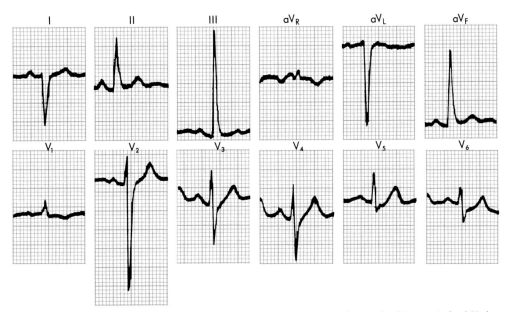

**FIGURE 6-8**    A tall R wave with an inverted T wave caused by right ventricular overload is seen in lead $V_1$ from a patient with tetralogy of Fallot. Marked right axis deviation is also present. (The R wave in lead III is taller than the R wave in lead II.)

Factors that cause RVH, such as congenital heart disease or lung disease, also often cause right atrial overload. So, not uncommonly, signs of RVH are accompanied by tall P waves. (The major condition in which signs of RVH are accompanied by left atrial abnormality is mitral stenosis, as illustrated in Figure 23-1.)

The presence of a right bundle branch block (RBBB) pattern by itself does not indicate RVH. A complete or incomplete RBBB pattern with RAD should, however, raise strong consideration of a right ventricular enlargement syndrome.

In summary, with RVH, the ECG may show tall R waves in the right chest leads and the R wave may be taller than the S wave in lead $V_1$.*

In addition, RAD and right precordial T wave inversions are often present. Some cases of RVH are more subtle, and the ECG may show only one of these patterns.

The appearance of all three patterns—tall right precordial R waves, RAD, and right precordial T wave inversions—is very strong evidence of marked RVH.

RVH may occur in a variety of clinical settings. An important cause is congenital heart disease, such as pulmonic stenosis, atrial septal defect,[†] tetralogy of Fallot, or Eisenmenger's syndrome. Patients with long-standing severe pulmonary disease may have pulmonary artery hypertension and RVH. As noted, mitral stenosis can produce a combination of LAA and RVH. T wave inversions in leads $V_1$ to $V_3$ due to right ventricular overload may also occur

---

*With RVH, the chest leads to the left of leads showing tall R waves may display a variable pattern. Sometimes the middle and left chest leads show poor R wave progression, with rS or RS complexes all the way to lead $V_6$ (see Fig. 6-9). In other cases, normal R wave progression is preserved and the left chest leads also show R waves (see Fig. 6-8).

---

[†]Patients with right ventricular enlargement from the most common type of atrial septal defect often exhibit a right bundle branch block pattern (RSR' in lead $V_1$) with a vertical or rightward QRS axis.

## Right Ventricular Hypertrophy

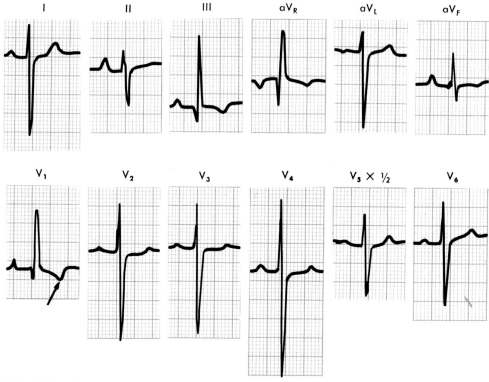

**FIGURE 6-9**   With right ventricular hypertrophy, lead $V_1$ sometimes shows a tall R wave as part of the qR complex. Because of right atrial enlargement, peaked P waves are seen in leads II, III, and $V_1$. The T wave inversion in lead $V_1$ (*arrow*) and the ST depressions in leads $V_2$ and $V_3$ are due to right ventricular overload. The PR interval is also prolonged (0.24 sec).

without other ECG signs of RVH, as in acute pulmonary embolism (see Chapter 11).

In patients who have right ventricular overload associated with emphysema, the ECG may not show any of the patterns just described. Instead of tall R waves in the right precordial leads, poor R wave progression is seen. RAD is also commonly present (see Figure 11-6).

## LEFT VENTRICULAR HYPERTROPHY

The ECG changes produced by LVH, like those from RVH, are predictable (see Fig. 6-7). Nor-

mally, the left ventricle, due its relatively larger mass, is electrically predominant over the right ventricle. As a result, prominent negative (S) waves are produced in the right chest leads, and tall positive (R) waves are seen in the left chest leads. When LVH is present, the balance of electrical forces is tipped even farther to the left. Thus with LVH, abnormally tall positive (R) waves are usually seen in the left chest leads, and abnormally deep negative (S) waves are present in the right chest leads.

The following criteria and guidelines have been established to help in the ECG diagnosis of LVH:

## Left Ventricular Hypertrophy

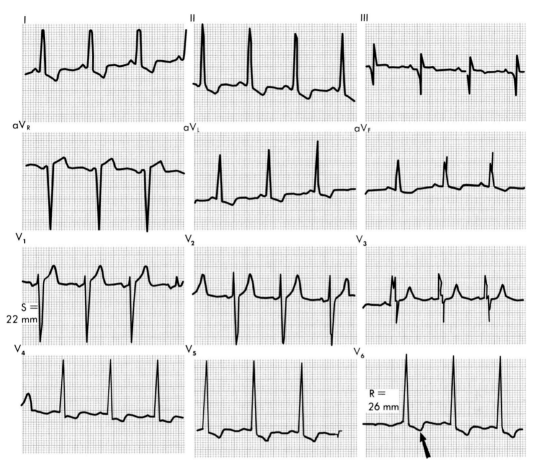

**FIGURE 6-10**   Pattern of left ventricular hypertrophy in a patient with severe hypertension. Tall voltages are seen in the chest leads and lead aV$_L$ (R = 17 mm). A repolarization (ST-T) abnormality (*arrow*), formerly referred to as a "strain" pattern, is also present in these leads. Similar ST-T changes may occur with ischemia, digitalis effect, and so on. In addition, enlargement of the left atrium is indicated by a biphasic P wave in lead V$_1$ and a broad, notched P wave in lead II.

1. If the sum of the depth of the S wave in lead V$_1$ (S$_{V1}$) and the height of the R wave in either lead V$_5$ or V$_6$ (R$_{V5}$ or R$_{V6}$) exceeds 35 mm (3.5 mV), LVH should be considered (Fig. 6-10). High voltage in the chest leads is a common normal finding, however, particularly in athletic or thin young adults. Consequently, high voltage in the chest leads (S$_{V1}$ + R$_{V5}$ or R$_{V6}$ > 35 mm) is not a *specific* indicator of LVH* (Fig. 6-11).

---

*Other LVH criteria (the Cornell voltage criteria) based on voltages in leads V$_3$ and aV$_L$ have been suggested: for men, S$_{V3}$ + R$_{aVL}$ > 28 mm; for women, S$_{V3}$ + R$_{aVL}$ > 20 mm.

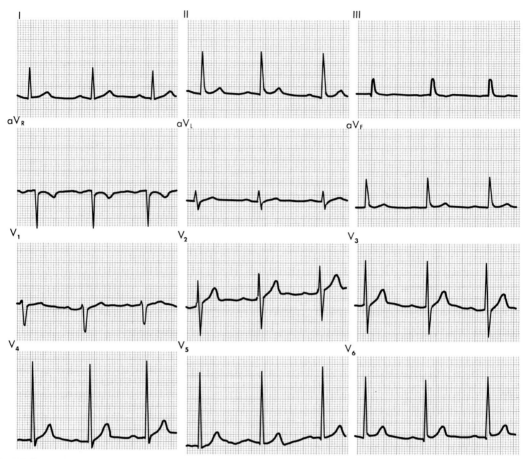

**FIGURE 6-11**　Tall voltages in the chest leads ($S_{V_1} + R_{V_5}$ = 36 mm) from a 20-year-old man represent a common normal ECG variant, particularly in athletic or thin young adults. The ST-T complexes are normal, without evidence of repolarization (ST-T) abnormalities or left atrial abnormality.

2. Sometimes LVH produces tall R waves in lead $aV_L$. An R wave of 11 to 13 mm (1.1 to 1.3 mV) or more in lead $aV_L$ is another sign of LVH* (see Fig. 6-9). Sometimes a tall R wave in lead $aV_L$ is the only ECG sign of LVH, and the voltage in the chest leads is normal. In other cases, the chest voltages are abnormally high, with a normal R wave seen in lead $aV_L$.

3. Just as RVH is sometimes associated with repolarization abnormalities, so ST-T changes are often seen in LVH. Figure 6-12 illustrates the characteristic shape of the ST-T complex with LVH. Notice that the complex usually has a distinctively asymmetric appearance, with a slight ST segment depression followed by a broadly inverted T wave. In some cases, these T wave inversions are very deep. This LVH-related repolarization abnormality is usually best seen in leads with tall R waves (see Fig. 6-10).

4. With LVH, the electrical axis is usually horizontal. Actual left axis deviation (i.e., an axis

*Occasionally, LVH develops with an electrically vertical axis. In this situation, a qR pattern with a tall R wave (exceeding 20 mm) may appear in lead $aV_F$. An LVH pattern with a vertical or especially a more rightward QRS axis should suggest biventricular hypertrophy.

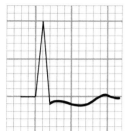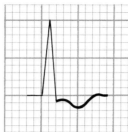

**FIGURE 6-12** Repolarization abnormalities associated with left ventricular hypertrophy were formerly referred to as the "strain" pattern, an imprecise but still sometimes used term. Notice the characteristic slight ST depression with T wave inversion in the leads that show tall R waves. These repolarization changes can be referred to as "LVH-related ST-T changes" or "ST-T changes due to LV overload." Similar findings may occur with ischemia or other factors.

$-30°$ or more negative) may also be seen. In addition, the QRS complex may become wider. Not uncommonly, patients with LVH eventually develop an incomplete or complete left bundle branch block (LBBB) pattern. Indeed, most patients with LBBB have underlying LVH (see Chapter 7).

5. Finally, signs of LAA (broad P waves in the limb leads or wide biphasic P waves in lead $V_1$) are often seen in patients with ECG evidence of LVH. Most conditions that lead to LVH ultimately produce left atrial overload as well.

In summary, the diagnosis of LVH can be made with reasonable certainty from the ECG if you find high QRS voltages and associated ST-T changes. In addition, signs of LAA are often present. Because high voltage in the chest or limb leads can sometimes be seen in normal people, especially athletes and young adults, the diagnosis of LVH should not be made on this finding alone.* ST-T changes resulting from left ventricular overload can also occur without other evidence of LVH.

The recognition of LVH is clinically important for two reasons:

*The voltage criteria used in this chapter to diagnose LVH in the chest and limb leads are by no means absolute numbers. In fact, many different criteria have been proposed (see Bibliography).

1. Diagnostically, LVH is a clue to the presence of a potentially life-threatening *pressure* or *volume* overload state. The two most common and important pressure overload states are systemic hypertension and aortic stenosis. The three major clinical conditions associated with left ventricular volume overload are aortic regurgitation, mitral regurgitation, and dilated cardiomyopathy. LVH patterns may also occur with hypertrophic cardiomyopathies.

2. Prognostically, patients with LVH from any cause are at increased risk for major cardiovascular complications, including congestive heart failure and serious atrial or ventricular arrhythmias.

## THE ECG IN CARDIAC ENLARGEMENT: A PERSPECTIVE

The ECG findings associated with enlargement of each of the four cardiac chambers have been presented. In some cases, combined patterns are seen on the same tracing (e.g., LAA and RVH in mitral stenosis, LAA and LVH in systemic hypertension). If hypertrophy is present in both ventricles, the ECG usually shows mainly evidence of LVH. Another pattern that may provide an important clue to *biventricular hypertrophy* is LVH with right axis deviation.

Always remember that in the assessment of cardiac size, the ECG is only an indirect laboratory test and not an absolute measurement. A person may have underlying cardiac enlargement that does not show up on the ECG. Conversely, the ECG may show high voltage in a normal person who does not have cardiac enlargement.

When the presence or degree of cardiac chamber enlargement must be determined with more precision, an *echocardiogram* should be obtained.*

*The diagnostic limitations of the ECG are discussed further in Chapter 23.

# REVIEW

Cardiac *dilation* refers to the stretching of muscle fibers, with enlargement of one or more of the cardiac chambers. Cardiac *hypertrophy* refers to an abnormal increase in the actual size of the heart muscle fibers. The ECG can indicate either right or left atrial dilation or hypertrophy but generally only right or left ventricular hypertrophy.

Right atrial abnormality (RAA), or right atrial overload, may be associated with tall peaked P waves exceeding 2.5 mm in height. These waves are usually best seen in leads II, III, $aV_F$, and sometimes $V_1$ or $V_2$.

*Left atrial abnormality (LAA),* or left atrial enlargement, is manifested by wide, sometimes notched P waves of 0.12 second or more duration in one or more of the limb leads. A biphasic P wave with a prominent, wide negative deflection may be seen in lead $V_1$.

Right ventricular hypertrophy may produce any or all of the following:

1. A tall R wave in lead $V_1$, equal to or larger than the S wave in that lead

2. Often, right axis deviation

3. T wave inversions in the right to middle chest leads.

With left ventricular hypertrophy (LVH), any or all of the following may occur:

1. The voltage of the S wave in lead $V_1$ plus the voltage of the R wave in lead $V_5$ or $V_6$ often exceeds 35 mm ($S_{V_1} + R_{V_5}$ or $R_{V_6} > 35$ mm).

2. A high-voltage R wave (11 to 13 mm or more) is seen in lead $aV_L$ when the QRS axis is horizontal. (More rarely, when the axis is vertical, lead $aV_F$ may show a tall R wave exceeding 20 mm as part of a qR complex.)

3. Repolarization abnormalities include inverted T waves in leads with tall R waves. (Similar findings may occur with ischemia.)

4. Other findings often include LAA, left axis deviation, and left ventricular conduction delay (wide QRS), which may eventually progress to incomplete or complete left bundle branch block.

The diagnosis of LVH should *not* be made solely on the basis of high voltage in the chest leads because these high voltages may occur normally, particularly in young adults, athletes, and thin individuals. In addition, enlargement of any of the four cardiac chambers can be present *without* diagnostic ECG changes. Echocardiograms are more sensitive and more specific in assessing chamber enlargement than the ECG is.

## QUESTIONS

1. Examine the ECG shown below and answer the following questions:

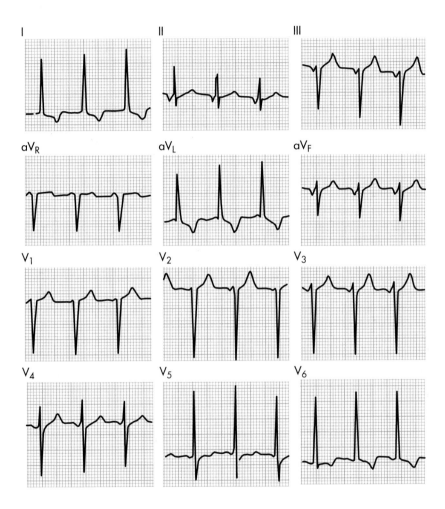

   a. What is the heart rate?

   b. Name two abnormal findings.

2. *True or false*: Echocardiography is more sensitive and specific than the ECG in assessing chamber enlargement.

## CHAPTER 7

# Ventricular Conduction Disturbances

Bundle branch blocks

Recall that in the normal process of ventricular activation the electrical stimulus reaches the ventricles from the atria by way of the atrioventricular (AV) junction (see Chapter 4). The first part of the ventricles to be stimulated (depolarized) is the left side of the ventricular septum. Soon after, the depolarization spreads to the main mass of the left and right ventricles by way of the left and right bundle branches. Normally, the entire process of ventricular depolarization is completed within about 0.1 second (100 msec). This is the reason the normal width of the QRS complex is less than or equal to 100 ms* (two and a half small boxes on the ECG graph paper). Any process that interferes with the normal stimulation of the ventricles may prolong the QRS width. This chapter focuses on the effects that blocks within the bundle branch system have on the QRS complex.

---

* Some references give the upper normal limits of QRS duration as 110 ms, especially when using computer-derived measurements based on multiple leads.

## RIGHT BUNDLE BRANCH BLOCK

Consider first the effect of cutting the right bundle branch, or markedly slowing conduction in this structure. Obviously, right ventricular stimulation will be delayed and the QRS complex will be widened. The shape of the QRS with a right bundle branch block (RBBB) can be predicted on the basis of some familiar principles.

Normally, the *first* part of the ventricles to be depolarized is the interventricular septum (see Fig. 4-6A). The left side of the septum is stimulated first (by a branch of the left bundle). On the normal ECG, this septal depolarization produces a small septal r wave in lead $V_1$ and a small septal q wave in lead $V_6$ (Fig. 7-1A). Clearly, RBBB should not affect the septal phase of ventricular stimulation because the septum is stimulated by a part of the left bundle.

The *second* phase of ventricular stimulation is the simultaneous depolarization of the left and right ventricles (see Fig. 4-6B). RBBB should not affect this phase either, since the left ventricle is

## Right Bundle Branch Block

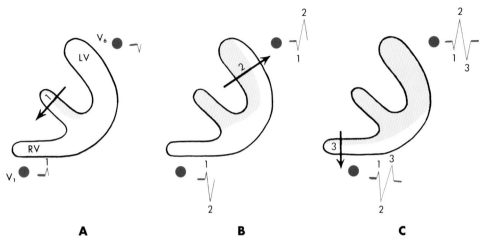

**FIGURE 7-1** Step-by-step sequence of ventricular depolarization in right bundle branch block (see text).

normally electrically predominant, producing deep S waves in the right chest leads and tall R waves in the left chest leads (Fig. 7-1*B*). The change in the QRS complex produced by RBBB is a result of the delay in the total time needed for stimulation of the right ventricle. This means that after the left ventricle has completely depolarized, the right ventricle continues to depolarize.

This delayed right ventricular depolarization produces a *third* phase of ventricular stimulation. The electrical voltages in the third phase are directed to the right, reflecting the delayed depolarization and slow spread of the depolarization wave outward through the right ventricle. Therefore a lead placed over the right side of the chest (e.g., lead $V_1$) records this phase of ventricular stimulation as a positive wide deflection (R′ wave). The rightward spread of the delayed and slow right ventricular depolarization voltages produces a wide negative (S wave) deflection in the left chest leads (e.g., lead $V_6$) (Fig. 7-1*C*).

Based on an understanding of this step-by-step process, the pattern seen in the chest leads with RBBB can be derived. With RBBB, lead $V_1$ typically shows an rSR′ complex with a broad R′ wave. Lead $V_6$ shows a qRS-type complex with a broad S wave. The tall wide R wave in the right chest leads and the deep terminal S wave in the left chest leads represent the same event viewed from opposite sides of the chest—the slow spread of delayed depolarization voltages through the right ventricle.

To make the initial diagnosis of RBBB, look at leads $V_1$ and $V_6$, in particular. The characteristic appearance of QRS complexes in these leads makes the diagnosis simple. (Figure 7-1 shows how the delay in ventricular depolarization with RBBB produces the characteristic ECG patterns.)

In summary, the ventricular stimulation process in RBBB can be divided into three phases. The first two phases are normal septal and left ventricular depolarization. The third phase is delayed stimulation of the right

## Right Bundle Branch Block

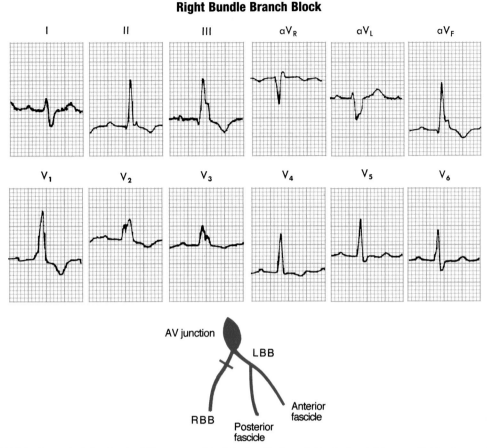

**FIGURE 7-2** Instead of the classic rSR′ pattern with right bundle branch block, the right precordial leads sometimes show a wide notched R wave (seen here in leads $V_1$ to $V_3$). Notice the *secondary* T wave inversions in leads $V_1$ to $V_3$, II, III, and $aV_F$, all of which show rSR′-type complexes. The abnormal ST-T changes in leads $V_4$ and $V_5$ are *primary*, however, because they are present in leads without an R′ wave. AV, atrioventricular; LBB, left bundle branch; RBB, right bundle branch.

ventricle. These three phases of ventricular stimulation with RBBB are represented on the ECG by the triphasic complexes seen in the chest leads:

- Lead $V_1$ shows an rSR′ complex with a wide R′ wave.

- Lead $V_6$ shows a qRS pattern with a wide S wave.

With an RBBB pattern, the QRS complex in lead $V_1$ generally shows an rSR′ pattern (Fig. 7-2). Occasionally, however, the S wave never quite makes its way below the baseline. Consequently, the complex in lead $V_1$ has the appearance of a large notched R wave (Fig. 7-3).

Figures 7-2 and 7-3 are typical examples of RBBB. Do you notice anything abnormal about the ST-T complexes in these tracings? If you

## Right Bundle Branch Block

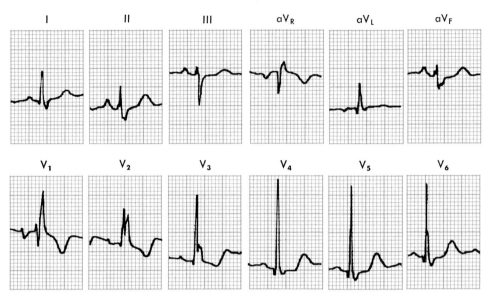

**FIGURE 7-3**  Notice the wide rSR' complex in lead $V_1$ and the qRS complex in lead $V_6$. Inverted T waves in the right precordial leads (in this case $V_1$ to $V_3$) are common with right bundle branch block and are called *secondary* T wave inversions.

look carefully, you can see that the T waves in the right chest leads are inverted. T wave inversions in the right chest leads are a characteristic finding with RBBB. These inversions are referred to as *secondary changes* because they reflect just the delay in ventricular stimulation. By contrast, *primary T wave abnormalities* reflect an actual change in repolarization, independent of any QRS change. Examples of primary T wave abnormalities include T wave inversions resulting from ischemia (see Chapters 8 and 9), hypokalemia and certain other electrolyte abnormalities (see Chapter 10), and drugs such as digitalis (see Chapter 10).

Some ECGs show both primary and secondary ST-T changes. In Figure 7-3, the T wave inversions in leads $V_1$ to $V_3$ and leads II, III, and $aV_F$ can be explained solely on the basis of the RBBB because the inversions occur in leads with an rSR'-type complex. The T wave inversions or ST depressions in other leads ($V_4$ and $V_5$),

however, represent a primary change, perhaps resulting from ischemia or a drug effect.

### COMPLETE AND INCOMPLETE RBBB

RBBB can be subdivided into complete and incomplete forms, depending on the width of the QRS complex. Complete RBBB is defined by a QRS that is 0.12 second or more in duration with an rSR' in lead $V_1$ and a qRS in lead $V_6$. Incomplete RBBB shows the same QRS patterns, but its duration is between 0.1 and 0.12 second.

### CLINICAL SIGNIFICANCE

RBBB may be caused by a number of factors. First, some normal people have this finding without any underlying heart disorder. Therefore RBBB itself is not necessarily abnormal. In many people, however, RBBB is associated with organic heart disease. It may occur with virtually any condition that affects the right side of the heart, including atrial septal defect with left-to-right shunting of blood, chronic pulmonary disease with pulmonary artery hypertension, and valvular lesions such as pulmonic stenosis. In some people (particularly older individuals), RBBB is related to chronic degenerative changes in the conduction system. It may also occur with acute or chronic coronary artery disease.

Pulmonary embolism, which produces acute right-sided heart overload, may cause a right ventricular conduction delay. When RBBB occurs after coronary artery bypass graft surgery, it does not seem to have any special clinical implications.

RBBB may be permanent or transient. Sometimes it appears only when the heart rate exceeds a certain critical value (rate-related RBBB).

By itself, RBBB does not require any specific treatment. In patients with acute anterior wall infarction, however, a new RBBB may indicate an increased risk of complete heart block (see Chapter 17), particularly when the RBBB is associated with left anterior or posterior hemiblock.

## LEFT BUNDLE BRANCH BLOCK

Left bundle branch block (LBBB) also produces a pattern with a widened QRS complex. The QRS complex with LBBB is very different, however, from that with RBBB. The major reason for this difference is that RBBB affects mainly the terminal phase of ventricular activation, whereas LBBB also affects the early phase.

Recall that the first phase of ventricular stimulation—depolarization of the left side of the septum—is started by a branch of the left bundle. LBBB therefore blocks this normal pattern. When LBBB is present, the septum depolarizes from *right* to *left* and not from left to right. Thus the first major ECG change produced by LBBB is a loss of the normal septal r wave in lead $V_1$ and the normal septal q wave in lead $V_6$ (Fig. 7-4A). Furthermore, the total time for left ventricular depolarization is prolonged with LBBB. As a result, the QRS complex is abnormally wide. Lead $V_6$ shows a wide, entirely positive (R) wave (Fig. 7-4B). The right chest leads (e.g., $V_1$) record a negative QRS (QS) complex because the left ventricle is still electrically predominant with LBBB and therefore produces greater voltages than the right ventricle.

Thus with LBBB the entire process of ventricular stimulation is oriented toward the left chest leads; that is, the septum depolarizes from right to left, and stimulation of the electrically predominant left ventricle is prolonged. Figure

### Left Bundle Branch Block

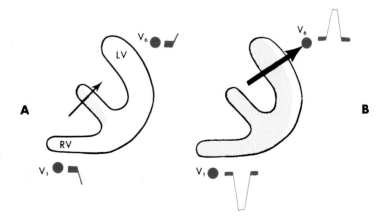

**FIGURE 7-4** The sequence of ventricular depolarization in left bundle branch block produces a wide QS complex in lead $V_1$ and a wide R wave in lead $V_6$. LV, left ventricle; RV, right ventricle.

7-4 illustrates the sequence of ventricular activation in LBBB.*

With LBBB, the QS wave in lead $V_1$ sometimes shows a small notching at its point, giving the wave a characteristic W shape. Similarly, the R wave in lead $V_6$ may show a notching at its peak, giving it a distinctive M shape. (An example of an LBBB pattern is presented in Figure 7-5.)

Just as *secondary* T wave inversions occur with RBBB, they also occur with LBBB. As Figure 7-5 shows, the T waves in the leads with tall R waves (e.g., the left precordial leads) are inverted; this is characteristic of LBBB. T wave inversions in the right precordial leads cannot, however, be explained solely on the basis of LBBB. If present, these T wave inversions reflect some *primary* abnormality such as ischemia (see Fig. 8-21).

In summary, the diagnosis of complete LBBB pattern can be made simply by inspection of leads $V_1$ and $V_6$:

- Lead $V_1$ usually shows a wide, entirely negative QS complex (rarely, a wide rS complex).

- Lead $V_6$ shows a tall wide R wave without a q wave.

You should have no problem differentiating LBBB and RBBB patterns (Fig. 7-6). Occasionally, an ECG shows wide QRS complexes that are not typical of an RBBB or LBBB pattern. In such cases, the general term *intraventricular delay* is used (Fig. 7-7).

## COMPLETE AND INCOMPLETE LBBB

LBBB, like RBBB, has complete and incomplete forms. With complete LBBB, the QRS complex has the characteristic appearance described pre-

viously and is 0.12 second or wider. With incomplete LBBB, the QRS is between 0.1 and 0.12 second wide.

## CLINICAL SIGNIFICANCE

Unlike RBBB, which is occasionally seen without evident cardiac disease, LBBB is usually a sign of organic heart disease. LBBB may develop in patients with long-standing hypertensive heart disease, a valvular lesion (e.g., calcification of the mitral annulus, aortic stenosis, or aortic regurgitation), or different types of cardiomyopathy (see Chapter 11). It is also seen in patients with coronary artery disease and often correlates with impaired left ventricular function. Most patients with LBBB have underlying left ventricular hypertrophy (see Chapter 6). Degenerative changes in the conduction system may lead to LBBB, particularly in the elderly. Often, more than one contributing factor may be identified (e.g., hypertension and coronary artery disease). Rarely, otherwise normal individuals have an LBBB pattern without evidence of organic heart disease by examination, echocardiogram, or even invasive studies.

LBBB, like RBBB, may be permanent or transient. It may also appear only when the heart rate exceeds a certain critical value (rate- or acceleration-dependent LBBB).[†]

*Important clinical consideration: LBBB may be the first clue to four previously undiagnosed but clinically important abnormalities. These are advanced coronary artery disease, valvular heart disease, hypertensive heart disease, and cardiomyopathy.*

## PACEMAKER PATTERNS

Pacemakers are battery-operated devices designed to stimulate the heart electrically. A pacemaker is used primarily when a patient's own heart rate is not adequate (e.g., in complete

---

*A variation of this pattern sometimes occurs: Lead $V_1$ may show an rS complex with a very small r wave and a wide S wave. This superficially suggests that the septum is being stimulated normally from left to right. Lead $V_6$, however, shows an abnormally wide and notched R wave *without* an initial q wave.

---

[†] Less commonly, LBBB occurs only when the heart decelerates below some critical value.

## Left Bundle Branch Block

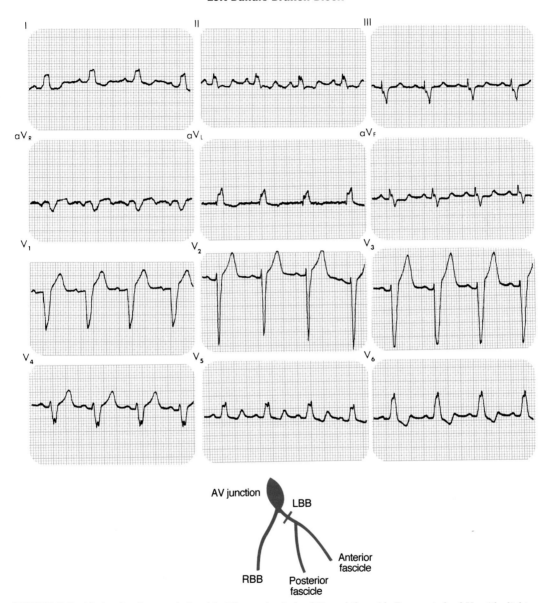

**FIGURE 7-5** Notice the characteristic wide QS complex in lead $V_1$ and the wide R wave in lead $V_6$ with slight notching at the peak. The inverted T waves in leads $V_5$ and $V_6$ (secondary T wave inversions) are also characteristic of left bundle branch block. AV, atrioventricular; LBB, left bundle branch; RBB, right bundle branch.

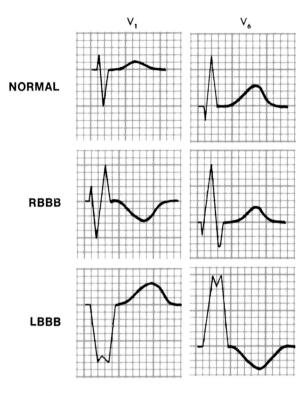

**FIGURE 7-6** Comparison of leads $V_1$ and $V_6$, with normal conduction, right bundle branch block (RBBB), and left bundle branch block (LBBB). Normally, lead $V_1$ shows an rS complex and lead $V_6$ shows a qR complex. With RBBB, lead $V_1$ shows a wider rSR' complex and lead $V_6$ shows a qRS complex. With LBBB, lead $V_1$ shows a wide QS complex and lead $V_6$ shows a wide R wave.

heart block or sick sinus syndrome). In most cases, the pacemaker electrode is inserted into the right ventricle. Therefore the ECG shows an LBBB pattern, which reflects delayed activation of the left ventricle.

Figure 7-8 is an example of a pacemaker tracing. The vertical spike preceding each QRS complex is the pacemaker spike. This spike is followed by a wide QRS complex with an LBBB morphology (QS in lead $V_1$ with a wide R wave in lead $V_6$). (Pacemakers are discussed in greater detail in Chapter 21.)

## FASCICULAR BLOCKS (HEMIBLOCKS)

*Fascicular blocks*, or *hemiblocks*, are a slightly more complex but important topic. To this point, the chapter has described the left bundle branch system as if it were a single pathway. Actually, this system has been known for many years to be subdivided into an *anterior fascicle* and a *posterior fascicle* (from the Latin *fasciculus*, meaning "small bundle"). The right bundle branch, by contrast, is a single pathway and consists of just one main fascicle or bundle. This revised concept of the bundle branch system as a *trifascicular* highway (one right lane and two left lanes) is illustrated in Figure 7-9.

In summary, the bundle of His divides into a right bundle branch and a left main bundle branch. The left main bundle branch then subdivides into an anterior and a posterior fascicle.

It makes sense to suppose that a block can occur at any single point (or at multiple points) in this trifascicular system. The ECG pattern with RBBB has already been presented (see Figs. 7-2 and 7-3). The pattern of LBBB can occur in one of two ways: by a block in the left main bundle before it divides or by blocks in both subdivisions (anterior and posterior fascicles).

What happens if a block occurs in just the anterior or just the posterior fascicle of the left

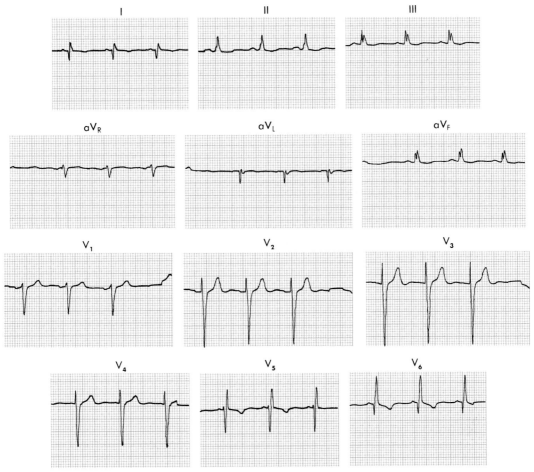

**FIGURE 7-7** In nonspecific intraventricular conduction delay, the QRS complex is abnormally wide (0.11 sec). Such a pattern is not typical of left or right bundle branch block, however. In this patient, the pattern was caused by an anterolateral wall myocardial infarction (see Chapter 8).

bundle? A block in either fascicle of the left bundle branch system is called a *hemiblock* or *fascicular block*. Recognition of fascicular blocks on the ECG is intimately related to the subject of axis deviation (see Chapter 5). Somewhat surprisingly, a fascicular block (unlike a full LBBB or RBBB) does not markedly widen the QRS complex. Experiments have shown that the main effect of cutting these fascicles is a change in the QRS axis. Specifically, *left anterior* fascicular block results in marked left axis deviation (−45° or more); *left posterior* fascicular block pro-

duces marked right axis deviation (+120° or more).*

In summary, fascicular blocks are partial blocks in the left bundle branch system and involve either the anterior or posterior fascicle.

_____

*Left anterior fascicular block shifts the QRS axis to the left by delaying activation of the more superior and leftward portions of the left ventricle. Left posterior fascicular block shifts it to the right by delaying activation of the more inferior and rightward portions of the left ventricle. In both cases, the QRS axis therefore is shifted *toward* the direction of delayed activation.

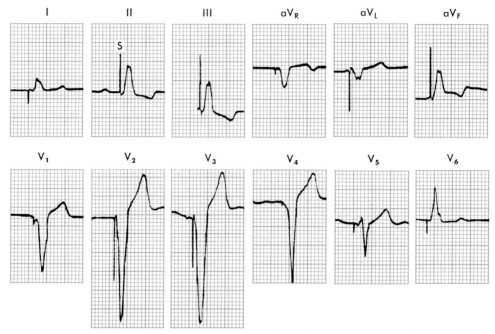

**FIGURE 7-8** A pacemaker inserted in the right ventricle generally produces a pattern resembling that of left bundle branch block, with a wide QS in lead $V_1$ and a wide R wave in lead $V_6$. This pattern is caused by delayed depolarization of the left ventricle. Notice the pacemaker spike in each lead preceding the QRS complex. In some leads (e.g., II), the spike (S) is positive; in others ($V_1$ to $V_6$), it is negative.

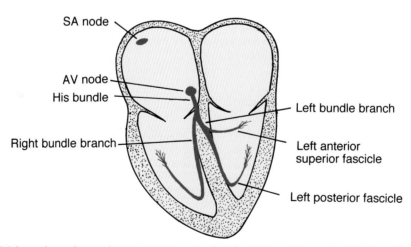

**FIGURE 7-9** With a trifascicular conduction system, notice that the left bundle branch subdivides into a left anterior fascicle and a left posterior fascicle. This diagram is a more detailed version of the original depiction of the conduction system (see Fig. 1-1). AV, atrioventricular; SA, sinoatrial.

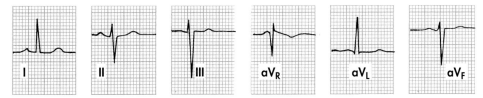

**FIGURE 7-10**   Left anterior fascicular block (hemiblock). Notice the marked left axis deviation without significant widening of the QRS duration. Compare this with Figure 9-8B, which shows left posterior fascicular (hemiblock).

The diagnosis of a fascicular block is made from the mean QRS axis in the limb (frontal plane) leads. This is in contrast to the diagnosis of complete (or incomplete) RBBB or LBBB, which is made primarily from the QRS patterns in the chest (horizontal plane) leads. Complete bundle branch blocks, unlike fascicular blocks, do not cause a characteristic shift in the mean QRS axis.

## LEFT ANTERIOR FASCICULAR BLOCK

Isolated left anterior fascicular block (LAFB) is diagnosed by finding a mean QRS axis of –45° or more negative and a QRS width of less than 0.12 second. A mean QRS axis of –45° or more negative can be easily recognized because the S wave in lead $aV_F$ equals or exceeds the R wave in lead I* (Fig. 7-10). Lead $aV_L$ usually shows a qR complex, with rS complexes in leads II, III, and $aV_F$ (or QS waves if an inferior myocardial infarction is also present).

## LEFT POSTERIOR FASCICULAR BLOCK

Isolated left fascicular block (LPFB) (see Fig. 9-8B) is diagnosed by finding a mean QRS axis of +120° or more, with a QRS width of less than 0.12 second. Usually, an rS complex is seen in lead I, and a qR complex is seen in leads II, III, and $aV_F$. *The diagnosis of left posterior fascicular block can be considered, however, only after other, more common causes of right axis deviation (RAD) have been excluded* (see Chapter 24). These causes can include right ventricular hypertrophy

(RVH), normal variant, emphysema, lateral wall infarction (see Fig. 8-11), and acute pulmonary embolism (or other causes of acute right ventricular overload).

Although left anterior fascicular block is relatively common, isolated left posterior fascicular block is quite rare. Most often it occurs with RBBB, as shown in Figure 17-8. In general, the finding of isolated left anterior fascicular block is not of much clinical significance. *Bifascicular and trifascicular* blocks are considered further in the discussion of complete heart block in Chapter 17.

## ECG PATTERNS IN VENTRICULAR CONDUCTION DISTURBANCES: GENERAL PRINCIPLES

A unifying theme to predicting what the ECG will show with a bundle branch block or hemiblock is the following.

*The last (and usually dominant) component of the QRS vector will be shifted in the direction of the last part of the ventricles to be depolarized. In other words, the major QRS vector shifts toward the regions of the heart that are most delayed in being stimulated:*

- RBBB: late QRS forces point toward the right ventricle (positive in $V_1$ and negative in $V_6$).

- LBBB: late QRS forces point toward the left ventricle (negative in $V_1$ and positive in $V_6$).

- LAFB: late QRS forces point in a leftward and superior direction (negative in II and positive in I and $aV_L$).

---

*Some authors use an axis of –30° or more negative. The original description of this pattern used a cutoff of –45° or more negative.

- LPFB: late QRS forces point in a rightward and inferior direction (negative in I and positive in II and III).

## DIAGNOSIS OF HYPERTROPHY IN THE PRESENCE OF BUNDLE BRANCH BLOCKS

The ECG diagnosis of hypertrophy (see Chapter 6) in the presence of bundle branch blocks may pose special problems. A few general guidelines are helpful.

When RVH occurs with RBBB, RAD is often present. A tall peaked P wave with RBBB should also suggest underlying RVH.

The usual voltage criteria for left ventricular hypertrophy (LVH) can be used in the presence of RBBB. Unfortunately, RBBB often masks these typical voltage increases. The presence of LAA with RBBB suggests underlying LVH.

The finding of LBBB, regardless of the QRS voltage, is highly suggestive of underlying LVH. Finding LBBB with prominent QRS voltages *and* evidence of left atrial abnormality virtually ensures the diagnosis of LVH (see Chapter 6).

Finally, it should be emphasized that the *echocardiogram* is much more accurate than the ECG in the diagnosis of cardiac enlargement (see Chapter 6).

## DIAGNOSIS OF MYOCARDIAL INFARCTION IN THE PRESENCE OF BUNDLE BRANCH BLOCKS

The ECG diagnosis of myocardial infarction in the presence of bundle branch blocks is discussed in Chapter 8.

# REVIEW

Right bundle branch block (RBBB) shows the following characteristic patterns: an rSR' with a prominent wide final R' wave in lead $V_1$, a qRS with a wide final S wave in lead $V_6$, and a QRS width of 0.12 second (three small time boxes) or more. *Incomplete RBBB* shows the same chest lead patterns, but the QRS width is between 0.1 and 0.12 second.

Left bundle branch block (LBBB) shows the following characteristic patterns: a deep wide QS (occasionally an rS with a wide S wave) in lead $V_1$, a prominent (often notched) R wave *without* a preceding q wave in lead $V_6$, and a QRS width of 0.12 second or more. *Incomplete LBBB* shows the same chest lead patterns as LBBB, but the QRS width is between 0.1 and 0.12 second.

*Pacemaker patterns* produced by an electrode in the right ventricle generally resemble LBBB but have a pacemaker spike before each QRS complex.

*Fascicular blocks (hemiblocks)* can occur because the left bundle splits into two subdivisions (fascicles): the left anterior fascicle and the left posterior fascicle. Conduction through either or both of these bundles can be blocked.

*Left anterior fascicular block* or *hemiblock* is characterized by a mean QRS axis of −45° or more negative. (When the mean QRS axis is −45°, left axis deviation is present and the height of the R wave in lead I ($R_I$) is equal to the depth of the S wave in lead $aV_F$ ($S_{aVF}$). When the mean QRS axis is more negative than −45°, $S_{aVF}$ becomes larger than $R_I$.)

*Left posterior fascicular block* or *hemiblock* is characterized by marked right axis deviation (RAD). Before the diagnosis of left posterior hemiblock is made, however, other more common causes of RAD must be excluded, including lead reversal (left/right arm electrodes), normal variants, right ventricular overload syndromes (including chronic lung disease), and lateral wall infarction (see Chapter 24).

## QUESTIONS

1. Draw the shape of the QRS complexes in leads $V_1$ and $V_6$ that would be expected with right and left bundle branch blocks.

2. Examine the chest leads shown below and then answer these questions:

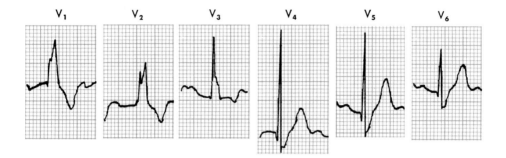

a. What is the approximate QRS width?
b. What conduction disturbance is present?
c. Why are the T waves in leads $V_1$ to $V_3$ inverted?

3. Examine the following 12-lead ECG and lead II rhythm strip carefully. Can you identify the major conduction abnormality?

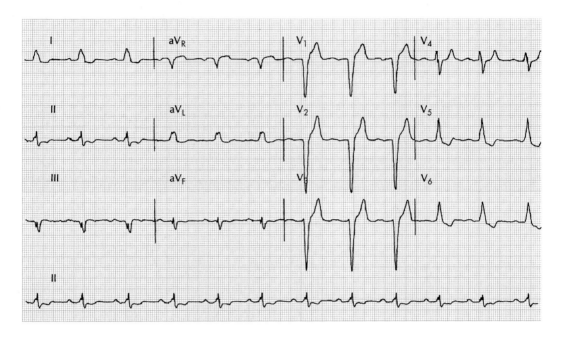

4. Define the terms *primary* and *secondary* T wave abnormality.

*True or false* (Questions 5 to 8):

5. Left anterior hemiblock does not markedly widen the QRS complex.

6. Left bundle branch block is generally seen in patients with organic heart disease.

7. Bundle branch blocks may occur transiently.

8. An electronic pacemaker stimulating the left ventricle will produce a left branch block pattern.

## CHAPTER 8

# Myocardial Ischemia and Infarction  Section I

## ST segment elevation ischemia and Q wave infarct patterns

This chapter and the next examine one of the most important topics of clinical electrocardiography: the diagnosis of myocardial ischemia and infarction (ischemic heart disease). Basic terms are discussed first.

### MYOCARDIAL ISCHEMIA

Myocardial cells require oxygen and nutrients to function. Oxygenated blood is supplied by the coronary arteries. If severe narrowing or complete blockage of a coronary artery causes the blood flow to become inadequate, ischemia of the heart muscle develops. *Ischemia* means literally to hold back blood.

Myocardial ischemia may occur transiently. For example, patients who experience angina pectoris with exercise are having transient myocardial ischemia. If the ischemia is more severe, necrosis of a portion of heart muscle may occur. *Myocardial infarction* (MI) refers to myocardial necrosis ("heart attack"), which is usually caused by severe ischemia.

This discussion focuses primarily on ischemia and infarction of the left ventricle, the predominant chamber of the heart. Right ventricular infarction is also discussed briefly.

### TRANSMURAL AND SUBENDOCARDIAL ISCHEMIA

A cross-sectional diagram of the left ventricle is presented in Figure 8-1. Notice that the left ventricle consists of an outer layer *(epicardium)* and an inner layer *(subendocardium)*. This distinction is important because myocardial ischemia may be limited to just the inner layer, or it may affect virtually the entire thickness of the ventricular wall (transmural ischemia).

### MYOCARDIAL BLOOD SUPPLY

Certain basic facts about the blood supply to the left ventricle are also important. The cardiac blood supply is delivered by the three main coronary arteries (Fig. 8-2). The right coronary

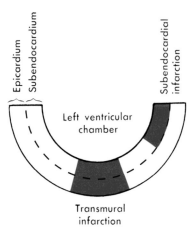

**FIGURE 8-1**   Cross section of the left ventricle showing the difference between a *subendocardial* infarct, which involves the inner half of the ventricular wall, and a *transmural* infarct, which involves the full thickness (or almost the full thickness) of the wall. As discussed in the text, pathologic Q waves may be a marker of transmural infarction. Not all transmural myocardial infarctions, however, produce abnormal Q waves; in some cases, subendocardial (nontransmural) infarctions are associated with Q waves.

artery supplies both the inferior (diaphragmatic) portion of the heart and the right ventricle. The left anterior descending coronary artery generally supplies the ventricular septum and a large part of the left ventricular free wall. The left circumflex coronary artery supplies the lateral wall of the left ventricle. This circulation pattern may be variable. Sometimes, for example, the circumflex artery also supplies the inferior-posterior portion of the left ventricle. MIs tend to be *localized* to the region (anterior or inferior) of the left ventricle supplied by one of these arteries or their branches.

## TRANSMURAL ISCHEMIA WITH MYOCARDIAL INFARCTION

This chapter examines the effect of a classic transmural MI on the ECG. Chapter 9 discusses the ECG patterns of subendocardial ischemia and non–Q wave infarction.

Transmural infarction is characterized by ischemia and ultimately necrosis of a portion of the entire (or nearly entire) thickness of the left ventricular wall. Not surprisingly, large transmural infarctions generally produce changes in both myocardial depolarization (QRS complex) and myocardial repolarization (ST-T complex).

The earliest ECG changes seen with an acute transmural infarction usually occur in the ST-T complex in two sequential phases. The *acute* phase is marked by the appearance of ST segment elevations and sometimes tall positive (hyperacute) T waves in certain leads. The *evolving* phase occurs hours or days later and is characterized by deep T wave inversions in the leads that previously showed ST elevations.

Transmural MIs can also be described in terms of the location of the infarct. *Anterior* means that the infarct involves the anterior and/or lateral wall of the left ventricle, whereas *inferior* indicates involvement of the inferior (diaphragmatic) wall of the left ventricle (Fig. 8-3). The anatomic location of the infarct determines the leads in which the typical ECG patterns appear. For example, with an acute anterior wall MI, the ST segment elevations and tall hyperacute T waves appear in one or more of the anterior leads (chest leads $V_1$ to $V_6$ and limb leads I and $aV_L$) (Fig. 8-4). With an inferior wall MI the ST segment elevations and tall hyperacute T waves are seen in inferior leads II, III, and $aV_F$ (Fig. 8-5).

One of the most important characteristics of the ST-T changes seen with MI is their *reciprocity*. The anterior and inferior leads tend to show inverse patterns. Thus in an anterior infarction with ST segment elevations in leads $V_1$ to $V_6$, I, and $aV_L$, ST segment depression is often seen in leads II, III, and $aV_F$. Conversely, with an acute inferior wall infarction, leads II, III, and $aV_F$ show ST segment elevation, with reciprocal ST depressions often seen in one or more of leads $V_1$ to $V_3$, I, and $aV_L$. (These reciprocal changes are illustrated in Figures 8-4 and 8-5.)

The ST segment elevation seen with acute MI is called a *current of injury* and indicates that

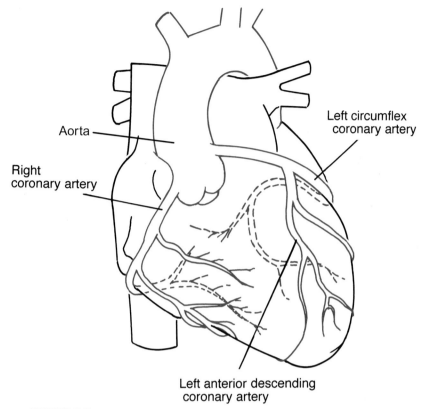

**FIGURE 8-2**  The three major coronary arteries that supply blood to the heart.

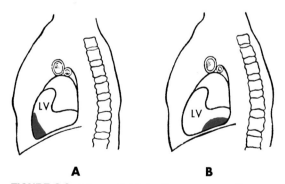

**FIGURE 8-3**  Myocardial infarctions are generally localized to either **(A)**, the anterior portion of the left ventricle (LV) or **(B)**, the inferior (diaphragmatic) portion of the walls of this chamber.

damage has occurred to the epicardial layer of the heart with a transmural ischemia. The exact reasons acute MI produces ST segment elevation are complex and not fully understood. Normally, the ST segment is isoelectric (neither positive nor negative) because no net current flow is occurring at this time. MI alters the electrical charge on the myocardial cell membranes. As a result, current flow becomes abnormal (current of injury) and produces ST segment deviations.

The ST segment elevation seen with acute MI may have different shapes and appearances (Fig. 8-6). Notice that the ST segment may be plateau shaped or dome shaped. Sometimes it is obliquely elevated.

### ECG Sequence with Anterior Wall Q Wave Infarction

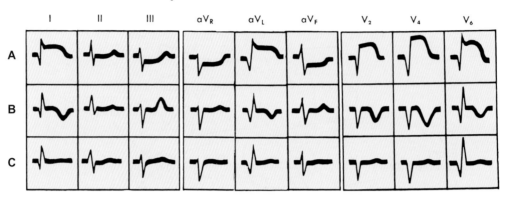

**FIGURE 8-4   A,** Acute phase of an anterior wall infarction: ST elevations and new Q waves. **B,** Evolving phase: deep T wave inversions. **C,** Resolving phase: partial or complete regression of ST-T changes (and sometimes of Q waves). In **A** and **B,** notice the reciprocal ST-T changes in the inferior leads (II, III, and aV$_F$).

### ECG Sequence with Inferior Wall Q Wave Infarction

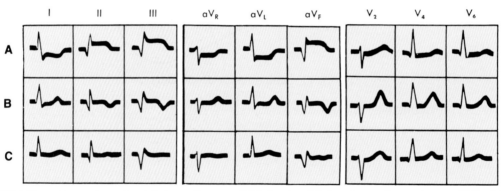

**FIGURE 8-5   A,** Acute phase of an inferior wall myocardial infarction: ST elevations and new Q waves. **B,** Evolving phase: deep T wave inversions. **C,** Resolving phase: partial or complete regression of ST-T changes (and sometimes of Q waves). In **A** and **B,** notice the reciprocal ST-T changes in the anterior leads (I, aV$_L$, and V$_2$).

The ST segment elevations (and reciprocal ST depressions) are the *earliest* ECG signs of infarction, and are generally seen within minutes of the infarct. Tall positive (hyperacute) T waves may also be seen at this time (Figs. 8-7 and 8-8). These T waves have the same significance as the ST elevations. In some cases, hyperacute T waves actually precede the ST elevations.

After a variable time lag (hours to days), the elevated ST segments start to return to the baseline. At the same time, the T waves become inverted in leads that previously showed ST segment elevations. This phase of T wave inversions is called the *evolving phase* of the infarction. Thus, with an anterior wall infarction, the T waves become inverted in one or more of the anterior leads (V$_1$ to V$_6$, I, aV$_L$). With an *inferior* wall infarction, the T waves become inverted in one or more of the inferior leads (II, III, aV$_F$). (These T wave inversions are illustrated in Figures 8-4 and 8-5.)

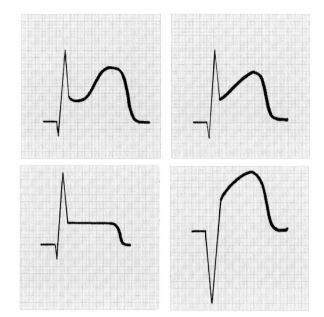

**FIGURE 8-6**  Variable shapes of ST segment elevations seen with acute myocardial infarctions.

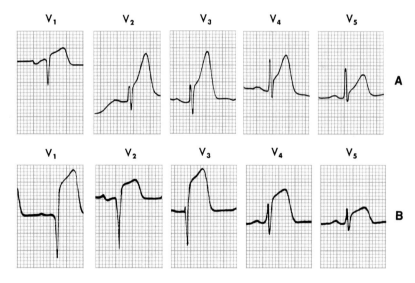

**FIGURE 8-7**  Chest leads from a patient with acute anterior wall infarction. **A,** In the earliest phase of the infarction, tall positive (hyperacute) T waves are seen in leads $V_2$ to $V_5$. **B,** Several hours later, marked ST segment elevation is present in the same leads (current of injury pattern), and abnormal Q waves are seen in leads in $V_1$ and $V_2$.

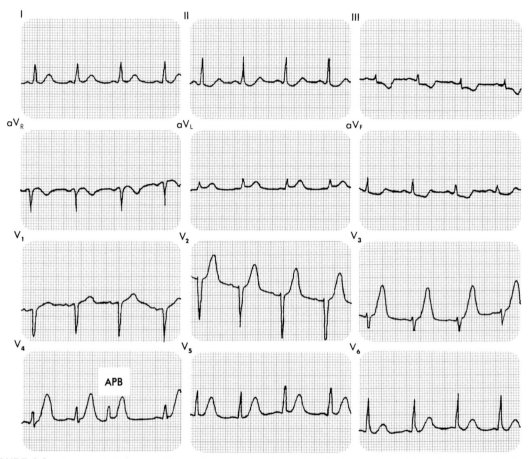

**FIGURE 8-8** Hyperacute T waves with anterior wall infarction. This patient was complaining of severe chest pain. Notice the very tall (hyperacute) T waves in the chest leads. In addition, slight ST segment elevations are present in lead $aV_L$ and reciprocal ST depressions are seen in leads II, III, and $aV_F$. Notice the atrial premature beat (*APB*) in lead $V_4$.

*Clinical correlate:* Of major importance is the finding that emergency reperfusion with percutaneous coronary intervention or with thrombolytic therapy has only been shown to be efficacious for acute MI associated with ST segment elevations. The earlier such therapy is given after the onset of the acute ST segment elevation MI (STEMI), the more likely it is to reduce the size of the infarct and the risk of major complications, including heart failure and death. Furthermore, successful reperfusion therapy for STEMI is generally associated with a prompt decrease in the amplitude of the ischemic ST elevations.

## QRS CHANGES: Q WAVES OF INFARCTION

MI, particularly when large and transmural, often produces distinctive changes in the QRS (depolarization) complex. The characteristic depolarization sign is the appearance of new Q waves.

Why do certain MIs lead to Q waves? Recall that a Q wave is simply an initial negative deflection of the QRS complex. If the entire QRS complex is negative, it is called a *QS complex*:

A Q wave (initial negative QRS deflection) in any lead indicates that the electrical voltages are directed away from that particular lead. With a transmural infarction, necrosis of heart muscle occurs in a localized area of the ventricle. As a result, the electrical voltages produced by this portion of the myocardium disappear. Instead of positive (R) waves over the infarcted area, Q waves are often recorded (either a QR or QS complex).

As discussed in the next chapter, the common clinical tendency to equate pathologic Q waves with transmural necrosis is an over-simplification. *Not all transmural infarcts lead to Q waves, and not all Q wave infarcts correlate with transmural necrosis.*

In summary, abnormal Q waves are characteristic markers of infarction. They signify the loss of positive electrical voltages caused by the death of heart muscle.

The new Q waves of an MI generally appear within the first day or so of the infarct. With an anterior wall infarction, these Q waves are seen in one or more of leads $V_1$ to $V_6$, I, and $aV_L$ (see Fig. 8-4). With an inferior wall MI, the new Q waves appear in leads II, III, and $aV_F$ (see Fig. 8-5).

## LOCALIZATION OF INFARCTIONS

As mentioned, MIs are generally localized to a specific portion of the left ventricle, affecting either the anterior or the inferior wall. Anterior infarctions are sometimes designated as *antero-septal, strictly anterior,* or *antero-lateral/apical,* depending on the leads that show signs of the infarction (Figs. 8-9 to 8-11).

### ANTERIOR WALL Q-WAVE INFARCTIONS

The characteristic feature of an anterior wall Q-wave infarct is *the loss of normal R wave progression in the chest leads.* Recall that normally the height of the R wave increases progressively as you move from lead $V_1$ to lead $V_6$. An anterior infarct interrupts this progression, and the result may be pathologic Q waves in one or

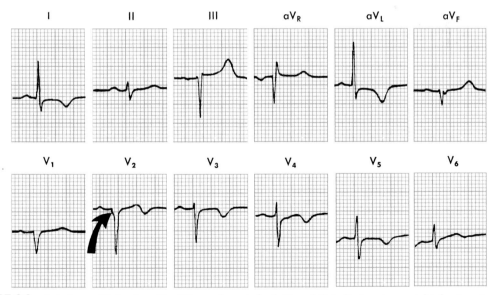

**FIGURE 8-9** Anterior wall infarction. The QS complexes in leads $V_1$ and $V_2$ indicate anteroseptal infarction. A characteristic notching of the QS complex, often seen with infarcts, is present in lead $V_2$ *(arrow).* In addition, the diffuse ischemic T wave inversions in leads I, $aV_L$, and $V_2$ to $V_5$ indicate generalized anterior wall ischemia or non–Q wave myocardial infarction.

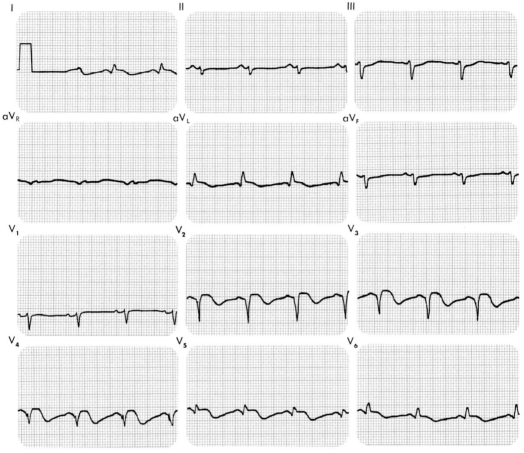

**FIGURE 8-10**   Evolving extensive anterior Q wave infarction. The patient sustained the infarct 1 week earlier. Notice the abnormal Q waves (leads I, $aV_L$, and $V_2$ to $V_5$) with slight ST segment elevations and deep T wave inversions. Left axis deviation resulting from left anterior fascicular block is also present (see Chapter 7).

more of the chest leads. In clinical practice, cardiologists often subdivide anterior MIs into a number of subsets depending on the leads showing Q waves.

### Anteroseptal Infarcts

Remember from Chapter 4 that the ventricular septum is depolarized from left to right and that leads $V_1$ and $V_2$ show small positive (r) waves (septal r waves). Now consider the effect of damaging the septum. Obviously, septal depolarization voltages are lost. Thus the r waves in leads $V_1$ and $V_2$ may disappear and an entirely negative (QS) complex appears.

The septum is supplied with blood by the left anterior descending coronary artery. Septal infarction generally suggests this artery or one of its branches is occluded.

### "Strictly" Anterior Infarcts

Normally, leads $V_3$ and $V_4$ show RS- or Rs-type complexes. If an infarction occurs in the anterior wall of the left ventricle, the positive R waves that reflect the voltages produced by this

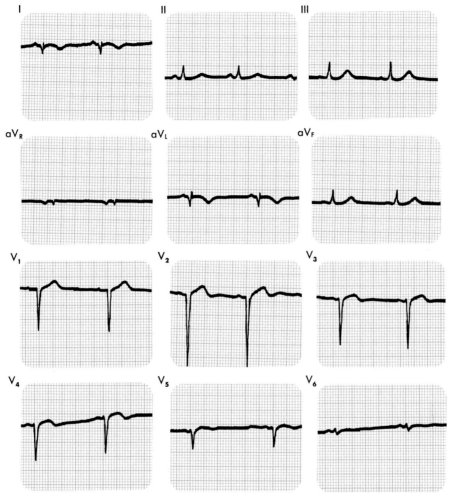

**FIGURE 8-11** Evolving anterior wall infarction. The infarct occurred 1 week earlier. Notice the slow R wave progression in leads $V_1$ to $V_5$ with Q waves in leads I and $aV_L$. The T waves are slightly inverted in these leads. In this ECG, right axis deviation is the result of loss of lateral wall forces, with Q waves seen in leads I and $aV_L$.

muscle area are lost. Instead, Q waves (as part of QS or QR complexes) are seen in leads $V_3$ and $V_4$. A strictly anterior infarct generally results from occlusion of the left anterior descending coronary artery.

### Anterolateral or Anteroapical Infarcts

An infarction of the anterolateral or apical wall of the left ventricle produces changes in the more laterally situated chest leads ($V_5$ and $V_6$).

With such infarctions, abnormal Q waves, as part of QS or QR complexes, appear in leads $V_5$ and $V_6$ (see Fig. 7-7). The infarcts are often caused by occlusion of the left circumflex coronary artery, but they may also result from occlusion of the left anterior descending coronary artery or even a branch of a dominant right coronary artery. ST elevations and pathologic Q waves localized to leads I and $aV_L$ are often ascribed to a "high lateral" MI.

### Differentiating Anterior Wall Infarcts: Some Cautions

The foregoing classification of anterior infarctions is not absolute, and infarct types often overlap. Q wave MIs may be most usefully described by simply referring to any infarct that shows ECG changes in one or more of leads I, $aV_L$, and $V_1$ to $V_6$ as *anterior* and then specifying the leads that show Q waves and ST-T changes.

Of note, anterior infarctions associated with large Q waves in leads $V_1$ to $V_5$ or $V_6$ usually represent extensive damage and substantially reduced left ventricular function (ejection fraction) (see Fig. 8-11).

### INFERIOR WALL INFARCTIONS

Infarction of the inferior (diaphragmatic) portion of the left ventricle is indicated by changes in leads II, III, and $aV_F$ (Figs. 8-12 to 8-14). These three leads, as shown in the diagram of the frontal plane axis, are oriented downward or inferiorly (see Fig. 5-1). Thus, they record voltages from the inferior portion of the ventricle. An inferior wall infarction may produce abnormal Q waves in leads II, III, and $aV_F$. This type of infarction is generally caused by occlusion of the right coronary artery. Less commonly, it occurs because of a left circumflex coronary obstruction.

### POSTERIOR INFARCTIONS

Infarctions can occur in the posterior (back) surface of the left ventricle. These infarctions may be difficult to diagnose because characteristic abnormal ST elevations may not appear in any of the 12 conventional leads. Instead, tall R waves and ST depressions may occur in leads $V_1$ and $V_2$ (reciprocal to the Q waves and ST segment elevations that would be recorded at the back of the heart). During the evolving phase of these infarctions, when deep T wave inversions appear in the posterior leads, the anterior chest leads show reciprocally tall positive T waves (Fig. 8-15).

In most cases of posterior MI, the infarct extends either to the lateral wall of the left ventricle, producing characteristic changes in lead $V_6$, or to the inferior wall of that ventricle, producing characteristic changes in leads II, III, and $aV_F$ (see Fig. 8-15). Because of the overlap between *inferior* and *posterior* infarctions, the more general term *inferoposterior* can be used when the ECG shows changes consistent with either inferior or posterior infarction.

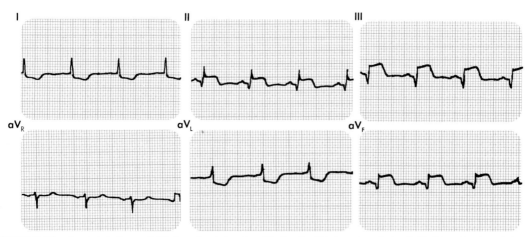

**FIGURE 8-12** Acute inferior wall ST elevation infarction. Notice the ST elevations in leads II, III, and $aV_F$ and the reciprocal ST depressions in leads I and $aV_L$. Abnormal Q waves are also present in leads II, III, and $aV_F$.

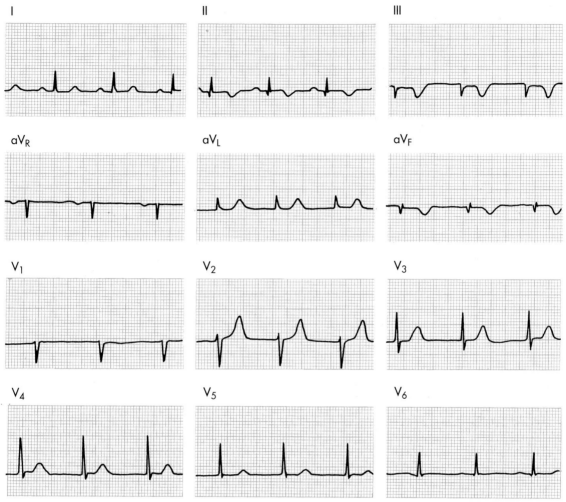

**FIGURE 8-13**   Inferior wall infarction. This patient sustained a myocardial infarction 1 month previously. Notice the abnormal Q waves and symmetric T wave inversions in leads II, III, and aV$_F$. In addition, T wave flattening is seen in lead V$_6$. After infarction, Q waves and ST-T changes may persist indefinitely or may resolve partially or completely.

## RIGHT VENTRICULAR INFARCTIONS

A related topic is right ventricular infarction. Clinical and autopsy studies have shown that patients with an inferoposterior infarct not uncommonly have associated right ventricular involvement. Right ventricular infarction in 30% or more of cases of inferoposterior MI but not in cases of anterior MI. Clinically, patients with a right ventricular infarct may have ele- vated central venous pressure (distended neck veins) because of the abnormally high diastolic filling pressures in the right side of the heart. If the damage to the right ventricle is severe, hypotension and even cardiogenic shock may result. Atrioventricular (AV) conduction distur- bances are not uncommon in this setting. The presence of jugular venous distension in patients with acute inferoposterior wall MIs

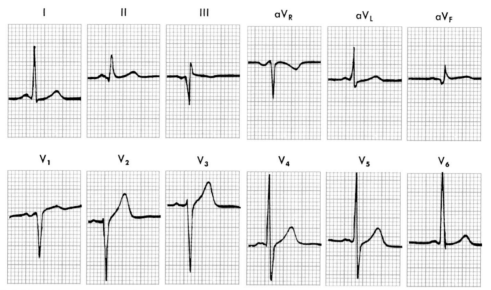

**FIGURE 8-14**   Old inferior wall infarction. Notice the prominent Q waves in leads II, III, and aV$_F$ from a patient who had a myocardial infarction 1 year previously. The ST-T changes have essentially reverted to normal.

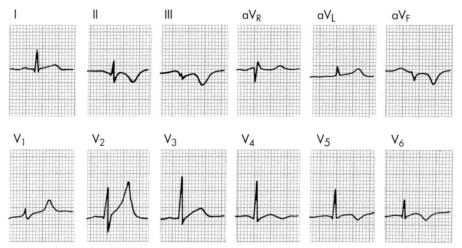

**FIGURE 8-15**   Posterior infarction. Notice the tall R waves in leads V$_1$ and V$_2$. This patient had a previous inferior infarction (Q waves in leads II, III, aV$_F$) and probably a lateral infarction as well (T wave inversions in leads V$_4$ to V$_6$). Notice also the reciprocally tall positive T waves in anterior precordial leads V$_1$ and V$_2$. (From Goldberger AL: Myocardial Infarction: Electrocardiographic Differential Diagnosis, 4th ed, St. Louis, Mosby, 1991.)

should always suggest this diagnosis. Many of these patients also have ST elevations in leads reflecting the right ventricle, such as $V_1$ and $V_3R$ to $V_6R$, as shown in Figure 8-16 (see also Chapter 3).

Recognition of right ventricular infarction is of major clinical importance. Careful volume expansion may be critical in acutely improving cardiac output in patients who are hypotensive and have a low or normal pulmonary capillary wedge pressure.

## SEQUENCE OF Q WAVES AND ST-T CHANGES WITH EVOLVING MYOCARDIAL INFARCTIONS

To this point, the chapter has discussed the ventricular depolarization (QRS complex) and repolarization (ST-T complex) changes produced by an acute MI separately. As shown in Figures 8-4 and 8-5, these changes often occur sequentially.

Ordinarily, the earliest sign of transmural ischemia is ST segment elevations (with reciprocal ST depressions). The ST elevations (current of injury pattern) usually persist for hours to days. During this same period, Q waves often begin to appear in the leads that show ST elevations. Once these changes have occurred, the ST segments start to return to the isoelectric baseline and the T waves become inverted during the evolving phase.

In the weeks or months after an infarct, what should you expect to happen to the Q waves and the ST-T changes just described? The answer is that you cannot make any certain predictions. In most cases, the abnormal Q waves persist for months and even years after the acute infarction. Occasionally, however, the abnormal Q waves diminish in size and even disappear entirely. In some cases, abnormal T wave inversions persist indefinitely. In others, improvement occurs, but minor nonspecific ST-T abnormalities such as slight T wave flattening may persist (see Figs. 8-4 and 8-5).

## NORMAL AND ABNORMAL Q WAVES

A frequently encountered diagnostic problem is deciding whether Q waves are abnormal. Not all Q waves are indicators of MI. For example, a Q wave is normally seen in lead $aV_R$. Furthermore, small "septal" q waves are normally seen in the left chest leads ($V_4$ to $V_6$) and in one or more of leads I, $aV_L$, II, III, and $aV_F$. Recall from Chapter 4 the significance of these septal q waves. The ventricular septum depolarizes from left to right. Left chest leads record this spread of voltages toward the right as a small negative deflection (q wave) that is part of a qR complex in which the R wave represents the spread of left ventricular voltages toward the lead. When the electrical axis is horizontal, such qR complexes are seen in leads I and $aV_L$. When the electrical axis is vertical, qR complexes appear in leads II, III, and $aV_F$.

These normal septal q waves must be differentiated from the pathologic Q waves of infarction. Normal septal q waves are characteristically narrow and of low amplitude. As a rule, septal q waves are less than 0.04 second in duration. A Q wave is generally abnormal if its duration is 0.04 second or more in lead I, all three inferior leads (II, III, $aV_F$), or leads $V_3$ to $V_6$.

What if Q waves with duration of 0.04 second or more are seen in leads $V_1$ and $V_2$? A large QS complex can be a normal variant in lead $V_1$ and rarely in leads $V_1$ and $V_2$. QS waves in these leads may be the only evidence of an anterior septal MI, however. An abnormal QS complex resulting from infarction sometimes shows a notch as it descends, or it may be slurred instead of descending and rising abruptly (see Fig. 8-9). Further criteria for differentiating normal from abnormal Q waves in these leads lie beyond the scope of this book.

What if a wide Q wave is seen in lead $aV_L$ or Q waves are present in leads III and $aV_F$? These waveforms can also occur normally. Although a discussion of the precise criteria for differentiating normal from abnormal Q waves in these leads is beyond the scope of this book, the following can be taken as general rules:

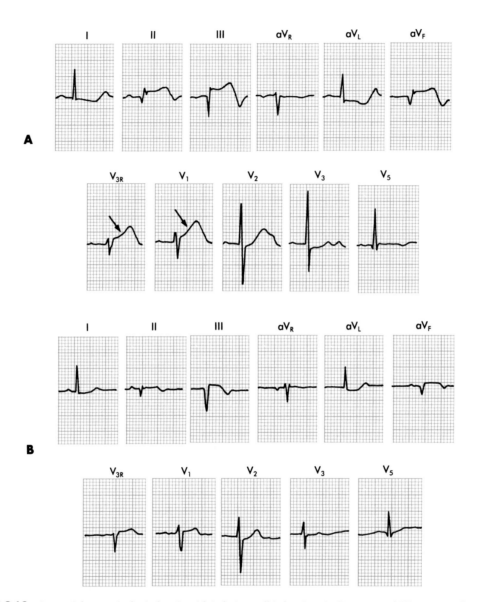

**FIGURE 8-16**   Acute right ventricular ischemia with inferior wall infarction. **A,** Q waves and ST segment elevations in leads II, III, and aV$_F$ are accompanied by ST elevations *(arrows)* in the right precordial leads (V$_{3R}$ and V$_1$). The ST-T changes in lead V$_6$ are consistent with lateral wall ischemia. The ST depressions in leads I and aV$_L$ are probably reciprocal to inferior lead ST elevations. **B,** Follow-up tracing obtained the next day, showing diminution of the ST changes. (From Goldberger AL: Myocardial Infarction: Electrocardiographic Differential Diagnosis, 4th ed, St. Louis, Mosby, 1991.)

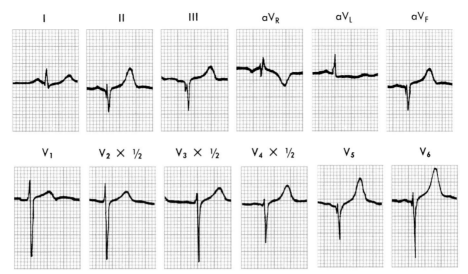

**FIGURE 8-17**   Hypertrophic obstructive cardiomyopathy (HOCM). Notice the prominent pseudoinfarction Q waves, which are the result of septal hypertrophy. Leads $V_2$ to $V_4$ are recorded at $^1/_2$, the usual voltage calibration. (From Goldberger AL: Myocardial Infarction: Electrocardiographic Differential Diagnosis, 4th ed, St. Louis, Mosby, 1991.)

- An inferior wall MI should be diagnosed with certainty only when abnormal Q waves are seen in leads II, III, and $aV_F$. If prominent Q waves appear only in leads III and $aV_F$, the likelihood of MI is increased by the presence of abnormal ST-T changes in all three inferior limb leads.

- An anterior wall MI should not be diagnosed from lead $aV_L$ alone. Look for abnormal Q waves and ST-T changes in the other anterior leads (I and $V_1$ to $V_6$).

Furthermore, *just as not all Q waves are abnormal, all abnormal Q waves are not the result of MI.* For example, slow R wave progression in the chest leads, sometimes with actual QS complexes in the right to middle chest leads (e.g., $V_1$ to $V_3$), may occur with left bundle branch block (LBBB), left ventricular hypertrophy, and chronic lung disease in the absence of MI. Prominent noninfarction Q waves are often a characteristic feature in the ECGs of patients with hypertrophic cardiomyopathy (Fig. 8-17). Noninfarction Q waves also occur with dilated

cardiomyopathy (see Fig. 11-4). As mentioned previously, the ECGs of normal people sometimes have a QS wave in lead $V_1$ and rarely in leads $V_1$ and $V_2$. Prominent Q waves in the absence of MI are sometimes referred to as a *pseudoinfarct pattern* (see Chapter 22).*

## VENTRICULAR ANEURYSM

After a large MI, a ventricular aneurysm develops in some patients. An aneurysm is a severely scarred portion of infarcted ventricular myocardium that does not contract normally. Instead, during ventricular systole, the aneurysmic portion bulges outward while the rest of the ventricle is contracting. Ventricular aneurysm may occur on the anterior or inferior surface of the heart.

---

*For a more complete discussion of this subject, see Goldberger AL: Myocardial Infarction: Electrocardiographic Differential Diagnosis, 4th ed, St. Louis, Mosby, 1991.

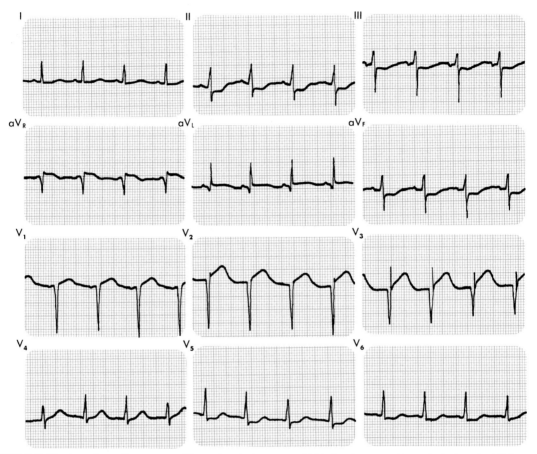

**FIGURE 8-18** Anterior wall aneurysm. The patient had a myocardial infarction several months before this ECG was taken. Notice the prominent Q waves in leads $V_1$ to $V_3$ and $aV_L$, the persistent ST elevations in these leads, and the reciprocal ST depressions in the inferior leads (II, III, and $aV_F$). The persistence of ST elevations more than 2 to 3 weeks after an infarction suggests the presence of a ventricular aneurysm.

The ECG may be helpful in making the diagnosis of ventricular aneurysm subsequent to an MI. Patients with ventricular aneurysm frequently have persistent ST segment elevations after an infarct. As mentioned earlier, the ST segment elevations seen with acute infarction generally resolve within several days. The persistence of ST segment elevations for several weeks or more is suggestive of a ventricular aneurysm (Fig. 8-18). The absence of persisting ST segment elevations, however, does not rule out the possibility of an aneurysm.

Ventricular aneurysms are of clinical importance for several major reasons. They may lead to congestive heart failure. They may be associated with serious ventricular arrhythmias. A thrombus may form in an aneurysm and break off, resulting in a stroke or some other embolic complication.

## MULTIPLE INFARCTIONS

Not infrequently, patients may have two or more MIs at different times. For example, a new

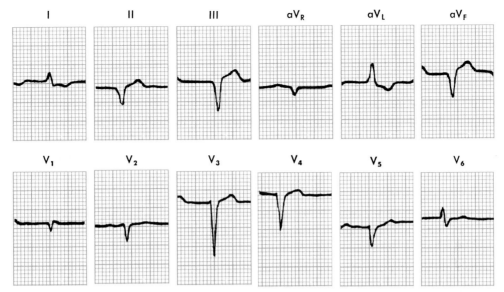

**FIGURE 8-19**   Multiple myocardial infarctions. This ECG shows evidence of previous anterior wall and inferior wall infarcts. Notice the slow R wave progression and QS complexes in chest leads $V_1$ to $V_5$, as well as the QS waves in leads II, III, and $aV_F$.

anterior wall infarct may develop in a patient with a previous inferior wall infarction. In such cases the ECG initially shows abnormal Q waves in leads II, III, and $aV_F$. During the anterior infarct, new Q waves and ST-T changes appear in the anterior leads. (The ECG of a patient with multiple infarcts [anterior and inferior] is presented in Figure 8-19.)

## "SILENT" MYOCARDIAL INFARCTION

Most patients with an acute MI have symptoms. They may experience the classic syndrome of crushing substernal chest pain, or they may have atypical pain (e.g., a sensation like indigestion, upper back pain, or jaw pain). Sometimes, however, patients may experience few if any symptoms ("silent" MI). Therefore it is not unusual for an ECG to show abnormal Q waves that indicate a previous infarction in a patient without a clinical history of definite MI.

## DIAGNOSIS OF MYOCARDIAL INFARCTION IN THE PRESENCE OF BUNDLE BRANCH BLOCK

The diagnosis of infarction is more difficult when the patient's baseline ECG shows a bundle branch block pattern or a bundle branch block develops as a complication of the MI. Then the ECG picture becomes more complex.

### RIGHT BUNDLE BRANCH BLOCK WITH MYOCARDIAL INFARCTION

The diagnosis of a Q wave MI can be made relatively easily in the presence of right bundle branch block (RBBB). Remember that RBBB affects primarily the terminal phase of ventricular depolarization, producing a wide R' wave in the right chest leads and a wide S wave in the left chest leads. MI affects the initial phase of ventricular depolarization, producing abnormal Q waves. When RBBB and an infarct occur together, a combination of these patterns is seen: The QRS complex is abnormally wide (0.12 second or more) as a result of the bundle branch block, lead $V_1$ shows a terminal positive deflection, and lead $V_6$ shows a wide S wave. If the infarction is anterior, the ECG shows a loss of R wave progression with abnormal Q waves in the anterior leads and characteristic ST-T changes. If the infarction is inferior, pathologic Q waves and ST-T changes are seen in leads II, III, and $aV_F$. (An anterior wall infarction with the RBBB pattern is shown in Figure 8-20.)

## LEFT BUNDLE BRANCH BLOCK WITH MYOCARDIAL INFARCTION

The diagnosis of LBBB in the presence of MI is considerably more complicated and confusing than that of RBBB. The reason is that LBBB alters both the early and the late phases of ventricular stimulation (see Chapter 7). It also produces secondary ST-T changes. As a general rule, LBBB hides the diagnosis of an infarct. *Thus a patient with a chronic LBBB pattern who develops an acute MI may not show the characteristic changes of infarction described in this chapter.*

Occasionally, patients with LBBB manifest primary ST-T changes indicative of ischemia or actual infarction. The secondary T wave inversions of uncomplicated LBBB are seen in leads $V_4$ to $V_6$ (with prominent R waves). The appearance of T wave inversions in leads $V_1$ to $V_3$ (with prominent S waves) is a primary abnormality that cannot be ascribed to the bundle branch block itself (Fig. 8-21).

The problem of diagnosing infarction with LBBB is further complicated by the fact that the LBBB pattern has several features that resemble those seen with infarction. Thus LBBB patterns can mimic infarct patterns. As discussed in Chapter 7, LBBB typically shows slow R wave progression in the chest leads because of the reversed way the ventricular septum is activated (i.e., from right to left, the opposite of what happens normally). Consequently, with LBBB, a loss of the normal septal R waves is seen in the right chest leads. This loss of normal R wave progression simulates the pattern seen with an anterior wall infarct.

Figure 7-5 shows an example of LBBB with slow R wave progression. In this case, anterior wall infarction was not present. Notice that the ST segment elevations in the right chest leads resemble the pattern seen during the hyperacute or acute phase of an infarction. ST segment elevation in the right chest leads is also commonly seen with LBBB in the absence of infarction.

As a general rule, a patient with an LBBB pattern should not be diagnosed as having had an MI simply on the basis of slow R wave progression in the right chest leads or ST elevations in those leads. The presence of Q waves as part of QR complexes in the left chest leads ($V_5$ and $V_6$) with LBBB, however, generally indicates an underlying MI (Fig. 8-22). In addition, the appearance of ST *elevations* in the left chest leads or in other leads with prominent R waves suggests ischemia (see Fig. 8-22, lead $V_5$), as does the appearance of ST segment *depressions* in the right leads or other leads with an rS or a QS morphology. (The discussion of the ECG with ischemia and infarction continues in Chapter 9, which focuses on *subendocardial* ischemia and non–Q wave MI patterns.)

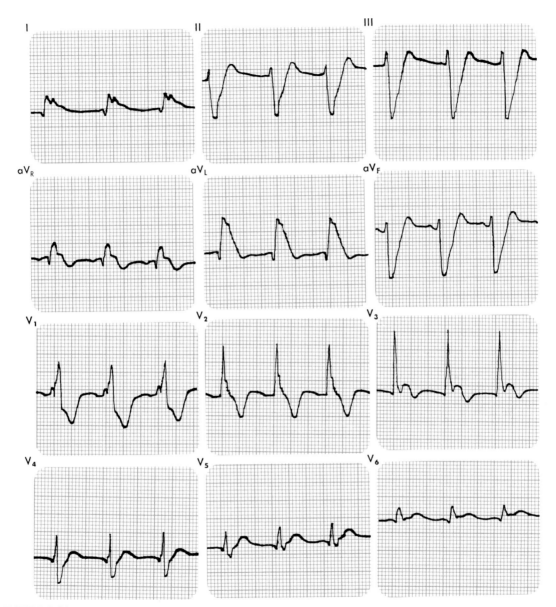

**FIGURE 8-20** Acute anterior wall infarction and the right bundle branch block (RBBB) pattern. The wide QRS complexes with an rSR' wave in lead $V_1$ and a qRS pattern in lead $V_5$ indicate the presence of RBBB. A pattern of acute anterior wall infarction is indicated by the Q waves and ST elevations in leads I and $aV_L$ and the marked reciprocal ST depressions in leads II, III, and $aV_F$. Finally, notice the left axis deviation caused by the left anterior fascicular block. This combination—left anterior fascicular block and RBBB—is an example of bifascicular block and may herald complete (trifascicular) heart block in patients with an acute anterior wall infarction (see Chapter 17).

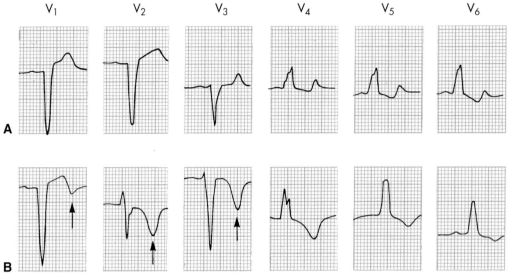

**FIGURE 8-21** **A,** Typical left bundle branch block (LBBB) pattern. Notice the slow R wave progression in the right precordial leads and the discordance of QRS and ST-T vectors reflected by the ST elevations in the right precordial leads and the ST depressions with T wave inversions in the left precordial leads. **B,** LBBB with ischemia. Subsequently, the ECG from this patient showed the development of primary T wave inversions in leads $V_1$ to $V_3$ *(arrows)* caused by anterior ischemia and probable infarction. (From Goldberger AL: Myocardial Infarction: Electrocardiographic Differential Diagnosis, 4th ed, St. Louis, Mosby, 1991.)

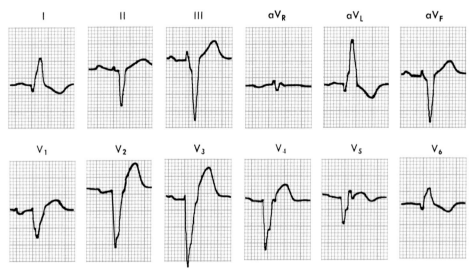

**FIGURE 8-22** Anterior wall infarction with left bundle branch block. Notice the prominent Q waves in the left chest leads as part of QR complexes (see text). (From Goldberger AL: Myocardial Infarction: Electrocardiographic Differential Diagnosis, 4th ed, St. Louis, Mosby, 1991.)

# REVIEW

Myocardial ischemia occurs when the blood supply to the myocardium is not adequate. *Myocardial infarction (MI)* refers to necrosis of the myocardium caused by severe ischemia.

Myocardial ischemia or infarction may affect the entire thickness of the ventricular muscle (*transmural* injury) or may be localized to the inner layer of the ventricle (*subendocardial* ischemia or infarction). Transmural MI, especially when large, often (but not always) produces a typical sequence of ST-T changes and abnormal Q waves. The ST-T changes can be divided into two phases:

1. The *acute* phase is marked by ST segment elevations (*current of injury* pattern) and sometimes tall positive T waves (hyperacute T waves).

2. The *evolving* phase is characterized by the appearance of deeply inverted T waves in leads that showed the hyperacute T waves and ST elevations.

These ST-T changes occur during a period of hours or days and usually resolve over weeks or months. During the first day or so after an MI, new abnormal Q waves may appear in one or more leads.

Thrombolytic therapy has only been found efficacious in the treatment of acute ST segment elevation MI (STEMI).

The persistence of ST segment elevations for more than 2 or 3 weeks after an acute MI may signify that a ventricular aneurysm has developed. The abnormal Q waves tend to persist, but may become smaller with time and, rarely, may even disappear.

A Q wave MI can also be described in terms of its location. With an *anterior* infarction, ST segment elevations and abnormal Q waves occur in one or more of leads $V_1$ to $V_6$, I, and $aV_L$. Reciprocal ST depressions may be seen in leads II, III, and $aV_F$. With an *inferior* infarction, ST elevations and Q waves appear in leads II, III, and $aV_F$, and reciprocal ST depressions may be seen in one or more of the anterior leads.

Right ventricular MI is a common complication of inferoposterior infarcts. In acute cases, the ECG may also show elevated ST segments in the right chest leads.

The pathologic Q waves of infarction must be distinguished from normal Q waves. For example, small normal "septal" q waves as part of qR complexes may be seen in the left chest leads ($V_4$ to $V_6$), in leads II, III, and $aV_F$ (with a vertical electrical axis), and in leads I and $aV_L$ (with a horizontal axis). These septal q waves are normally less than 0.04 second in width.

A QS wave may be seen normally in lead $V_1$ and occasionally in leads $V_1$ and $V_2$. Q waves may also be seen as normal variants in leads $aV_F$, III, and $aV_L$.

Multiple MIs can occur. In such cases, the ECG may show old Q waves from the preceding infarct and new Q waves and/or ST-T changes from the current infarct.

When *right bundle branch block (RBBB)* complicates an acute MI, the diagnosis of both conditions is possible. The RBBB prolongs the QRS width, and lead $V_1$ shows a tall positive final deflection. In addition, abnormal Q waves and ST segment elevations resulting from the acute MI are present in the chest leads with an anterior MI and in leads II, III, and $aV_F$ with an inferior MI.

When *left bundle branch block (LBBB)* complicates an acute MI, the infarction may be difficult to diagnose because the LBBB may mask both the abnormal Q waves of the infarction and the ST segment elevations and T wave inversions of the ischemia. In addition, LBBB may produce QS waves in the right chest leads with ST segment elevations and slow R wave progression across the chest *without* MI. The presence of QR complexes in the left chest leads with LBBB is suggestive of underlying MI. Ischemia with underlying LBBB is suggested by the presence of T wave inversions in the right chest leads, ST segment elevations in the left chest leads (or in other leads with prominent R waves), or ST segment depression in the right precordial leads (or other leads with rS or QS waves).

## QUESTIONS

See the end of Chapter 9.

# Myocardial Ischemia and Infarction Section II

## ST segment depression ischemia and non–Q wave infarct patterns

**M**yocardial infarction (MI) may be associated with abnormal Q waves and the typical progression of ST-T changes described in Chapter 8. In other cases, however, myocardial ischemia (with or without actual infarction) may be limited primarily to the *subendocardium* (inner layer) of the ventricle.

### SUBENDOCARDIAL ISCHEMIA

How can subendocardial ischemia occur without transmural ischemia or infarction? The subendocardium is particularly vulnerable to ischemia because it is most distant from the coronary blood supply and closest to the high pressure of the ventricular cavity. This inner layer of the ventricle can become ischemic while the outer layer (epicardium) remains normally perfused with blood.

The most common ECG change with subendocardial ischemia is ST segment depression (Fig. 9-1). The ST depression may be limited to the anterior leads (I, aV$_L$, and V$_1$ to V$_6$) or to the inferior leads (II, III, and aV$_F$), or it may be seen more diffusely in both groups of leads. As shown in Figure 9-1, the ST depression with subendocardial ischemia has a characteristic squared-off shape. (ST segment elevation is usually seen in lead aV$_R$.)

Recall from the previous chapter that acute transmural ischemia produces ST segment elevation, a current of injury pattern. This results from epicardial injury. With pure subendocardial ischemia, just the opposite occurs; that is, the ECG shows ST segment depression (except in lead aV$_R$, which typically shows ST elevation).

In summary, myocardial ischemia involving primarily the subendocardium usually produces ST segment depression, whereas acute ischemia involving the epicardium usually produces ST elevation. (This difference in the direction of the injury current vector is depicted in Figure 9-2.)

### ECG CHANGES WITH ANGINA PECTORIS

The term *angina pectoris* refers to transient attacks of chest discomfort caused by myocardial ischemia. Angina is a symptom of coronary

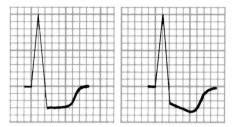

**FIGURE 9-1** Subendocardial ischemia may produce ST depressions.

artery disease. The classic attack of angina is experienced as a dull, burning, or boring substernal pressure or heaviness. It is typically precipitated by exertion, stress, exposure to cold, and other factors, and it is relieved by rest and nitroglycerin.

Many (but not all) patients with classic angina have an ECG pattern of subendocardial ischemia, with ST depressions seen during an attack. When the pain disappears, the ST segments generally return to the baseline. (Figure 9-3 shows ST depressions during a spontaneous episode of angina.)

The ECGs of some patients with angina do not show ST depressions during chest pain. Consequently, the presence of a normal ECG does not rule out underlying coronary artery

disease. The appearance of transient ST depressions in the ECG of a patient with chest pain is, however, a very strong indicator of myocardial ischemia.

## EXERCISE TESTING AND CORONARY ARTERY DISEASE

Many patients with coronary artery disease have a normal ECG while at rest. During exercise, however, ischemic changes may appear because of the extra oxygen requirements imposed on the heart by exertion. To assist in diagnosing coronary artery disease, the cardiologist can record the ECG while the patient is being exercised under controlled conditions. *Stress electrocardiography* is usually performed while the patient walks on a treadmill or pedals a bicycle. The test is stopped when the patient develops angina, fatigue, or diagnostic ST changes or when the heart rate reaches 85% to 90% of a maximum predetermined rate predicted from the patient's age. This approach is known as *submaximal testing*.

Figure 9-4*A* is the normal resting ECG of a patient, whereas Figure 9-4*B* shows the marked ST depressions recorded while the patient was exercising. The appearance of ST segment depressions constitutes a positive (abnormal) result. Most cardiologists accept horizontal or

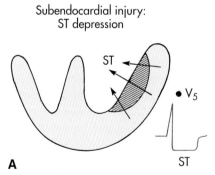

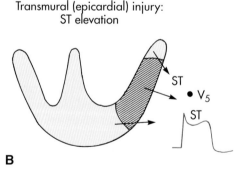

**FIGURE 9-2** **A,** With acute subendocardial ischemia the electrical forces *(arrows)* responsible for the ST segment are deviated toward the inner layer of the heart, causing ST depressions in lead V₅, which faces the outer surface of the heart. **B,** With acute transmural (epicardial) ischemia, electrical forces *(arrows)* responsible for the ST segment are deviated toward the outer layer of the heart, causing ST elevations in the overlying lead.

Lead V₄

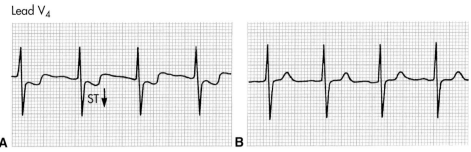

**FIGURE 9-3**  **A,** Marked ST depressions are seen in the ECG from a patient who complained of chest pain while being examined. **B,** Five minutes later, after the patient was given sublingual nitroglycerin, the ST segments have reverted to normal, with relief of angina.

Rest                                    Exercise

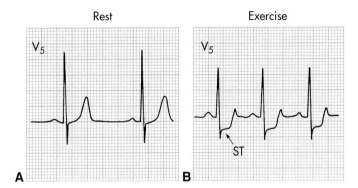

**FIGURE 9-4**  **A,** Baseline rhythm strip from the positive exercise test of a patient with coronary artery disease. **B,** Notice the marked ST depressions with increased heart rate.

downward ST depressions of at least 1 mm or more, lasting at least 0.08 second (2 small boxes) as a positive (abnormal) test result (see Fig. 9-4*B*). ST depressions of less than 1 mm (or depressions of only the J point) with a rapid upward sloping of the ST segment are considered a negative (normal) test response (Fig. 9-5).

The finding of prominent ischemic ST changes, with or without symptoms, occurring at a low level of activity is particularly ominous.

Exercise electrocardiography is often helpful in diagnosing coronary artery disease. Like all tests, however, it may give both false-positive and false-negative results. For example, up to 10% of normal men and an even higher percentage of normal women may have false-positive exercise tests.

False-positive tests (defined as ST depressions without obstructive coronary disease) can also be seen in patients who are taking digitalis and in patients who have hypokalemia, left ventricular hypertrophy (LVH), ventricular conduction disturbances, or Wolff-Parkinson-White patterns (see Chapter 12).

False-negative tests can occur despite the presence of significant underlying coronary artery disease. *A normal "negative" exercise test does not exclude coronary artery disease.* The diagnostic accuracy of exercise tests may be increased in selected patients by simultaneous imaging studies, using echocardiography or nuclear medicine scans.

In summary, subendocardial ischemia, such as occurs with typical angina pectoris (and as may be elicited with stress testing), often

Lead V₅

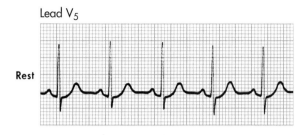

Rest

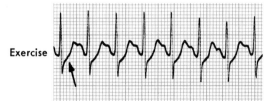

Exercise

**FIGURE 9-5** Lead V₅ shows physiologic ST segment depression that may occur with exercise. Notice the J junction depression *(arrow)* with sharply upsloping ST segments. (From Goldberger AL: Myocardial Infarction: Electrocardiographic Differential Diagnosis, 4th ed, St. Louis, Mosby, 1991.)

produces ST segment depressions in multiple leads.

## "SILENT" MYOCARDIAL ISCHEMIA

A patient with coronary artery disease may have episodes of myocardial ischemia *without* angina, hence the term *silent ischemia*. Silent ischemia is sometimes detected during exercise testing. Ambulatory ECG (Holter) monitoring is another useful way to assess silent myocardial ischemia (see Chapter 3). 24-hour ECG monitoring of patients with coronary artery disease reveals a surprisingly high frequency of ST depressions *not* associated with angina. This important topic is discussed again later in this chapter.

## SUBENDOCARDIAL INFARCTION

If ischemia of the subendocardial region is severe enough, actual infarction may occur. In such cases, the ECG may show more persistent ST depressions instead of the transient depressions seen with reversible subendocardial ischemia.

Figure 9-6 shows an example of a non–Q wave infarction with persistent ST depressions. Is it possible for Q waves to appear with pure subendocardial infarction? The answer is that if only the inner half of the myocardium is infarcted, abnormal Q waves usually do not appear. Subendocardial infarction generally affects ventricular repolarization (ST-T complex) and not depolarization (QRS complex). As discussed at the end of this chapter, however, important exceptions may occur, and so-called *nontransmural* infarctions, particularly larger ones, may be associated with Q waves.

Another ECG pattern sometimes seen in non–Q wave infarction is T wave inversions with or without ST segment depressions. Figure 9-7 shows an infarction pattern with deep T wave inversions. (T wave inversions may also be seen in some cases of noninfarctional ischemia.)

In summary, non–Q wave infarction can be associated with persistent ST depressions and/or T wave inversions.

## VARIETY OF ECG CHANGES SEEN WITH MYOCARDIAL ISCHEMIA

Myocardial ischemia clearly can produce a wide variety of ECG changes. For example, infarction may cause abnormal Q waves in association with ST segment elevations followed by T wave inversions. Ventricular aneurysm may be associated with persistent ST segment elevations. Subendocardial ischemia (e.g., during an anginal attack or a stress test) may produce transient ST depressions. In other cases, infarction may be associated with ST depressions or T wave inversions without Q waves.

### ECG CHANGES ASSOCIATED WITH NONINFARCTION ISCHEMIA

Myocardial ischemia does not always cause diagnostic ST-T changes. Several other patterns

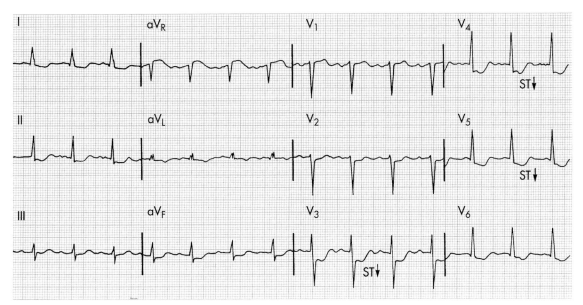

**FIGURE 9-6**  Non–Q wave infarction in a patient who complained of severe chest pain. Subsequently, the patient's cardiac enzyme levels were elevated. Notice the marked, diffuse ST depressions in leads I, II, III, aV$_L$, aV$_F$, and V$_2$ to V$_6$, in conjunction with the ST elevation in lead aV$_R$. These findings are consistent with severe subendocardial ischemia. Other abnormalities include a prolonged PR interval (0.28 sec) and left atrial abnormality.

may be seen. In some patients, the ECG may remain entirely normal during episodes of ischemia. In others, the ST-T complex may display only subtle changes. For example, you may see just slight T wave flattening or minimal T wave inversions. These are *nonspecific ST-T changes* (see Chapter 10).

Nonspecific ST-T changes may be abnormal, but they are not definite indicators of ischemia. They may be a sign of ischemic heart disease, but they may also be caused by many other conditions, including drug effects, hyperventilation, and electrolyte abnormalities. Therefore you should *not* make a definite diagnosis of myocardial ischemia solely on the basis of nonspecific ST-T changes.

Prinzmetal's angina is another form of noninfarction ischemia. Recall that the ECG with classic or typical angina often shows the pattern of subendocardial ischemia with ST segment depressions. An atypical form of angina (first reported by Dr. M. Prinzmetal) is seen in a small but important group of patients. Their angina is atypical because, during episodes of chest pain, they have ST segment elevations, a pattern described previously with acute transmural MI. In Prinzmetal's angina, the ST segment elevations are transient. After the episode of chest pain, the ST segments usually return to the baseline, without the characteristic evolving pattern of Q waves and T wave inversions that occur with acute transmural MI. Thus Prinzmetal's angina is atypical because the ECG shows ST elevations rather than the ST depressions seen with typical angina.

Patients with Prinzmetal's angina are also atypical because their chest pain often occurs at rest or at night. (In contrast, patients with classic angina pectoris usually have chest pain with exertion or emotional stress.) Prinzmetal's angina pattern is significant because it is a marker of coronary artery *spasm* that causes

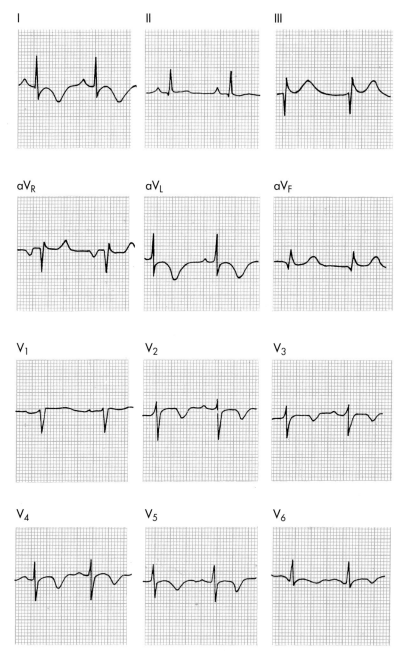

**FIGURE 9-7** Non–Q wave infarction in a patient who complained of chest pain and also had elevated cardiac enzyme levels. Notice the deep T wave inversions in leads I, aV$_L$, and V$_2$ to V$_6$. (Prominent Q waves in III and aV$_F$ represent an old inferior wall infarction.) Patients with acute myocardial infarction may have ST segment depressions or T wave inversions without Q waves.

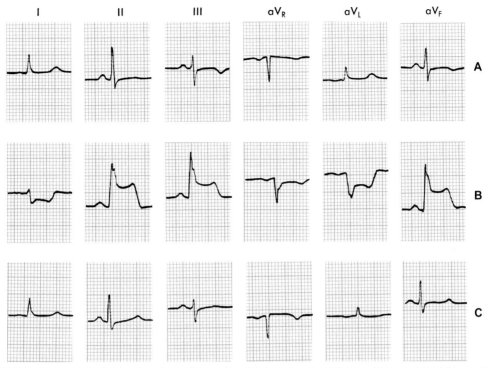

**FIGURE 9-8**  Prinzmetal's (variant) angina with transient ST elevations in a 30-year-old man with a history of angina with exertion and at rest. **A,** The baseline resting ECG shows nonspecific inferior lead ST-T changes. **B,** With chest pain, marked ST segment elevations occur in leads II, III, and aV$_F$, and reciprocal ST depressions are seen in leads I and aV$_L$. The rightward axis shift and slight widening of the QRS complex are consistent with left posterior fascicular block. **C,** The ST segments return to baseline after the patient is given nitroglycerin. Cardiac catheterization showed severe right coronary obstruction with intermittent spasm producing total occlusion and transient ST elevations. (From Goldberger AL: Myocardial Infarction: Electrocardiographic Differential Diagnosis, 4th ed, St. Louis, Mosby, 1991.)

transient transmural ischemia. These episodes of spasm may occur in patients with otherwise normal coronary arteries. In most cases, spasm is associated with high-grade coronary obstruction (Fig. 9-8). Increasing evidence implicates cocaine as another cause of coronary spasm, sometimes leading to MI.

At this point, the diverse ECG changes seen with ischemic heart disease can be summarized. These changes may include Q waves, ST segment elevations or depressions, tall positive T waves or deep T wave inversions, nonspecific ST-T changes, and even a normal ECG (Fig. 9-9).

## ST SEGMENT ELEVATIONS: DIFFERENTIAL DIAGNOSIS

ST segment elevations (current of injury pattern) are the earliest sign of acute transmural ischemia with infarction. Transient elevations are also seen with Prinzmetal's angina. ST segment elevations persisting for several weeks after an acute MI may be a sign of a ventricular aneurysm.

In Figure 9-10 (the ECG of a *normal* young adult), notice the marked elevation of the ST segments. This is a benign variant known as the

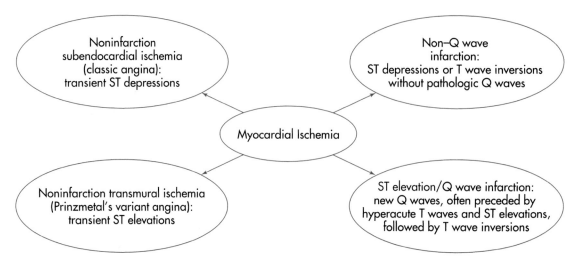

**FIGURE 9-9** Myocardial ischemia produces diverse ECG changes. T wave inversions may also occur with noninfarctional ischemia. Sometimes the ECG may be normal or show only nonspecific ST-T changes. ST elevation infarction is not always followed by Q waves.

## Early Repolarization

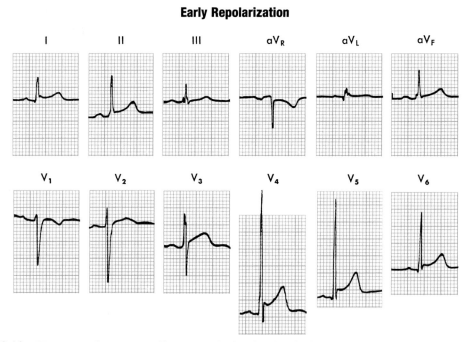

**FIGURE 9-10** ST segment elevation, usually most marked in the chest leads, is sometimes seen as a normal variant. This so-called early repolarization pattern may be confused with the ST segment elevations of acute myocardial infarction or pericarditis.

*early repolarization pattern*. With early repolarization, the ST segments in the chest leads may rise to 2 to 3 mm above the baseline. Although most common in young people, these ST elevations can also occur in older persons, simulating the pattern seen with acute pericarditis or MI. The elevations are stable, however, and do not undergo the evolutionary sequence seen with *acute pericarditis* (Chapter 11). Furthermore, they are not associated with reciprocal ST depressions (except in lead $aV_R$), contrary to what is often observed with acute MI.

ST segment elevations, resembling myocardial infarction or pericarditis, may also be seen with acute myocarditis (Chapter 11). Chronic ST elevations are often seen in leads $V_1$ and $V_2$ in association with the patterns of LVH or left bundle branch block (LBBB) (Chapter 7). Other causes of ST elevations include systemic hypothermia (J waves or Osborn waves, Chapter 10) and the Brugada pattern (Chapter 19). A comprehensive "instant review" summary of the differential diagnosis of ST segment elevations is given in Chapter 24.

## ST SEGMENT DEPRESSIONS: DIFFERENTIAL DIAGNOSIS

Subendocardial ischemia is usually characterized by ST segment depression. Not all ST depressions are indicative of subendocardial ischemia, however. For example, the ST-T changes associated with LVH (formerly referred to as the "strain" pattern) were discussed in Chapter 6. As shown in Figure 6-12, the ST segment may be slightly depressed with LVH. *Acute transmural ischemia* is another cause of ST segment depressions.

Remember that acute anterior wall ischemia may be associated with reciprocal ST depressions in one or more of leads II, III, and $aV_F$. Conversely, acute inferior wall ischemia may be associated with reciprocal ST depressions in one or more of the anterior leads (I, $aV_L$, $V_1$ to $V_3$). Therefore whenever you see ST depressions,

you need to look at all the leads and evaluate these changes in context.

The ST segment may also be depressed by two important and common factors: *digitalis effect* and *hypokalemia* (see Chapter 10). Digitalis may produce scooping of the ST-T complex with slight ST depression (see Fig. 10-1). The ST segment may also be somewhat depressed in the ECGs of patients with a low serum potassium level (see Fig. 10-8). Prominent U waves may also appear. In some cases, it may be difficult to sort out which factors are responsible for the ST depressions you are seeing. For example, a patient with LVH may be taking digitalis and may also be having acute subendocardial ischemia.

A comprehensive "instant review" summary of the differential diagnosis of ST segment depressions is given in Chapter 24.

## DEEP T WAVE INVERSIONS: DIFFERENTIAL DIAGNOSIS

Deep T wave inversions, as described previously, usually occur during the evolving phase of a Q wave MI (see Fig. 8-4*B*) and also sometimes with a non–Q wave MI (see Fig. 9-7). These deep inversions are the result of a delay in regional repolarization produced by the ischemic injury.

Just as not all ST segment elevations reflect ischemia, however, not all deep T wave inversions are abnormal. For example, T wave inversions may be seen normally in leads with a *negative QRS complex* (e.g., in lead $aV_R$). In adults, the T wave may be normally negative in lead $V_1$ and sometimes also in lead $V_2$. Furthermore, as mentioned in Chapter 4, some adults have a persistent *juvenile T wave inversion pattern*, with negative T waves in the right and middle chest leads (typically $V_1$ to $V_3$).

In addition, not all abnormal T wave inversions are caused by MI. T wave inversions in the right chest leads may be caused by right ventricular overload and in the left chest leads by

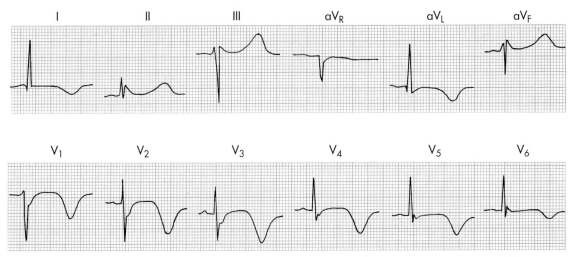

**FIGURE 9-11**    The ECG of a patient with acute subarachnoid hemorrhage shows giant T wave inversions. Heart rate was about 40/min. Subarachnoid hemorrhage may cause deeply inverted T waves, usually with markedly prolonged QT intervals, simulating the pattern seen in myocardial infarction. Bradycardia is often present. (From Goldberger AL: Myocardial Infarction: Electrocardiographic Differential Diagnosis, 4th ed, St. Louis, Mosby, 1991.)

left ventricular overload (Chapter 6). Diffusely inverted T waves are seen during the evolving phase of pericarditis.

Very deep, widely splayed T wave inversions (with a long QT interval and sometimes prominent U waves) have been described in some patients with cerebrovascular accident (CVA), particularly subarachnoid hemorrhage *(CVA T wave pattern)* (Fig. 9-11). The cause of these marked repolarization changes in some types of cerebrovascular injury is not certain, but they probably reflect changes in the autonomic nervous system.

As described in Chapter 7, secondary T wave inversions (resulting from abnormal depolarization) are seen in the right chest leads with right bundle branch block (RBBB) and in the left chest leads with LBBB. Deep T wave inversions also occur after electronic ventricular pacing ("postpacemaker" T wave pattern).

This list of noninfarctional factors that cause T wave inversions is by no means complete; however, it should convey the point that *T wave inversions are not always indicative of myocardial ischemia.* In some cases, deep diffuse *(global)* T wave inversions may occur without any identifiable cause.

A comprehensive "instant review" summary of the differential diagnosis of T wave inversions is given in Chapter 24.

## COMPLICATIONS OF MYOCARDIAL INFARCTION

The major complications of MI can be either mechanical/structural or electrical. The *mechanical* complications include heart failure, cardiogenic shock, left ventricular aneurysm, rupture of the heart, pericarditis, papillary muscle dysfunction, infarct extension and expansion, and embolism. The *electrical* complications include the arrhythmias and conduction disturbances that occur as a consequence of ischemia or infarction. MI can cause virtually any arrhythmia, including sustained ventricular tachycardia or ventricular fibrillation leading to cardiac arrest. (The general subject of arrhythmias is discussed in Part II.) The conduction disturbances include atrioventricular block (heart block) and intraventricular block (bundle branch block) (see Chapters 7 and 17).

## ECG AFTER CORONARY REPERFUSION

ECG recognition of acute MIs is important because such patients are generally candidates for emergency coronary reperfusion with catheterization/angioplasty-related procedures or with intravenous thrombolytic therapy. As noted in Chapter 8, thrombolytic therapy has only proved helpful in cases of ST elevation MI (STEMI). Current evidence suggests that acute angioplasty, when feasible, is even more efficacious in this setting and it may also be useful in selected patients with non–ST elevation MI.

Acute reperfusion therapies may alter the usual ECG evolution. Immediate successful reperfusion very early after an acute MI may be marked by the return of elevated ST segments toward the baseline, without new Q waves. Deep T wave inversions may evolve in leads that showed ST elevations. Q waves often appear even after successful reperfusion, however, although the intervention may lessen the amount of myocardium that is affected by the infarction. As a rule, the longer the time after the onset of ischemia or infarction, the less effect reperfusion has on acute or evolving ECG changes.

## THE ECG IN MYOCARDIAL INFARCTION: A CLINICAL PERSPECTIVE

One final note of caution should be emphasized: The ECG is a reasonably sensitive but hardly perfect indicator of acute MI. Most patients with an acute MI or severe ischemia show the ECG changes described in Chapter 8. The ECG may be relatively nondiagnostic or even normal, however, particularly during the early minutes or hours after an infarction. Furthermore, an LBBB or pacemaker pattern may completely mask the changes of an acute infarct.

*The ECG therefore must always be considered in clinical perspective, and the diagnosis of myocardial ischemia or infarction should not be dismissed simply because the ECG does not show the classic changes.*

In addition, as noted earlier, the traditional distinction between transmural and subendocardial (nontransmural) MIs on the basis of the ECG findings is an oversimplification and often invalid. In some patients, extensive infarction may occur without Q waves; in others, nontransmural injury may occur with Q waves. Furthermore, substantial evidence indicates that subendocardial infarction may have as ominous a long-term prognosis as transmural infarction. For these reasons, cardiologists have appropriately abandoned the terms *transmural* and *subendocardial* when describing a clinically diagnosed infarction and instead more appropriately use the more descriptive terms: *Q wave* and *non–Q wave MI.*

# REVIEW

Subendocardial ischemia generally produces ST segment depressions, which may appear only in the anterior leads (I, $aV_L$, and $V_1$ to $V_6$), only in the inferior leads (II, III, and $aV_F$), or diffusely in both groups of leads. (Lead $aV_R$ usually shows ST segment elevations.)

These ischemic ST segment depressions may be seen during attacks of typical *angina pectoris.* Similar ST segment depressions may develop during exercise (with or without chest pain) in patients with ischemic heart disease. The presence of ischemic heart disease may be determined by recording the ECG during exercise *(stress electrocardiography).* ST segment depression of 1 mm or more, lasting 0.08 second or more, is generally considered a *positive (abnormal)* response. *False-negative (normal)* results can occur, however, in patients with ischemic heart disease and *false-positive* results can occur in normal people.

Ischemic ST segment changes may also be detected during ambulatory ECG (Holter) monitoring. Analysis of these records has shown that many episodes of myocardial ischemia are not associated with angina pectoris *(silent ischemia).*

With *non–Q wave infarction,* the ECG may show persistent ST segment depressions or T wave inversions. Abnormal Q waves do not usually occur with subendocardial infarction limited to the inner half of the ventricular wall.

With *Prinzmetal's angina,* transient ST segment elevations suggestive of epicardial or transmural ischemia occur during attacks of angina. Patients with Prinzmetal's angina often have atypical chest pain that occurs at rest or at night. In contrast, patients with classic angina, typically have exertional pain that is associated with ST segment depressions. Prinzmetal's (variant) angina pattern is generally a marker of coronary artery spasm with or without underlying coronary obstruction.

The ST segment elevations of acute transmural MI can be simulated by the ST elevations of Prinzmetal's angina, the normal variant ST elevations seen in some healthy people *(early repolarization pattern),* the ST elevations of acute pericarditis (see Chapter 11), along with a number of other conditions summarized in Chapter 24.

The abnormal ST depressions of subendocardial ischemia may be simulated by the repolarization abnormalities of left ventricular hypertrophy, digitalis effect (see Chapter 10), or hypokalemia (see Chapter 10), as well as other conditions summarized in Chapter 24.

T wave inversions can be a sign of ischemia or infarction, but they may also occur in a variety of other settings (see Chapter 24), such as in normal variants, with ventricular hypertrophy or subarachnoid hemorrhage, after ventricular pacing, or as part of secondary ST-T changes from bundle branch block.

# QUESTIONS—CHAPTERS 8 AND 9

1. Answer these questions about the ECG shown below:

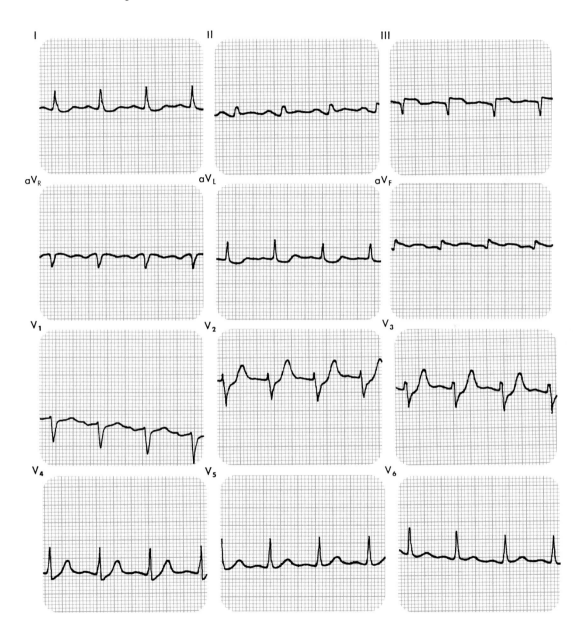

a. What is the approximate heart rate?
b. Are ST segment elevations present?
c. Are abnormal Q waves present?
d. What is the diagnosis?

2. Answer these questions about the ECG shown below:

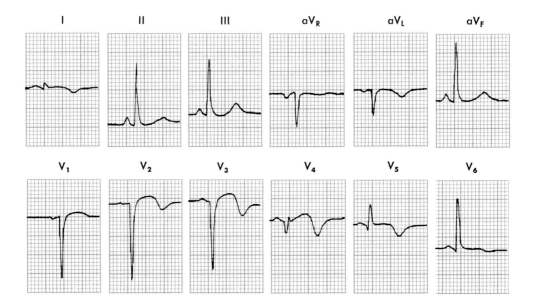

a. What is the approximate mean QRS axis?
b. Is the R wave progression in the chest leads normal?
c. Are the T waves normal?
d. What is the diagnosis?

3. With acute transmural *anterior wall* ischemia, the ST segments in leads II, III, and aV$_F$ are likely to be _____.

4. Persistent ST elevations several weeks or more after an infarction may be a sign of _____.

5. A patient with severe chest pain has prominent ST segment depressions in leads I, II, aV$_L$, aV$_F$, and V$_2$ to V$_5$, with abnormal elevations of cardiac enzymes. Which of the listed conditions is the most likely diagnosis?
a. Prinzmetal's angina
b. Non–Q wave infarction
c. Hyperacute phase of infarction
d. Angina pectoris

6. What ECG abnormality is shown below, and what symptoms might this patient be having?

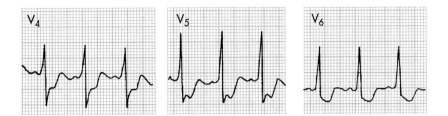

7. What conduction disturbance is present in the ECG below? What other major abnormality is present?

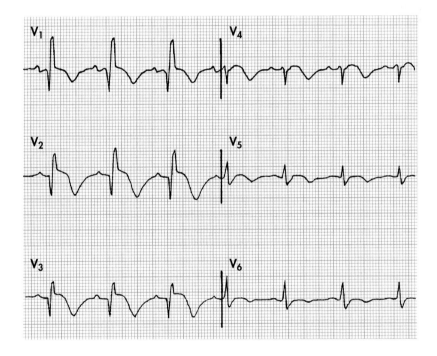

8. *True or false:* Thrombolytic therapy is equally effective for acute ST segment elevation MI and ST segment depression MI.

## CHAPTER 10

# Drug Effects, Electrolyte Abnormalities, and Metabolic Factors

The ECG is importantly affected by a number of factors, including drug effects, certain electrolyte abnormalities, and a variety of other metabolic conditions. Indeed, the ECG may be the major initial indicator of a life-threatening abnormality such as hyperkalemia or tricyclic antidepressant toxicity. This chapter introduces these topics and provides a brief review of nonspecific versus more specific ST-T changes.

## DRUG EFFECTS

### CARDIAC DRUGS

Numerous drugs can affect the ECG. Generally, the ECG changes are slight and nonspecific. Distinctive changes can be produced, however, by a number of commonly used classes of drugs, including digitalis glycosides, cardiac antiarrhythmic agents, and psychotropic agents.

Digitalis is used in the treatment of heart failure and certain arrhythmias. One of its effects is to shorten repolarization time in the ventricles. This shortens the QT interval and is associated with a characteristic scooping of the ST-T complex *(digitalis effect)*, as shown in Figures 10-1 and 10-2. Notice that when digitalis effect occurs, the ST segment and T wave are fused together and it is impossible to tell where one ends and the other begins. Digitalis effect can be seen in patients taking therapeutic or toxic doses of any digitalis preparation (e.g., digoxin). Digitalis effect must be distinguished from *digitalis toxicity*, which refers to arrhythmias, conduction disturbances, and systemic side effects produced by excessive amounts of digitalis (see Chapter 18).

Quinidine, procainamide, and disopyramide are antiarrhythmic drugs with similar properties. In contrast to digitalis, they prolong ventricular repolarization, due to blocking of a potassium channel. Therefore they may prolong the QT interval and flatten the T wave. In toxic doses, they may also prolong ventricular depolarization, leading to a widening of the QRS complexes. Occasionally, these agents produce prominent U waves resembling those seen with hypokalemia (discussed later in this chapter).

In selected cases, these drugs may actually cause sudden cardiac arrest due to the torsades de pointes type of ventricular tachycardia, as described in Chapter 16. This *proarrhythmic* effect is most likely to occur with prolonged QT intervals and/or prominent U waves (Fig. 10-3).

Prolongation of the QT(U) interval with a risk of torsades de pointes can occur with other cardiac antiarrhythmic drugs, notably ibutilide, dofetilide, sotalol, and amiodarone (Fig. 10-4). This effect is also related to blocking of potassium channel function with prolongation of myocardial cellular repolarization.

Other drugs used to treat cardiac arrhythmias can have important effects on the ECG. Drugs such as flecainide and propafenone, used to treat atrial fibrillation and other supraventricular tachycardias, may produce widening of the QRS complex (intraventricular conduction delay). This effect is due to blocking of sodium channels in the ventricular conduction system and myocardium.

### OTHER DRUGS

Psychotropic drugs (e.g., phenothiazines and tricyclic antidepressants) can markedly alter the ECG and, in toxic doses, can induce syncope or cardiac arrest due to a ventricular tachyarrhythmia or asystole. They may also prolong the QRS interval, causing a bundle branch block–like pattern, or they may lengthen repolarization (long QT-U intervals), predisposing patients to develop torsades de pointes. Figure 10-5 presents the typical ECG findings of tricyclic antidepressant overdose, in this case, in

### Digitalis Effect

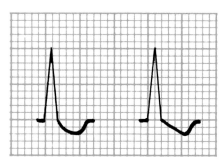

**FIGURE 10-1** Characteristic scooping of the ST-T complex produced by digitalis. (Not all patients taking digitalis exhibit these changes.)

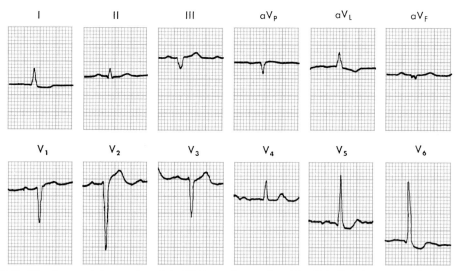

**FIGURE 10-2** The characteristic scooping of the ST-T complex produced by digitalis is best seen in leads $V_5$ and $V_6$. (Low voltage is also present, with total QRS amplitude of 5 mm or less in all six limb leads.)

## Quinidine Effects and Early Toxicity

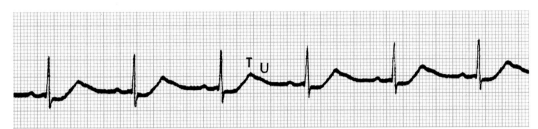

**FIGURE 10-3**   Lead V$_6$ from the ECG of a patient with a quinidine blood level of 2.9 μg/mL (therapeutic range). Notice the prolonged repolarization with prominent T-U waves, similar to the pattern of hypokalemia. Patients in whom quinidine and other drugs causes marked repolarization (QT) prolongation (often with large U waves) are at increased risk for polymorphic ventricular tachycardia (torsades de pointes, see Chapter 16). This patient did, in fact, subsequently develop torsades de pointes.

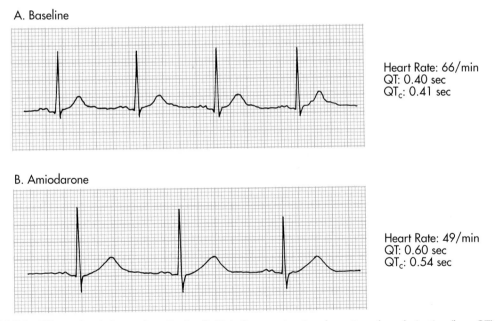

A. Baseline

Heart Rate: 66/min
QT: 0.40 sec
QT$_c$: 0.41 sec

B. Amiodarone

Heart Rate: 49/min
QT: 0.60 sec
QT$_c$: 0.54 sec

**FIGURE 10-4**   Effects of amiodarone (monitor lead). Note the prominent prolongation of repolarization (long QT) produced by a therapeutic dose of amiodarone in this patient as therapy for atrial fibrillation. The heart rate also slowed due to the beta-blocking effect of the drug.

## Tricyclic Antidepressant Overdose

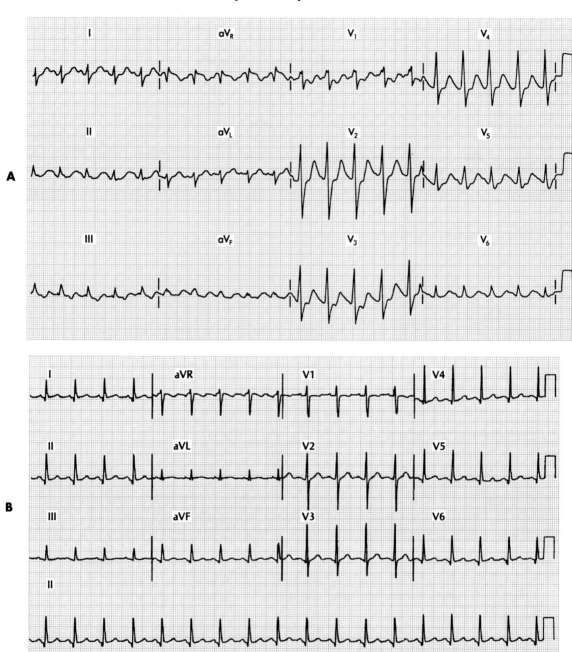

**FIGURE 10-5** **A,** This ECG from a patient with tricyclic antidepressant overdose shows three major findings: sinus tachycardia (from anticholinergic and adrenergic effects), prolongation of the QRS complex (from slowed ventricular conduction), and prolongation of the QT interval (from delayed repolarization). **B,** A repeat ECG obtained 4 days later shows persistent sinus tachycardia but normalization of the QRS complex and QT interval.

a young adult. Notice the prolonged QRS and QT intervals, as well as sinus tachycardia.

Lithium carbonate may cause nonspecific ST-T changes. Occasionally, especially in toxic doses, it may cause sinus node dysfunction and severe bradycardia.

A variety of noncardiac drugs can prolong the QT interval, predisposing the development of the torsades de pointes type of ventricular tachycardia. This topic is discussed further in Chapter 16 and is summarized in a review in Chapter 24.

## ELECTROLYTE DISTURBANCES

Abnormal serum concentrations of potassium and calcium can produce marked effects on the ECG. Hyperkalemia can, in fact, be lethal because of its cardiac toxicity.

### HYPERKALEMIA

As shown in Figure 10-6, progressive hyperkalemia produces a distinctive sequence of ECG changes affecting both depolarization (QRS complex) and repolarization (ST-T segments). The normal serum potassium concentration is between 3.5 and 5 mEq/L. The first change seen

with abnormal elevation of the serum potassium concentration is narrowing and peaking of the T waves. As Figure 10-6 demonstrates, the T waves with hyperkalemia have a characteristic "tented" or "pinched" shape, and they may become quite tall. With further elevation of the serum potassium concentration, the PR intervals become prolonged and the P waves are smaller and may disappear entirely. Continued elevations produce an intraventricular conduction delay, with widening of the QRS complexes (see Figs. 10-6 and 10-7). As the serum potassium concentration rises further, the QRS complexes continue to widen, leading eventually to a large undulating (sine-wave) pattern and asystole.

Because hyperkalemia can be fatal, recognition of the earliest signs of T wave peaking may prove lifesaving. Hyperkalemia can be seen in several clinical settings. The most common is kidney failure, in which the excretion of potassium is reduced.

### HYPOKALEMIA

Hypokalemia produces distinctive changes in the ST-T complex. The most common pattern seen is ST depressions with prominent U waves

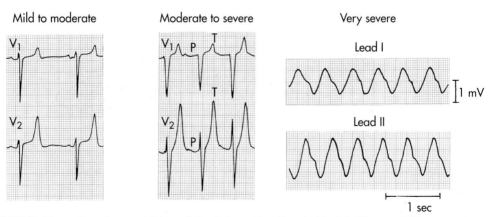

**FIGURE 10-6**   The earliest change with hyperkalemia is peaking ("tenting") of the T waves. With progressive increases in the serum potassium concentration, the QRS complexes widen, the P waves decrease in amplitude and may disappear, and finally a sine-wave pattern leads to asystole unless emergency therapy is given.

**Marked Hyperkalemia**

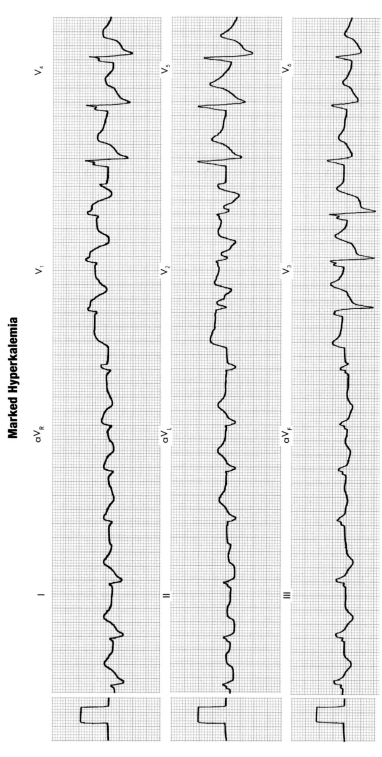

**FIGURE 10-7** ECG of a patient with a serum potassium concentration of 8.5 mEq/L. Notice the absence of P waves and the presence of bizarre wide QRS complexes.

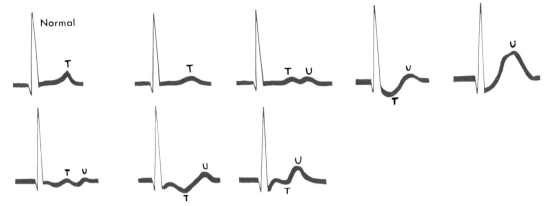

**FIGURE 10-8**   The ECG patterns that may be seen with hypokalemia range from slight T wave flattening to the appearance of prominent U waves, sometimes with ST depressions or T wave inversions. These patterns are not directly related to the specific level of serum potassium.

and prolonged repolarization* (Figs. 10-8 and 10-9). With hypokalemia, the U waves typically become enlarged and may even exceed the height of the T waves.

## HYPERCALCEMIA AND HYPOCALCEMIA

Ventricular repolarization is shortened by hypercalcemia and lengthened by hypocalcemia (Fig. 10-10). In hypercalcemia, the shortening of the QT interval is due to shortening of the ST segment. With marked hypercalcemia, the T wave appears to take off right from the end of the QRS complex. High serum calcium concentrations may lead to coma and death. A short QT interval in a patient with mental status changes is sometimes the first clue to the diagnosis of hypercalcemia. Hypocalcemia lengthens or prolongs the QT interval, usually by "stretching out" the ST segment. Note, however, that patients may have clinically significant hypocalcemia or hypercalcemia without diagnostic ECG changes.

---

*Technically the QT interval with hypokalemia may remain normal, whereas repolarization is prolonged (as shown by the prominent U waves). Because the T waves and U waves often merge, the QT intervals cannot always be accurately measured.

## OTHER METABOLIC FACTORS

### HYPOTHERMIA

Patients with systemic hypothermia may develop a distinctive ECG pattern in which a humplike elevation is usually localized to the junction of the end of the QRS complex and the beginning of the ST segment (J point) (Fig. 10-11). These pathologic J waves are sometimes called *Osborn waves*. This pattern disappears with rewarming. The basic mechanism of these prominent J waves appears to be related to the differential effects of systemic cooling on epicardial and endocardial repolarization in the ventricles.

### ENDOCRINE ABNORMALITIES

Most endocrine disorders do not produces specific changes on the ECG. In some instances, however, the ECG may play an important role in the diagnosis and management of hormonal abnormalities. For example, hyperthyroidism (most commonly due to Graves disease) is often associated with an inappropriately high resting sinus heart rate. The finding of a high sinus rate at rest should always lead to suspicion of hyperthyroidism, as should the finding of atrial fibrillation (see Chapter 15).

## Hypokalemia

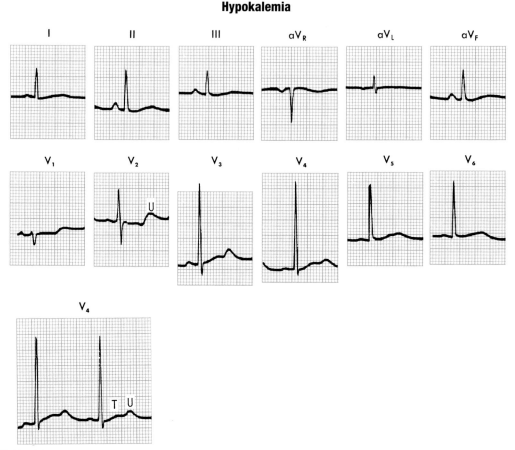

**FIGURE 10-9**   ECG leads from a patient with a markedly low serum potassium concentration of 2.2 mEq/L. Notice the prominent U waves, with flattened T waves.

In contrast, hypothyroidism is often associated with a slow resting heart (sinus bradycardia). Severe hypothyroidism (myxedema) may lead to pericardial effusion, thereby causing *low-voltage* QRS complexes. Low QRS voltage is said to be present when the total amplitude of the QRS complexes in each of the six limb leads is 5 mm or less, or 10 mm or less in the chest leads. Low QRS voltage is not a specific finding but can be related to a variety of mechanisms and causes (see Chapter 24). These include increased insulation of the heart by air (chronic obstructive pulmonary disease) or adipose tissue (obesity); replacement of myocardium, for example, by

fibrous tissue (in cardiomyopathy), amyloid, or tumor; or due to the abnormal accumulation of extracellular fluid (as with anasarca, or with pericardial or pleural effusions).

## ST-T CHANGES: SPECIFIC AND NONSPECIFIC

The concluding topic of this chapter is a brief review of the major factors that cause ST-T (repolarization) changes. The term *nonspecific ST-T change* (defined in Chapter 9) is commonly used in clinical electrocardiography. Many factors (e.g., drugs, ischemia, electrolyte

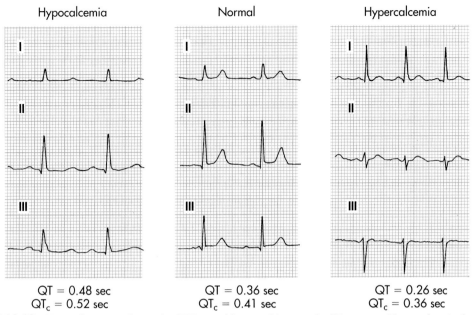

| Hypocalcemia | Normal | Hypercalcemia |
|---|---|---|
| QT = 0.48 sec | QT = 0.36 sec | QT = 0.26 sec |
| QT$_c$ = 0.52 sec | QT$_c$ = 0.41 sec | QT$_c$ = 0.36 sec |

**FIGURE 10-10** Hypocalcemia prolongs the QT interval by stretching out the ST segment. Hypercalcemia decreases the QT interval by shortening the ST segment so that the T wave seems to take off directly from the end of the QRS complex.

Systemic Hypothermia

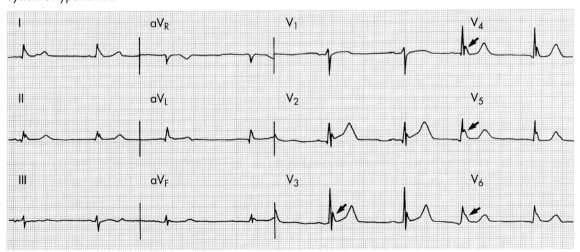

**FIGURE 10-11** Systemic hypothermia is associated with a distinctive bulging of the J point (the very beginning of the ST segment). The prominent J waves *(arrows)* with hypothermia are referred to as *Osborn waves.*

Normal T wave

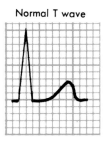

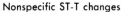

Nonspecific ST-T changes

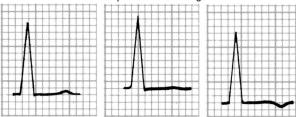

**FIGURE 10-12** Flattening of the T wave (*bottom left* and *middle*) and slight T wave inversion (*bottom right*) are abnormal but relatively nonspecific ECG changes that may be caused by numerous factors.

imbalances, infections, and pulmonary disease) can affect the ECG. As already mentioned, the repolarization phase (ST-T complex) is particularly sensitive to such effects and can show a variety of nonspecific changes as a result of multiple factors (Figs. 10-12 and 10-13). These changes include slight ST depressions, T wave flattening, and slight T wave inversions (see Fig. 10-12).

In contrast to these nonspecific ST-T changes, certain fairly specific changes are associated with particular conditions (e.g., the tall tented T waves of hyperkalemia). Some of these relatively specific ST-T changes are shown in Figure 10-14. Even such apparently specific changes can be misleading, however. For example, ST elevations are characteristic of acute transmural ischemia, but they are also seen in ventricular aneurysms, pericarditis, and benign (normal) early repolarization. Similarly, deep T wave inversions are most characteristic of ischemia but may occur in other conditions as well (see Chapters 9 and 24).

In summary, repolarization abnormalities can be grouped into two general categories. *Nonspecific* ST-T changes include slight ST segment deviation and flattening or inversion of the T wave. These changes are not diagnostic of any particular condition but must always be interpreted in clinical context. The relatively *specific* ST-T changes are more strongly but not always definitively diagnostic of some particular underlying cause (e.g., hyperkalemia or myocardial ischemia).

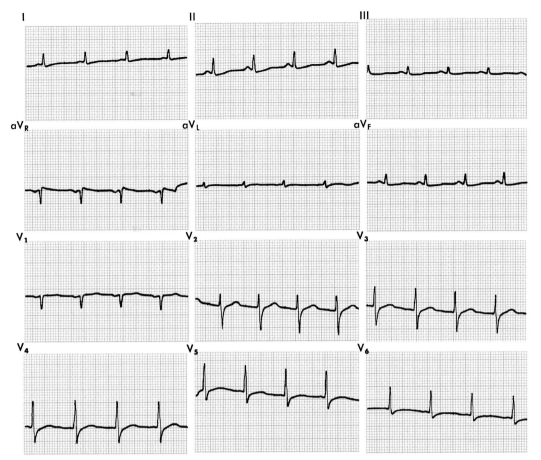

**FIGURE 10-13**  ECG showing nonspecific ST-T changes. Notice the diffuse T wave flattening.

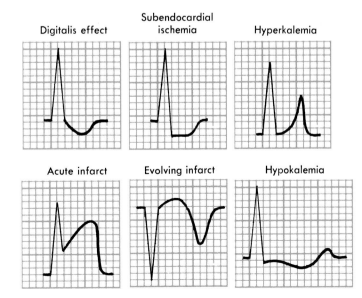

**FIGURE 10-14**  Examples of relatively specific ST-T changes. Note, however, that the changes are not absolutely specific for the abnormalities shown.

# REVIEW

The ECG can be influenced by numerous factors, including many *drugs. Digitalis effect* refers to the characteristic scooped-out depression of the ST segment produced by therapeutic doses of digitalis. (*Digitalis toxicity* refers to the arrhythmias and conduction disturbances produced by excessive doses of digitalis.) *Quinidine, procainamide, disopyramide, ibutilide, dofetilide, sotalol,* and certain *psychotropic drugs* can prolong the QT interval and may also induce a potentially lethal type of ventricular tachycardia called *torsades de pointes* (see Chapter 16). Patients likely to develop this complication usually show prominently prolonged QT intervals and/or large U waves. *Amiodarone* is an antiarrhythmic drug that typically prolongs the QT interval, even at therapeutic doses.

Electrolyte disturbances can also affect the ECG:

1. *Hyperkalemia* typically produces a sequence of changes. First the T wave narrows and peaks ("tents"). Further elevation of the serum potassium concentration leads to prolongation of the PR interval and then to loss of P waves and widening of the QRS complex, followed by a sine-wave pattern and asystole.

2. *Hypokalemia* may produce ST depressions and prominent U waves. The QT interval becomes prolonged. (In some cases, you are actually measuring the QU interval, and not the QT interval, because it may be impossible to tell where the T wave ends and the U wave begins.)

3. *Hypercalcemia* may shorten the QT interval, and *hypocalcemia* may prolong it.

With *systemic hypothermia,* the ECG shows a humplike elevation located at the junction (J point) of the end of the QRS complex and the beginning of the ST segment. The pattern disappears with rewarming.

# QUESTIONS

1. Which of the following factors can produce ST segment elevations?
   a. Hypokalemia
   b. Early repolarization pattern
   c. Digitalis effect
   d. Ventricular aneurysm
   e. Hypocalcemia
   f. Right bundle branch block
   g. Pericarditis

**2.** Match ECGs *A, B,* and *C* with the following causes:

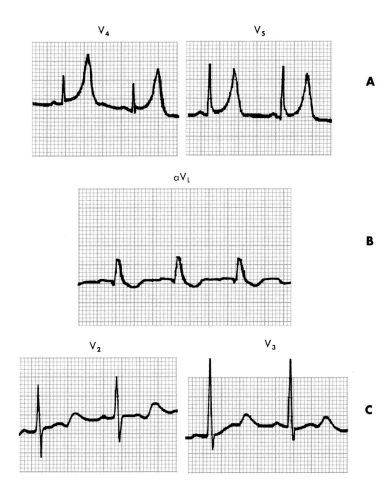

a. Digitalis effect
b. Hyperkalemia
c. Hypokalemia

**3.** Prominent U waves are characteristic of which one of the following:
a. Hyperkalemia
b. Hypokalemia
c. Hypercalcemia
d. Hypocalcemia
e. Digitalis effect

## CHAPTER 11

# Pericardial, Myocardial, and Pulmonary Syndromes

A wide variety of major disease processes may affect the ECG. Particularly important are conditions affecting the pericardium (pericarditis and pericardial effusion), the myocardium itself (not including ischemia and infarction, which are discussed in Chapters 8 and 9), and the lungs (acute pulmonary embolism and chronic obstructive pulmonary disease).

## PERICARDITIS AND PERICARDIAL EFFUSION

Pericarditis (inflammation of the pericardium) may be caused by a number of factors, including viral or bacterial infection, metastatic tumors, collagen vascular diseases, myocardial infarction (MI), cardiac surgery, and uremia.

As mentioned in Chapter 9, the ECG patterns of pericarditis resemble those seen with acute MI. The early phase of acute pericarditis is usually characterized by ST segment elevations. This type of current of injury pattern results from inflammation of the heart's surface (epicardium) that often accompanies pericardial inflammation. Figure 11-1 shows an example of the ST segment elevations with acute pericarditis. A major difference between these elevations and the ones occurring with acute MI is their distribution. The ST segment elevations with acute MI are characteristically limited to the anterior or inferior leads because of the localized area of the infarct. The pericardium envelops the heart, and the ST-T changes occurring with pericarditis are therefore usually more generalized. ST elevations are typically seen in both anterior and inferior leads. For example, in Figure 11-1, notice the elevations in leads I, II, $aV_L$, $aV_F$, and $V_2$ to $V_6$.

Not only does acute pericarditis affect ventricular repolarization (the ST segment), it also affects repolarization of the atria, which starts during the PR segment (the end of the P wave to the beginning of the QRS complex). In particular, pericardial inflammation often causes an atrial current of injury, reflected by elevation

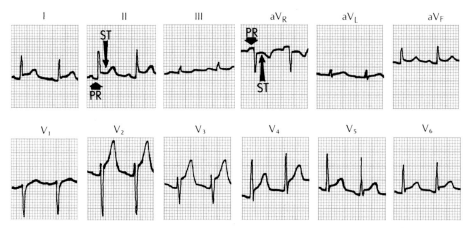

**FIGURE 11-1** Acute pericarditis causing diffuse ST segment elevations in leads I, II, aV$_F$, and V$_2$ to V$_6$, with reciprocal ST depressions in lead aV$_R$. By contrast, a concomitant atrial current of injury causes PR segment elevations in lead aV$_R$ with reciprocal PR depressions in the left chest leads and lead II. (From Goldberger AL: Myocardial Infarction: Electrocardiographic Differential Diagnosis, 4th ed. St. Louis, Mosby, 1991.)

of the PR in lead aV$_r$ and depression of the PR in other limb leads and the left chest leads (V$_5$ and V$_6$). Thus, with acute pericarditis, the PR and ST segments typically point in opposite directions, with the PR being elevated (often by only 1 mm, or so) in lead aV$_R$ and the ST usually being slightly depressed in that lead. Other leads may show PR depression and ST elevation.

Figure 11-1 illustrates the subtle but often helpful repolarization changes seen with acute pericarditis. The presence of PR changes may be a useful clue in the differential diagnosis of ST segment elevation, suggesting acute pericarditis as the cause.

The ST elevations seen with acute pericarditis are sometimes followed (after a variable time) by T wave inversions (Fig. 11-2). This sequence of elevations and inversions is the same as that described for MI. In some cases, the T wave inversions caused by pericarditis resolve completely with time and the ECG returns to normal. In other cases, the T wave inversions persist for long periods.

The similarity between the ECG patterns of acute pericarditis and acute MI has been emphasized because both conditions may produce ST segment elevations followed by T wave inversions. As noted, however, the ST-T changes with pericarditis tend to be more diffuse than the localized changes of MI. Another major difference is that pericarditis does not produce abnormal Q waves, such as those seen with certain infarcts. With MI, abnormal Q waves occur because of the death of heart muscle and the consequent loss of positive depolarization voltages (see Chapter 8). Pericarditis, on the other hand, generally causes only a superficial inflammation and does not produce actual myocardial necrosis. Thus abnormal Q waves never result from pericarditis alone.

*Pericardial effusion* refers to an abnormal accumulation of fluid in the pericardial sac. In most cases, this fluid accumulates as the result of pericarditis. In some cases, however, such as myxedema (hypothyroidism) or rupture of the heart, pericardial effusion may occur in the absence of pericarditis. The major clinical significance of pericardial effusion is the danger of cardiac tamponade, in which the fluid actually "chokes off" the heart, leading to a drop in

## Pericarditis: Evolving Pattern

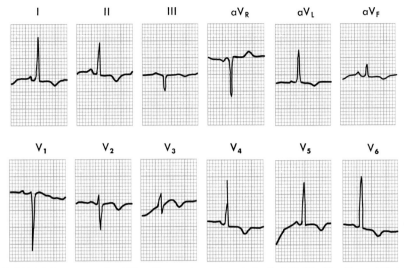

**FIGURE 11-2**  Notice the diffuse T wave inversions in leads I, II, III, aV$_L$, aV$_F$, and V$_2$ to V$_6$.

blood pressure and sometimes to cardiac arrest (see Chapter 19).

The most common ECG sign of pericardial effusion (with or without actual tamponade) is low voltage of the QRS complexes. In such cases, the low voltage is probably due to short-circuiting of cardiac voltages by the fluid surrounding the heart.

The criteria for high voltage were mentioned in the discussion of hypertrophy patterns (see Chapter 6). *Low voltage* is said to be present when the total amplitude of the QRS complexes in each of the six limb leads is 5 mm (0.5 mV) or less. (Low voltage in the limb leads may or may not be accompanied by low voltage in the chest leads, defined as a peak-to-peak QRS amplitude of 10 mm or less in each of leads V$_1$ to V$_6$.)

Figure 11-2 shows an example of low voltage. A listing of other factors that can produce low QRS voltage is presented in one of the review tables in Chapter 24.

For example, obesity can cause low voltage because of the fat tissue that lies between the heart and the chest wall. Patients with emphysema have increased inflation of the lungs. This extra air acts to insulate the heart. Of the causes of low voltage listed, obesity, anasarca (generalized edema), and emphysema are among the most common. When you see low voltage (particularly with sinus tachycardia), however, you always need to consider pericardial effusion because it can lead to fatal tamponade (see also Chapter 19).

*Electrical alternans* is another very important pattern that can occur with pericardial effusion and tamponade (Fig. 11-3). This pattern is characterized by a beat-to-beat shift in the QRS axis associated with mechanical swinging of the heart to and fro in a large accumulation of fluid. Electrical alternans with sinus tachycardia is virtually diagnostic of cardiac tamponade, although *not* every patient with tamponade shows this pattern.

## Electrical Alternans in Pericardial Tamponade

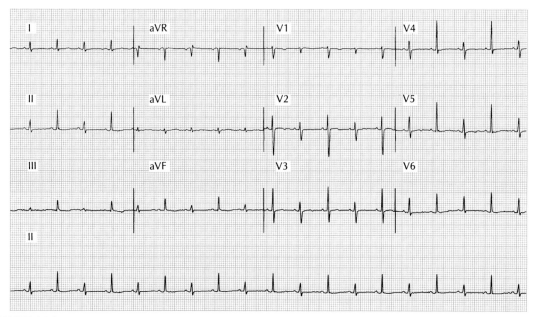

**FIGURE 11-3** Electrical alternans may develop in patients with pericardial effusion and cardiac tamponade. Notice the beat-to-beat alternation in the P-QRS-T axis; this is caused by the periodic swinging motion of the heart in a large pericardial effusion. Relatively low QRS voltage and sinus tachycardia are also present.

In summary, acute pericarditis causes a diffuse current of injury pattern with ST segment elevations in the anterior and inferior leads, sometimes followed by T wave inversions in those leads. Abnormal Q waves, however, are not seen with pericarditis alone. Pericardial effusion is one of the causes of low voltage on the ECG.

## MYOCARDITIS

A variety of conditions (e.g., certain viral infections) may be associated with inflammation of the heart muscle (myocarditis). Individuals with myocarditis may have a wide range of symptoms and presentations, ranging from those who are asymptomatic to those who have severe heart failure and even sudden death. In some cases, pericarditis and myocarditis occur together.

The ECG findings with myocarditis are also quite variable, ranging from nonspecific ST-T changes to the repolarization changes that occur with acute pericarditis. Occasionally, the ECG findings of severe myocarditis may exactly simulate those of acute MI, even with ST elevations initially and the development of pathologic Q waves. Atrial or ventricular arrhythmias can occur with myocarditis, as can atrioventricular (AV) or ventricular conduction disturbances.

## CONGESTIVE HEART FAILURE

Congestive heart failure (CHF) is a complex syndrome that can result from multiple causes, including extensive myocardial infarction, systemic hypertension, valvular heart disease, myocarditis, and cardiomyopathy The ECG may provide helpful clues to a specific diagnosis in some of these patients:

- Prominent Q waves and typical ST-T changes suggest underlying ischemic heart disease with extensive underlying infarction.

- Left ventricular hypertrophy patterns (see Chapter 6) may occur with hypertensive heart disease, aortic valve disease (stenosis or regurgitation), or mitral regurgitation.

- The combination of left atrial enlargement (or atrial fibrillation) and signs of right ventricular hypertrophy (RVH) strongly suggest mitral stenosis (see Fig. 23-1).

- Left bundle branch block (LBBB) (see Chapter 7) may occur with CHF caused by ischemic heart disease, valvular abnormalities, hypertension, or cardiomyopathy.

In some patients, marked enlargement and decreased function of the left (and often the right) ventricle occur without coronary artery disease, hypertension, or significant valvular lesions. In such cases, the term *dilated ("congestive") cardiomyopathy* is applied. Dilated car-

diomyopathy can be idiopathic, or it can be associated with chronic excessive alcohol ingestion (alcoholic cardiomyopathy), viral infection, hereditary factors, or a variety of other etiologies.

Patients with dilated cardiomyopathy from any cause may have a distinctive ECG pattern (the *ECG-CHF* triad), which is characterized by the following:

1. Relatively low voltages in the limb leads, such that the QRS in each of the six limb leads is 8 mm or less in amplitude

2. Relatively prominent QRS voltages in the chest leads, such that the sum of the S wave in either lead $V_1$ or lead $V_2$ plus the R wave in $V_5$ or $V_6$ is 35 mm or more

3. Very slow R wave progression defined by a QS- or rS-type complex in leads $V_1$ to $V_4$

When the ECG-CHF triad is present (Fig. 11-4), it strongly suggests underlying cardiomyopathy but does not indicate a specific etiology. The triad may occur not only with primary

**ECG-CHF Triad**

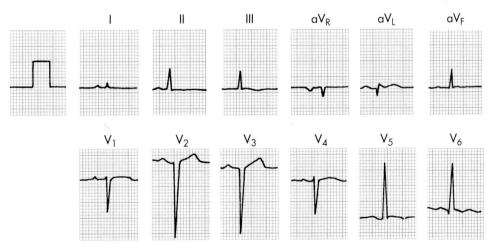

**FIGURE 11-4**  Severe idiopathic dilated cardiomyopathy in a 29-year-old man. The triad of (1) relatively low QRS voltages in the limb leads, (2) prominent precordial QRS voltages, and (3) very slow R wave progression in the chest leads (rS in V4) is highly suggestive of dilated cardiomyopathy. Poor precordial R wave progression simulates anterior wall infarction. (From Goldberger AL: Myocardial Infarction: Electrocardiographic Differential Diagnosis, 4th ed. St. Louis, Mosby, 1991.)

dilated cardiomyopathy but also with severe heart disease caused by previous infarction or significant valvular dysfunction. Furthermore, the ECG-CHF triad has only modest sensitivity; that is, its absence does not exclude underlying cardiomyopathy.

## PULMONARY EMBOLISM

The ECG is *not* a sensitive test for pulmonary embolism. In some cases, the obstruction produced by an embolus in the pulmonary artery system can lead to ECG changes, but generally no single pattern is always diagnostic. All of the following patterns may be seen (Fig. 11-5):

- Sinus tachycardia (Arrhythmias such as ventricular ectopy and atrial fibrillation also occur.)

- A right ventricular overload (formerly called "strain") pattern (inverted T waves in leads $V_1$ to $V_4$)

- The so-called $S_IQ_{III}T_{III}$ pattern, with an S wave in lead I and a new Q wave in lead III with T wave inversion in that lead (This pattern,

which may simulate that produced by acute inferior wall MI, is probably due to acute right ventricular dilation.)

- Shifting of the QRS axis to the right

- ST segment depressions indicative of subendocardial ischemia

- An incomplete or complete right bundle branch block (RBBB) pattern (wide rSR' in lead $V_1$)

The appearance of these changes, particularly in combination, is suggestive but not diagnostic of pulmonary embolism. Some patients with even massive pulmonary embolism have only minor, relatively nonspecific changes on their ECG. Thus both the diagnostic sensitivity and the specificity of the ECG with pulmonary embolism are limited. Figure 11-5 shows a classic example of the changes seen with pulmonary embolism. These findings may also be due to other causes of acute or subacute right ventricular overload (*cor pulmonale,* due, for example, to severe pneumonia or extensive pulmonary malignancy).

**Acute Pulmonary Embolism**

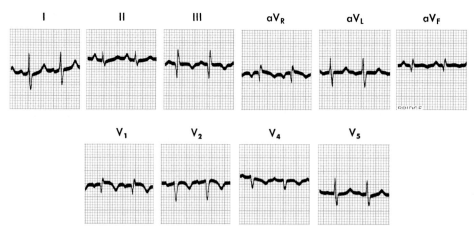

**FIGURE 11-5** Features occasionally seen with pulmonary embolism include sinus tachycardia, S waves in lead I with Q waves and T wave inversions in lead III ($S_IQ_{III}T_{III}$ pattern), and slow R wave progression with T wave inversions in chest leads $V_1$ to $V_4$ resulting from acute right ventricular overload.

## Chronic Lung Disease

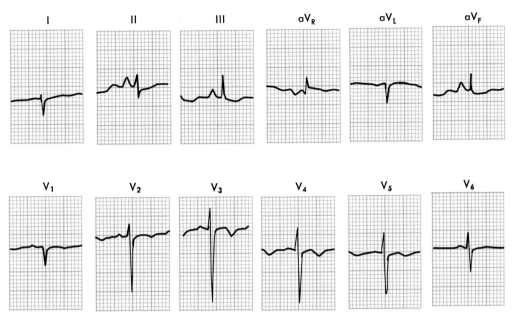

**FIGURE 11-6** Notice the characteristic combination of relatively low voltages in the limb leads, right axis deviation, right atrial overload pattern ("P pulmonale"), and slow R wave progression. The P wave axis is also more rightward than usual (almost +90°).

## CHRONIC LUNG DISEASE (EMPHYSEMA)

Patients with severe chronic obstructive lung disease from emphysema often have a relatively characteristic constellation of ECG findings (Fig. 11-6), including low QRS voltage, slow R wave progression in the chest leads, and a vertical or rightward QRS axis in the frontal plane. Excessive pulmonary air trapping causes the low voltage. The slow R wave progression results, in part, from the downward displace-ment of the diaphragm. Thus the chest leads are actually placed *relatively* higher than usual. In addition, right ventricular dilation may con-tribute to the delayed chest lead transition zone. Finally, the anatomically vertical position of the heart in the chest of a patient with emphysema (and sometimes right ventricular enlargement) causes the mean QRS axis to be vertical or even rightward (greater than +100°). Tall, relatively narrow P waves caused by right atrial overload (see Fig. 11-6) may also be present, with a ver-tical or rightward P wave axis (+90° or so).

# REVIEW

*Pericarditis* often produces diffuse ST segment elevations, usually in one or more of the chest leads and also in leads I, $aV_L$, II, and $aV_F$. PR segment elevation in lead $aV_r$ with PR depression in other leads may be caused by an atrial current of injury. Abnormal Q waves do not develop. After a variable period, the ST segment elevations may be followed by T wave inversions.

*Pericardial effusion* often produces *low voltage* of the QRS complex (amplitude of 5 mm or less in all six limb leads). Low voltage is not specific for pericardial effusion because it may also occur with obesity, emphysema, and diffuse myocardial injury or infiltration. In addition, low voltage may occur as a normal variant.

Pericardial effusion complicated by *cardiac tamponade* is usually associated with sinus tachycardia and low-voltage complexes. Some of these patients also have *electrical alternans,* a pattern characterized by a beat-to-beat shift in the QRS axis.

*Myocarditis* can produce ST-T changes that are nonspecific or that resemble the changes of pericarditis or myocardial infarction (MI). It may also be associated with serious atrial or ventricular arrhythmias.

The ECG may provide important clues to the etiology of *congestive heart failure,* including evidence of extensive myocardial infarction and ventricular hypertrophy. Patients with *dilated cardiomyopathy* from any cause may have a distinctive ECG pattern (the *ECG-CHF triad*):

1. Relatively low voltages in the limb leads, such that the QRS in each of the six limb leads is 8 mm or less in amplitude

2. Relatively prominent QRS voltages in the chest leads, such that the sum of the S wave in either lead $V_1$ or lead $V_2$ plus the R wave in $V_5$ or $V_6$ is 35 mm or more

3. Very slow R wave progression defined by a QS- or rS-type complex in leads $V_1$ to $V_4$

*Pulmonary embolism* may produce any of the following patterns:

1. Sinus tachycardia and various arrhythmias

2. Right ventricular strain T wave inversions

3. $S_I Q_{III} T_{III}$

4. Right axis shift

5. ST depressions resulting from subendocardial ischemia

6. Acute right bundle branch block

*Chronic obstructive lung disease* from emphysema often produces a relatively characteristic combination of ECG findings, including low QRS voltage, slow R wave progression in the chest leads, and a vertical or rightward QRS axis in the frontal plane. Peaked P waves (right atrial overload pattern) may also be present.

# QUESTIONS

1. Sinus tachycardia with electrical alternans is most indicative of which one of the following life-threatening conditions?
   a. Pericardial effusion with cardiac tamponade
   b. Acute myocardial infarction
   c. Acute pulmonary embolism
   d. Emphysema with respiratory failure
   e. Acute myocarditis

2. *True or false:* The ECG is a highly sensitive and specific test for acute pulmonary embolism.

## CHAPTER 12

# Wolff-Parkinson-White Preexcitation Patterns

T he Wolff-Parkinson-White (WPW) pre-excitation pattern is a distinctive and important ECG abnormality caused by *preexcitation* of the ventricles. Normally, the electrical stimulus passes to the ventricles from the atria via the atrioventricular (AV) junction. The physiologic lag of conduction through the AV junction results in the normal PR interval of 0.12 to 0.2 second. Consider the consequences of having an extra pathway between the atria and ventricles that would *bypass* or short-circuit the AV junction and *preexcite* the ventricles. This situation is exactly what occurs with the WPW pattern: an *atrioventricular bypass tract* connects the atria and ventricles, circumventing the AV junction (Fig. 12-1).

Bypass tracts (also called *accessory pathways*) represent persistent abnormal connections that form and fail to disappear during fetal development of the heart in certain individuals. These abnormal conduction pathways, composed of bands of heart muscle tissue, are located in the area around the mitral or tricuspid valves (AV rings) or interventricular

septum. An atrioventricular bypass tract is sometimes referred to as a bundle of Kent.

Preexcitation of the ventricles with the classic WPW pattern produces the following characteristic triad of findings on the ECG (Figs. 12-2 to 12-4):

1. The QRS is widened, giving the superficial appearance of a bundle branch block pattern. The wide QRS is caused, however, not by a delay in ventricular depolarization but by early stimulation of the ventricles. (The QRS is widened to the degree that the PR is shortened.)

2. The PR is shortened (often but not always to less than 0.12 second) because of the ventricular preexcitation.

3. The upstroke of the QRS complex is slurred or notched. This is called a *delta* wave.

The bypass tract initially activates the ventricular myocardium, rather than the faster-conducting specialized (His-Purkinje) system in the ventricles. This early myocardial con-

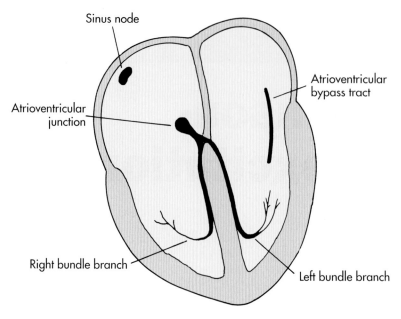

Sinus node

Atrioventricular bypass tract

Atrioventricular junction

Right bundle branch

Left bundle branch

**FIGURE 12-1** Anatomy of the ECG pattern of the Wolff-Parkinson-White (WPW) preexcitation pattern. In a small percentage of people, an accessory fiber (atrioventricular bypass tract) connects the atria and ventricles. (The consequences of this abnormal, extra conduction path are discussed in the text.)

duction imparts the distinctive notching or slurring (delta wave) to the very beginning of the QRS.

Figures 12-2 and 12-3 show the WPW pattern, with its classic triad of a widened QRS, a short PR interval, and a delta wave. Notice that the pattern superficially resembles a bundle branch block pattern because of the widened QRS complexes.

Bypass tracts can be located on the left lateral, posterior (septal or left ventricular),

### Wolff-Parkinson-White Preexcitation

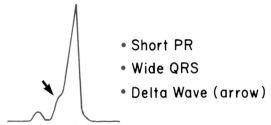

- **Short PR**
- **Wide QRS**
- **Delta Wave (arrow)**

**FIGURE 12-2** Preexcitation via the bypass tract in the Wolff-Parkinson-White (WPW) pattern is associated with a triad of findings.

right free wall, or anteroseptal regions of the ventricles. The most common locations are left lateral and posterior. Some patients have more than one bypass tract. Depending on which area of the ventricles (left or right side) is preexcited first, the ECG may show a pattern simulating that of either RBBB with tall R waves in the right chest leads or LBBB with a predominantly negative QRS in leads $V_1$ and $V_2$.

The 12-lead ECG with sinus rhythm may also provide important clues about the specific location of the bypass tract. With reasonable accuracy, you can often predict the insertion point of the bypass tract in the ventricles based on the polarity of the delta wave. *As a general rule: the initial QRS complex (delta wave) vector will point away from the area of the ventricles that is first to be stimulated by the bypass tract.*

If the bypass tract inserts into the lateral part of the left ventricle, the initial QRS vector will point from left to right. Thus the delta waves will be negative in leads I and/or aVL and positive in lead V1 (resembling a lateral wall MI pattern).

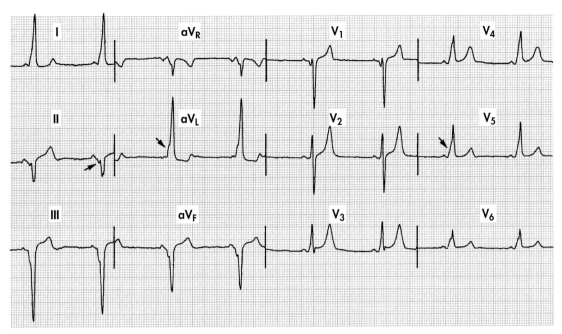

**FIGURE 12-3**   Notice the characteristic triad of the WPW pattern: wide QRS complexes, short PR intervals, and delta waves *(arrows)* that are negative in some leads (e.g., II, III, and aV$_R$) and positive in others (aV$_L$ and V$_2$ to V$_6$). The Q waves in leads II, III, and aV$_F$ are the result of abnormal ventricular conduction (negative delta waves) rather than an inferior myocardial infarction. This pattern is consistent with a bypass tract inserting into the posterior wall of the left ventricle.

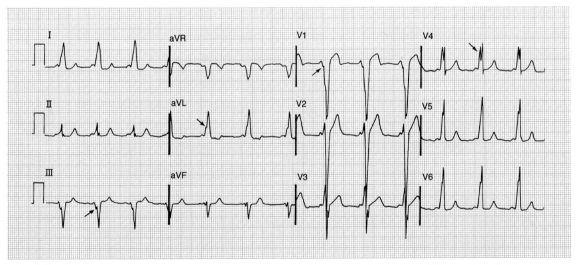

**FIGURE 12-4**   Another example of WPW with the triad of wide QRS complexes, short PR intervals, and delta waves *(arrows)*. The finding of delta waves that are predominantly negative in lead V$_1$ and positive in the lateral leads is consistent with a bypass tract inserting into the free wall of the right ventricle. This pattern simulates a left bundle branch block pattern.

If the bypass tract hooks into the posterior ventricular wall, the ECG usually shows positive delta waves in most of the precordial leads and negative delta waves in the inferior limb leads (resembling an inferior-posterior infarct; see Fig. 12-3).

With right free wall preexcitation, the QRS complexes are predominantly negative in V1 and V2 and the delta waves are typically positive in leads 1 and V6 (see Fig. 12-4).

Anteroseptal bypass tracts may be associated with negative delta waves in leads V1 and V2 (resembling an anteroseptal infarct).

## CLINICAL SIGNIFICANCE

Estimates of the frequency of this pattern in the general population vary widely, but the classic WPW appearance on ECG has been reported in roughly 1 to 2 per 1000 individuals. In some instances, familial occurrence is observed.

The significance of WPW preexcitation is twofold:

1. Individuals with this pattern are prone to arrhythmias, especially paroxysmal supraventricular tachycardia (PSVT) (see Fig. 12-4). Less commonly, they may also develop atrial fibrillation with a rapid ventricular rate. If the rate becomes extremely fast, atrial fibrillation may lead to ventricular fibrillation with sudden cardiac arrest. Fortunately, this occurrence is very rare. These important topics, introduced briefly in this chapter, are discussed further in Chapters 14 and 20. *Note on terminology:* Use the term *WPW syndrome* to apply to patients with the WPW pattern who also have arrhythmias related to the bypass tract.

2. The WPW pattern ECG is often mistaken for either a bundle branch block, due to the wide QRS, or for an MI, due to the negative delta waves simulating pathologic Q waves (see Fig. 12-3).

The WPW abnormality predisposes patients to PSVT because of the presence of the extra conduction pathway. For example, a premature impulse traveling down the AV junction may recycle up the accessory pathway and then back down the AV junction, and so on. This type of recirculating impulse is an example of *reentry.* The topic of reentry and PSVT is discussed further in Chapter 14.

When PSVT develops in a patient with the WPW preexcitation pattern, the QRS complex generally becomes narrow (Fig. 12-5). The widened QRS seen with WPW syndrome during normal sinus rhythm occurs because the stimulus travels concomitantly down the bypass tract and down the AV junction, resulting in a type of hybrid or *fusion* beat. When PSVT occurs, the impulse usually travels down the AV junction and back up the bypass tract in a retrograde fashion, resulting in a loss of the delta wave. (The delta wave and wide QRS will only be seen when an impulse travels down the bypass tract.)

Of note, some patients with bypass tracts do not show the classic WPW pattern during sinus rhythm but may develop reentrant types of PSVT. These patterns associated with a concealed bypass tract are described in Chapter 14.

Another type of preexcitation variant, the Lown-Ganong-Levine (LGL) syndrome, may be caused by a bypass tract that connects the atria and AV junction area. Bypassing the AV node results in a short PR interval (less than 0.12 second). The QRS width is not prolonged, however, because ventricular activation occurs normally. Therefore, the LGL pattern consists of a normal-width QRS complex with a short PR interval and no delta wave. In contrast, the WPW pattern consists of a wide QRS complex with a short PR interval and a delta wave (see Figs. 12-2 to 12-4).

Patients with the classic LGL syndrome also have intermittent reentrant-type PSVT or paroxysmal atrial fibrillation or flutter.

Most people with a short PR interval and normal QRS, however, do not actually have LGL preexcitation. For example, a relatively short PR interval may be seen as a normal

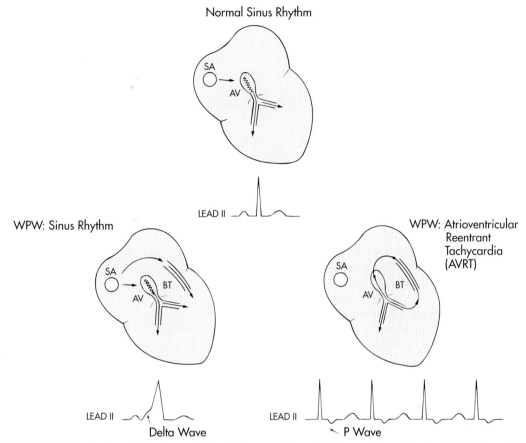

Normal Sinus Rhythm

WPW: Sinus Rhythm

WPW: Atrioventricular Reentrant Tachycardia (AVRT)

Delta Wave

P Wave

**FIGURE 12-5**  Conduction during sinus rhythm in the normal heart *(top)* spreads from the sinoatrial (SA) node to the atrioventricular (AV) node and then down the bundle branches. The *jagged line* indicates physiologic slowing of conduction in the AV node. With the WPW syndrome *(bottom left)*, an abnormal accessory conduction pathway called a bypass tract (BT) connects the atria and ventricles. With WPW, during sinus rhythm, the electrical impulse is conducted quickly down the bypass tract, preexciting the ventricles before the impulse arrives via the AV node. Consequently, the PR interval is short and the QRS complex is wide, with slurring at its onset (delta wave). WPW predisposes patients to develop an atrioventricular reentrant tachycardia (AVRT) *(bottom right)* in which a premature atrial beat may spread down the normal pathway to the ventricles, travel back up the bypass tract, and recirculate down the AV node again. This reentrant loop can repeat itself over and over, resulting in a tachycardia. Notice the normal QRS complex and often negative P wave in lead II during this type of bypass-tract tachycardia (see Chapter 14).

variant, without a bypass tract, because of accelerated AV conduction. Therefore, you should not "overread" an ECG on which the only noteworthy finding is a somewhat short PR interval, especially in an asymptomatic person. Such ECGs can be read as: "Short PR interval without evidence of preexcitation," or as: "Short PR interval, which may be seen as a physiologic variant (accelerated AV conduction pattern), although a preexcitation variant cannot be excluded."

Another relatively rare preexcitation variant is related to a slowly conducting bypass tract that typically connects the right atrium with the right bundle branch or right ventricle. These "atriofascicular" or "atrioventricular" fibers are sometimes referred to as Mahaim fibers. The 12-lead ECG in sinus rhythm may be normal or show a normal PR with a subtle delta wave. If PSVT develops, the impulse goes down the bypass tract, stimulates the right ventricle before the left and then reenters up the AV node. This sequence will produce a left bundle branch block pattern during the tachycardia.

## TREATMENT

Patients with WPW who have symptomatic tachycardias can usually be cured by a procedure during which the bypass tract is ablated using radiofrequency (RF) current. This highly successful treatment requires a cardiac electrophysiology (EP) procedure in which special catheters are inserted into the heart through peripheral veins and the bypass tract is located by means of ECG recordings (cardiac electrograms) made inside the heart. Patients who are not candidates for RF catheter ablation therapy can usually be treated with drug therapy.

Not all individuals with the WPW pattern have associated arrhythmias. Sometimes, the WPW pattern will be discovered in asymptomatic subjects who have an ECG ordered as part of a routine examination or for other indications. The major concern is the risk of the sudden onset of atrial fibrillation leading to ventricular fibrillation. Fortunately, the risk of sudden death from this mechanism is extremely low in completely asymptomatic subjects with the WPW pattern. Individuals in whom WPW is discovered as an incidental finding, therefore, usually do not require specific intervention. Disappearance of the WPW pattern during exercise (with the appearance of a normal QRS with sinus tachycardia) is particularly reassuring. Electrophysiologic evaluation and prophylactic ablation therapy in asymptomatic subjects is sometimes considered in special circumstances, for example, with competitive athletes, pilots, and those with a family history of sudden death.

## OVERVIEW: DIFFERENTIAL DIAGNOSIS OF WIDE QRS COMPLEX PATTERNS

Finding a wide QRS complex pattern is of importance because it is often indicative of an important abnormality with significant clinical implications. The major ECG patterns that produce a widened QRS complex can be divided into four major categories.

1. Bundle branch blocks (intrinsic conduction delays) including the classic RBBB and LBBB patterns

2. "Toxic" conduction delays caused by some extrinsic factor, such as hyperkalemia or drugs (e.g., quinidine, propafenone, flecainide, and other related antiarrhythmics, as well as phenothiazines and tricyclic antidepressants)

3. Beats arising in the ventricles, which may be ventricular escape beats or ventricular premature beats (Chapter 16), or electronic ventricular pacemaker beats (Chapters 7 and 21)

4. WPW-type preexcitation patterns

Differentiation among these possibilities is usually straightforward. The ECG effects of RBBB and LBBB have already been described in Chapter 7. Hyperkalemia produces widening of the QRS complex, often with loss of P waves (Chapter 10). Widening of the QRS complex in any patient who is taking an antiarrhythmic or a psychotropic agent should always suggest possible drug toxicity. Pacemakers generally produce an LBBB pattern with a pacemaker spike before each QRS complex. (An important exception is biventricular pacing used in the treatment of congestive heart failure in which an RBBB pattern is usually seen in conjunction with the left ventricular component of pacing; see Chapter 21.) The WPW pattern is recognized by the triad of a short PR interval, a wide QRS complex, and a delta wave, as discussed in this chapter.

# REVIEW

The Wolff-Parkinson-White (WPW) pattern is due to ventricular preexcitation from a bypass tract (accessory pathway) that connects the atria and ventricles, short-circuiting the AV node. As a result, the ECG shows a characteristic triad of findings consisting of (1) a short PR interval, (2) a wide QRS, and (3) slurring or notching of the initial part of the QRS, referred to as a delta wave.

Patients with the WPW pattern are particularly prone to attacks of reentrant-type paroxysmal supraventricular tachycardia (PSVT) that may cause palpitations, shortness of breath, or even syncope.

Less commonly, WPW may be associated with atrial fibrillation with a fast ventricular rate. If the rate becomes very rapid, atrial fibrillation may lead to ventricular fibrillation with sudden cardiac arrest.

The syndrome of symptomatic WPW is curable in most cases by radiofrequency catheter ablation of the accessory pathway during a cardiac electrophysiology procedure.

The differential diagnosis of ECG patterns with a wide QRS complex includes four major classes of abnormalities:

1. Right or left bundle branch block

2. "Toxic" conduction delays caused by hyperkalemia or certain drugs

3. Beats arising in the ventricles, such as ventricular premature beats or pacemaker beats

4. WPW preexcitation

# QUESTION

1. What caused the wide QRS complex in the ECG shown below?

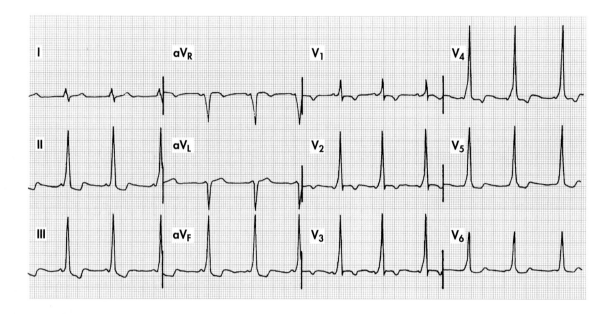

   a. Right bundle branch block
   b. Tricyclic antidepressant toxicity
   c. Posterolateral MI
   d. Wolff-Parkinson-White preexcitation pattern
   e. Hyperkalemia

# Cardiac Rhythm Disturbances

# TWO

# Sinus Rhythms

## NORMAL SINUS RHYTHM

Normal sinus rhythm is the reference physiologic rhythm of the heart. The diagnosis of normal sinus rhythm was described in Chapter 3. When the sinus (or sinoatrial [SA]) node is pacing the heart, atrial depolarization spreads from right to left and downward toward the atrioventricular (AV) junction. An arrow representing this depolarization wave points downward and toward the left. Therefore, with normal sinus rhythm, the P wave is negative in lead $aV_R$ and positive in lead II (Figs. 13-1 to 13-4; see also Fig. 4-3).

By convention, *normal sinus rhythm* is usually defined as sinus rhythm with a heart rate between 60 and 100 beats/min. Sinus rhythm with a heart rate of less than 60 beats/min is called *sinus bradycardia*.* Sinus rhythm with a heart rate greater than 100 beats/min is termed *sinus tachycardia*.

## REGULATION OF THE HEART RATE

The heart, like the other organs of the body, has a special nerve supply from the *autonomic nervous system*, which controls involuntary muscle action. The autonomic nerve supply to the heart (the SA and AV nodes in particular) consists of two opposing groups of fibers: the

---

*Some authors define sinus bradycardia based on a heart rate of less than 50 beats/min.

*sympathetic nerves* and the *parasympathetic nerves*. Sympathetic stimulation produces an increased heart rate and also increases the strength of myocardial contraction. Parasympathetic stimulation (from the vagus nerve) produces a slowing of the heart rate as well as a slowing of conduction through the AV nodal area. In this way, the autonomic nervous system exerts a counterbalancing control of the heart rate.

The sympathetic nervous system acts as a cardiac accelerator, whereas the parasympathetic (vagal) system produces a braking effect. For example, when you become excited or upset, increased sympathetic stimuli (and diminished parasympathetic tone) result in an increased heart rate and increased contractility, producing the familiar sensation of a pounding heart (palpitations). Palpitations may be associated with a normal heartbeat, isolated premature beats (atrial or ventricular), or an actual run of ectopic (nonsinus) heartbeats (e.g., from atrial fibrillation, paroxysmal supraventricular tachycardia, or ventricular tachycardia).

## SINUS TACHYCARDIA

*Sinus tachycardia* is simply sinus rhythm with a heart rate exceeding 100 beats/min. In adults, the heart rate with sinus tachycardia is generally between 100 and 180 beats/min. Somewhat faster rates, up to 200 beats/min or so, can be observed in healthy young adults during maximal exercise.

## Normal Sinus Rhythm

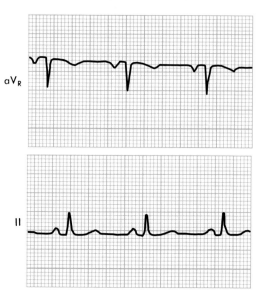

**FIGURE 13-1** Each QRS complex is preceded by a P wave that is negative in lead aV$_R$ and positive in lead II.

Aging decreases the capacity to generate very rapid sinus rates. Elderly individuals (more than 70 years) rarely show sinus tachycardia at rates above 140 to 150 beats/min. Indeed, heart rates above this range in the elderly usually indicate the presence of a nonsinus tachycardia (e.g., atrial fibrillation or flutter, or a paroxysmal supraventricular tachycardia).

Figure 13-2 shows an example of sinus tachycardia. Each QRS complex is preceded by a P wave. Notice that the P waves are positive in lead II. With sinus tachycardia at very fast rates, the P wave may merge with the preceding T wave and become difficult to distinguish.

In general, sinus tachycardia occurs with any condition that produces an *increase* in sympathetic tone or a *decrease* in vagal tone. The following conditions are commonly associated with sinus tachycardia:

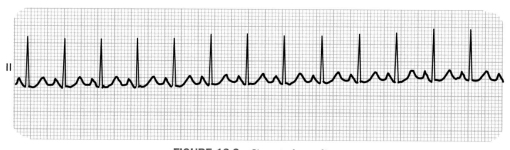

**FIGURE 13-2** Sinus tachycardia.

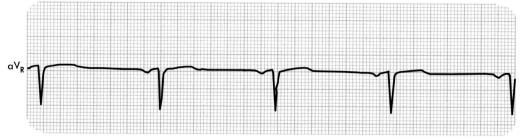

**FIGURE 13-3** Sinus bradycardia. Notice the negative P waves, because this is lead aV$_R$.

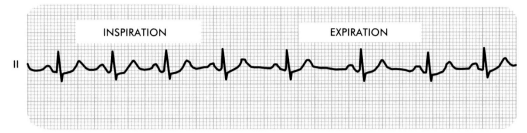

**FIGURE 13-4** Respiratory sinus arrhythmia. Normally, the heart rate increases slightly with inspiration and decreases slightly with expiration.

- Anxiety, excitement, exertion, and pain

- Drugs that increase sympathetic tone (e.g., epinephrine, dopamine, tricyclic antidepressants, isoproterenol, and cocaine)

- Drugs that block vagal tone (e.g., atropine and other anticholinergic agents)

- Fever, many infections, and septic shock

- Congestive heart failure (CHF) (Sinus tachycardia caused by increased sympathetic tone is generally seen with pulmonary edema.)

- Pulmonary embolism (As noted in Chapter 11, sinus tachycardia is the most common arrhythmia seen with acute pulmonary embolism.)

- Acute myocardial infarction (MI), which may produce virtually any arrhythmia (Sinus tachycardia persisting after an acute MI is generally a bad prognostic sign and implies extensive heart damage.)

- Hyperthyroidism (Sinus tachycardia occurring at rest may be an important diagnostic clue.)

- Pheochromocytoma

- Intravascular volume loss because of bleeding, vomiting, diarrhea, acute pancreatitis, dehydration, and related conditions

- Alcohol intoxication or withdrawal

Treatment of sinus tachycardia associated with a pathologic condition must be directed at the underlying cause (e.g., infection, hyperthyroidism, CHF, or alcohol withdrawal).*

## SINUS BRADYCARDIA

With sinus bradycardia, sinus rhythm is present and the heart rate is less than 60 beats/min (Fig. 13-3). This arrhythmia commonly occurs in the following conditions:

- Normal variant (Many people have a resting pulse rate of less than 60 beats/min, and trained athletes may have a resting or sleeping pulse rate as low as 35 beats/min.)

- Drugs that increase vagal tone (e.g., digitalis or edrophonium) or that decrease sympathetic tone (e.g., beta blockers) (In addition, calcium channel blockers such as diltiazem and verapamil may cause marked sinus bradycardia.)

- Hypothyroidism

- Hyperkalemia

---

*A small subset of patients who complain of palpitations (typically young adults) is found to have *inappropriate sinus tachycardia*. The causes of this syndrome are not certain. In some cases, autonomic factors may play a role; in others, a reentrant tachycardia originating in or very near the SA node is discovered.

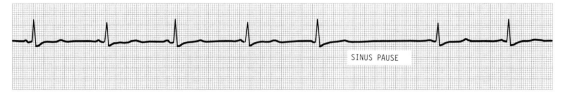

**FIGURE 13-5** Sinus pause in a patient with sick sinus syndrome. The monitor lead shows sinus bradycardia with a long pause (about 2.4 sec).

- Sick sinus syndrome (Some patients, particularly elderly ones, have marked sinus bradycardia without obvious cause, probably from degenerative disease of the SA node or surrounding tissue. Sick sinus syndrome is discussed further at the end of this chapter and in Chapter 20; see also Fig. 13-5.)

- Sleep apnea syndromes

- Carotid sinus hypersensitivity syndrome

- Vasovagal reactions

Moderate sinus bradycardia usually produces no symptoms. If the heart rate is very slow (especially if it is less than 40 to 50 beats/min), light-headedness and even syncope may occur. Treatment may require adjusting medication doses (e.g., beta blockers, calcium channel blockers). If inappropriate sinus bradycardia causes symptoms (as in sick sinus syndrome), or if severe sinus bradycardia is due to an essential medication, an electronic pacemaker is indicated (see Chapter 21).

## SINUS ARRHYTHMIA

In healthy people, especially younger subjects, the SA node does not pace the heart at a perfectly regular rate. Instead, a slight beat-to-beat variation is present (Fig. 13-4). When this variability is more accentuated, the term *sinus arrhythmia* is used.

The most common cause of sinus arrhythmia is respiration. *Respiratory sinus arrhythmia* (RSA) is a normal finding and may be quite marked (up to 10 to 20 beats/min or more), particularly in children and young adults. The heart rate normally increases with inspiration and decreases with expiration because of changes in vagal tone that occur during the different phases of respiration (see Fig. 13-4).

## SINUS PAUSES, SINUS ARREST, AND ESCAPE BEATS

Normal sinus rhythm, sinus tachycardia, sinus bradycardia, and sinus arrhythmia have been considered. Now suppose that the sinus node fails to stimulate the atria for one or more beats. Such dysfunction may occur intermittently, with simply a missed beat (no P wave or QRS complex) at occasional intervals, or it may be more extreme.* An example of the latter is *sinus pause* or *sinus arrest*, in which the SA node fails to stimulate the atria for a prolonged period (Fig. 13-5). This leads to syncope or even cardiac arrest with asystole unless the sinus node regains function or some other pacemaker (escape pacemaker) takes over. Fortunately, other parts of the cardiac conduction system are capable of producing electrical stimuli and functioning as an escape pacemaker in these circumstances. *Escape beats* may come from the atria, the AV node, or the ventricles. Figure

---

*The two distinct mechanisms for sinus node dysfunction are sinus pacemaker failure and SA block. The former is due to actual failure of the SA node to fire electrically (depolarize) for one or more beats. The latter results when the SA node fires but the impulse is apparently blocked from exiting the node and stimulating the atria. From a clinical viewpoint, distinguishing between SA pacemaker dysfunction and SA (exit) block is not usually essential.

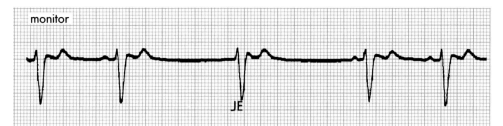

**FIGURE 13-6**  The monitor strip shows a sinus pause interrupted by a junctional escape (JE) beat. The wide QRS complex is due to an underlying bundle branch block.

13-6 shows a junctional escape beat. (The characteristics of escape beats are described in Chapter 14.)

SA block or arrest can be caused by numerous *acute* factors, including the following:

- Hypoxemia

- Myocardial ischemia or infarction

- Hyperkalemia

- Digitalis toxicity

- Toxic responses to drugs such as beta blockers and calcium channel blockers (e.g., diltiazem and verapamil)

- Vagal hyperreactivity (e.g., severe vasovagal episode)

Particularly in elderly persons, the SA node may undergo *chronic* degenerative changes, with periods of SA dysfunction and bradycardia leading at times to light-headedness and syncope. The term *sick sinus syndrome* refers to this type of irreversible SA node dysfunction (see Figs. 13-5 and 20-13).

The next few chapters describe important arrhythmias in which the cardiac pacemaker is located *outside* the SA node—in the atria, AV junction, or ventricles.

# REVIEW

With *normal sinus rhythm,* each heartbeat originates in the sinus (or sinoatrial [SA]) node. The P wave is always negative in lead $aV_R$ and positive in lead II. The heart rate is between 60 and 100 beats/min.

The heart rate is greater than 100 beats/min with *sinus tachycardia* and is less than 60 beats/min with *sinus bradycardia.* Sinus bradycardia and sinus tachycardia have multiple causes, and both rhythms may occur normally.

Beat-to-beat variation of the sinus rate occurs with *sinus arrhythmia.* The rate variation is typically phasic with respiration *(respiratory sinus arrhythmia).* SA node dysfunction (because of either pacemaker cell failure or exit block) may lead to sinus pauses or, in extreme cases, SA *arrest.* Prolonged sinus arrest causes fatal asystole unless normal sinus rhythm resumes or *escape beats* from other foci in the atria, AV junction, or ventricles take over. SA dysfunction may be seen, particularly in elderly people, as a consequence of *sick sinus syndrome.* Digitalis toxicity or toxic responses to other drugs (e.g., beta blockers, calcium channel blockers, amiodarone) must always be excluded in patients with marked sinus bradycardia, SA pauses, or sinus arrest.

# QUESTIONS

1. Is normal sinus rhythm present in the ECG shown below?

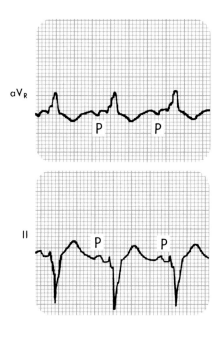

2. Is normal sinus rhythm present in this ECG?

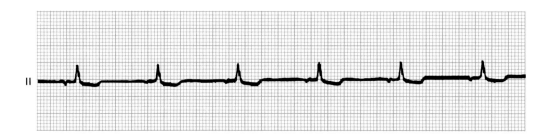

3. Which one of the following drugs is not a cause of sinus bradycardia?
   a. amiodarone
   b. metoprolol
   c. verapamil
   d. isoproterenol
   e. edrophonium

4. *True or false:* Respiratory sinus arrhythmia is a normal, expected finding in healthy young adults.

## CHAPTER 14

# Supraventricular Arrhythmias  Section I

Premature atrial and AV junctional beats, paroxysmal supraventricular tachycardias, and AV junctional rhythms

The sinus node, or sinoatrial (SA) node, is the physiologic, intrinsic pacemaker of the heart and normally initiates each heartbeat. Pacemaker stimuli can, however, arise from other parts of the heart, such as the atria muscle, the atrioventricular (AV) junction, or the ventricles. The terms *ectopy, ectopic pacemaker,* and *ectopic beat* are used to describe these nonsinus heartbeats.

Ectopic beats are often premature; that is, they come before the next sinus beat is due. Thus *atrial premature beats* (APBs), *AV junctional premature beats* (JPBs), and *ventricular premature beats* (VPBs) may occur. Ectopic beats can also come after a pause in the normal rhythm, as in the case of AV junctional or ventricular *escape* beats. Ectopic beats originating in the AV junction (node) or atria are referred to as *supraventricular* (i.e., coming from *above* the ventricles).

In this chapter and the next, ectopic atrial and AV junctional (supraventricular) rhythms are described. Chapter 16 discusses ventricular ectopy.

## ATRIAL AND AV JUNCTIONAL (NODAL) PREMATURE BEATS

APBs* result from ectopic stimuli; that is, these beats arise from somewhere in either the left or right atrium but not in the SA node. The atria therefore are depolarized from an ectopic site. After an atrial or junctional depolarization, the stimulus may spread normally through the His-Purkinje system into the ventricles. For this reason, ventricular depolarization (QRS complex) is generally not affected by APBs or JPBs.

APBs have the following major features (Figs. 14-1 to 14-3):

---

*The terms *atrial premature contractions, atrial premature beats, atrial premature depolarizations,* and *atrial extrasystoles* are used synonymously. Most cardiologists prefer the designations *premature beat, depolarization,* and *complex* because not every premature stimulus is associated with an actual mechanical contraction of the atria or ventricles.

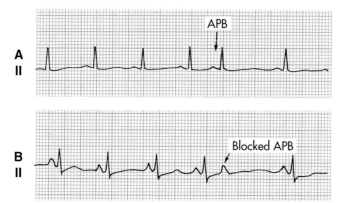

**FIGURE 14-1** **A,** Notice the atrial premature beat (APB) after the fourth sinus beat *(arrow).* **B,** Notice also the blocked atrial premature beat, again after the fourth sinus beat *(arrow).* The premature P wave falls on the T wave of the preceding beat and is not followed by a QRS complex because the atrioventricular node is still in a refractory state.

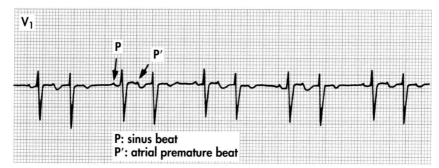

**FIGURE 14-2** Atrial bigeminy in which each sinus beat is followed by an atrial premature beat (or premature atrial complex).

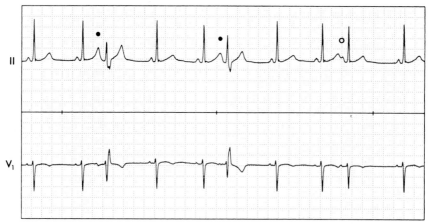

**FIGURE 14-3** This rhythm strip shows sinus rhythm with three atrial premature beats. The first two (marked •) are conducted with right bundle branch block aberrancy (rSR′ in lead V₁). The third atrial premature beat (○) is conducted with normal ventricular activation. Notice how the first two premature P waves come so early in the cardiac cycle that they fall on the T waves of the preceding sinus beats, making these T waves slightly taller.

1. The atrial depolarization is premature, occurring before the next normal P wave is due.

2. The QRS complex of the APB is often preceded by a visible P wave that usually has a slightly different shape and/or different PR interval from the P wave seen with normal sinus beats. The PR interval of the APB may be either longer or shorter than the PR interval of the normal beats. In some cases, the P wave may be "buried" in the T wave of the preceding beat.

3. After the APB, a slight pause generally occurs before the normal sinus beat resumes. This usually slight delay is due to "resetting" of the SA node pacemaker by the premature atrial stimulus. This slight delay contrasts with the longer, "compensatory" pause often (but not always) seen after VPBs (Fig. 16-7).

4. The QRS complex of the APB is usually identical or very similar to the QRS complex of the preceding beats. Remember that with APBs the atrial pacemaker is in an ectopic location, but the ventricles are usually depolarized in a normal way. This finding contrasts with VPBs, in which the QRS complex is usually very wide because of abnormal depolarization of the ventricles (see Chapter 16).

5. Occasionally, APBs result in *aberrant ventricular conduction,* so that the QRS complex is wider than normal. Figure 14-3 shows an example of such beats causing delayed depolarization of the right ventricle. Thus these APBs are associated with right bundle branch block *aberrancy.* APBs with left bundle branch block aberrancy may also occur.

6. Sometimes when an APB is very premature, the stimulus reaches the AV junction just after it has been stimulated by the preceding normal beat. Because the AV junction, like all other conductive tissues, requires time to

recover its capacity to conduct impulses, this premature atrial stimulus may reach the junction when it is still *refractory*. In this situation the APB may not be conducted to the ventricles and no QRS complex appears. The result is a *blocked* APB. The ECG shows a premature P wave *not* followed by a QRS complex (see Fig. 14-1B). After the blocked P wave, a brief pause occurs before the next normal beat resumes. The blocked APB therefore produces a slight irregularity of the heartbeat. (If you do not search carefully for these blocked APBs, you may overlook them.)

The APBs may occur frequently (e.g., five or more times per minute) or sporadically. Two APBs occurring consecutively are referred to as an *atrial couplet.* Sometimes, as shown in Figure 14-2, each sinus beat is followed by an APB. This pattern is referred to as *atrial bigeminy.*

## CLINICAL SIGNIFICANCE

APBs are very common. They may occur with a normal heart or virtually any type of organic heart disease. Thus the presence of APBs does not imply that an individual has cardiac disease. In normal people, these premature beats may be seen with emotional stress, excessive intake of caffeine, or the administration of sympathomimetic agents (epinephrine, isoproterenol, theophylline). APBs may also occur with hyperthyroidism. APBs may produce palpitations; in this situation, patients may complain of feeling a skipped beat or an irregular pulse. APBs may also be seen with various types of structural heart disease. Frequent APBs are sometimes the forerunner of atrial fibrillation or flutter (see Chapter 15) or other atrial tachyarrhythmias.

## PAROXYSMAL SUPRAVENTRICULAR TACHYCARDIAS (PSVTs)

Premature supraventricular beats may occur singly or repetitively. A sudden run of three or

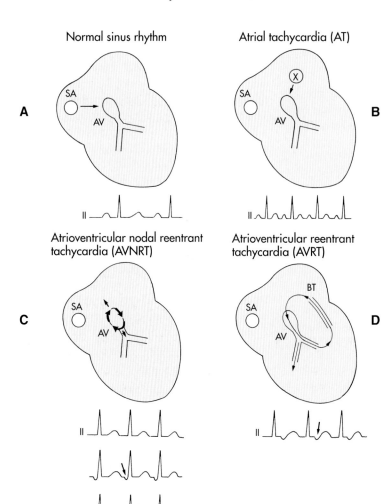

Normal sinus rhythm

**A**

Atrial tachycardia (AT)

**B**

Atrioventricular nodal reentrant tachycardia (AVNRT)

**C**

Atrioventricular reentrant tachycardia (AVRT)

**D**

**FIGURE 14-4**   Major types of paroxysmal supraventricular tachycardia. **A,** The reference is normal sinus rhythm. **B,** With atrial tachycardia (AT), a focus *(X)* outside the sinoatrial (SA) node fires off automatically at a rapid rate. **C,** With atrioventricular (AV) nodal reentrant tachycardia (AVNRT), the cardiac stimulus originates as a wave of excitation that spins around the AV nodal (junctional) area. As a result, retrograde P waves may be buried in the QRS or appear immediately before or just after the QRS complex *(arrows)* because of nearly simultaneous activation of the atria and ventricles. **D,** A similar type of reentrant (circus-movement) mechanism may occur with a bypass tract (BT) of the type found in Wolff-Parkinson-White syndrome (see Fig. 12-5). This mechanism is referred to as *atrioventricular reentrant tachycardia* (AVRT). Note the negative P wave *(arrow)* in lead II, somewhat after the QRS complex. (With AVRT, the P wave in lead II may be negative or isoelectric.)

more beats constitutes a paroxysmal supraventricular tachycardia (PSVT). Episodes of PSVT may be brief and nonsustained (i.e., lasting from three beats up to 30 sec). Sustained episodes (longer than 30 sec) may last minutes, hours, or longer. The topic of PSVTs is actually quite complex. Therefore the following brief discussion is intended to provide only an introduction and overview.*

*See the Bibliography for texts that describe this important area of cardiology in more detail.

The three major types of PSVT are *atrial tachycardia* (AT) and related rhythms, *atrioventricular nodal reentrant tachycardia* (AVNRT), and *AV reentrant tachycardia* (AVRT) involving a bypass tract of the type seen in the Wolff-Parkinson-White (WPW) syndrome (see Chapter 12). These arrhythmias are depicted schematically in Figure 14-4.

## ATRIAL TACHYCARDIA

Atrial tachycardia (AT) is defined simply as three or more consecutive APBs (Figs. 14-4*B* and

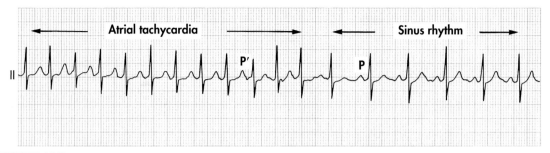

**FIGURE 14-5** Atrial tachycardia (a type of paroxysmal supraventricular tachycardia) terminating spontaneously with the abrupt resumption of sinus rhythm. The P waves of the tachycardia (rate: about 150 beats/min) are superimposed on the preceding T waves.

14-5). Most episodes appear to involve an ectopic (nonsinus) pacemaker located in either the left or right atrium that fires off "automatically" in a rapid way. A sustained episode that lasts 30 seconds or longer, particularly at a rapid rate, may cause light-headedness or even syncope (fainting) and, in susceptible individuals, can induce angina or congestive heart failure (CHF). The atrial rate with AT may be as high as 200 beats per minute or faster (usual range: 100 to 250 beats/min). AT has been observed in patients without apparent structural cardiac abnormality as well as in those with virtually any type of heart disease.* Short episodes may require no special therapy, but longer runs causing symptoms are usually treated with antiarrhythmic drugs or radiofrequency (RF) catheter ablation (see later discussion).

A special type of atrial tachycardia is related to multiple sites of atrial stimulation and is called *multifocal atrial tachycardia* (MAT). This arrhythmia is discussed in Chapter 20, a general review of bradycardias and tachycardias.

## AV NODAL REENTRANT TACHYCARDIA

AV nodal reentrant tachycardia (AVNRT), which was once mistakenly considered a variant of *paroxysmal atrial tachycardia*, is actu-

ally a distinct arrhythmia caused by a rapidly circulating impulse in the AV node area. The term *reentry* (introduced in Chapter 12) describes situations in which a cardiac impulse literally spins around and around and appears to "chase its own tail." Reentry can occur in virtually any part of the heart. Atrial flutter is due to a large reentrant circuit usually originating in the right atrium. (In the ventricles, reentry may lead to VPBs and sometimes ventricular tachycardia.)

AVNRT produces a very rapid and regular supraventricular rhythm with rates typically between 140 and 250 beats/min (Fig. 14-6). This arrhythmia may occur with otherwise normal hearts or with underlying heart disease. Runs of AVNRT are generally initiated by an APB.

With AVNRT, the reentrant rhythm originates in the AV nodal area and spreads simultaneously or nearly simultaneously up the atria and down the ventricles (see Fig. 14-4B). As a consequence, the P waves are usually hidden in the QRS complex because the atria and ventricles are activated simultaneously. In other cases, the P waves may appear just before or just after the QRS complex and therefore may be difficult to see. Because of this retrograde (bottom-to-top) activation of the atria, the P waves are negative in lead II. Episodes of AVNRT may cease spontaneously or may require treatment. The initial therapy usually involves attempts to increase vagal tone, since the vagus nerve slows

---

*See Chapter 18 for a brief discussion of AT *with block* resulting from digitalis toxicity.

## Paroxysmal Supraventricular Tachycardia

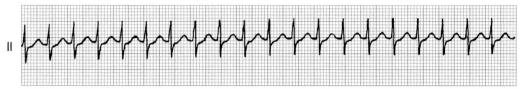

**FIGURE 14-6** Notice the marked regularity of rhythm in this paroxysmal supraventricular tachycardia (PSVT), which has a rate of about 170 beats/min. This tachycardia is probably due to a rapidly circulating impulse in the atrioventricular (AV) node (junction) and thus is referred to as an *AV nodal reentrant tachycardia.* No P waves are visible (see also Fig. 14-4C.).

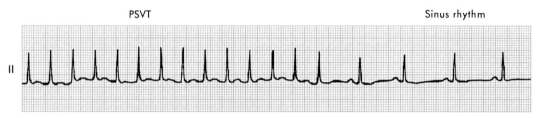

**FIGURE 14-7** Paroxysmal supraventricular tachycardia (PSVT) treated with carotid sinus massage. The first 14 beats in this rhythm strip show the tachyarrhythmia with a rate of about 140 beats/min and no visible P waves. Carotid sinus massage resulted in its abrupt termination, with the appearance of normal sinus rhythm. The PSVT here is probably an atrioventricular nodal reentrant tachycardia (AVNRT) (see Fig. 14-4C).

conduction in the AV node. This "braking effect" may interrupt the reentrant mechanism (Fig. 14-7). Vagal tone can be increased with the Valsalva maneuver (i.e., the patient is instructed to strain against a closed glottis by bearing down, as for a bowel movement) or with carotid sinus massage.

A variety of intravenous drugs are used to interrupt the reentrant mechanism in AVNRT. Clinically, adenosine and verapamil or diltiazem are the drugs most often enlisted in the acute setting. Beta blockers and digoxin also are useful in selected cases.*

Younger patients and individuals without significant underlying cardiovascular disease may tolerate heart rates up to 250 beats/min

with complaints of only palpitations or lightheadedness. In patients with limited cardiac reserve, however, a heart rate above 160 beats/min (or even less) can have disastrous consequences. In these patients, myocardial ischemia or even infarction may occur. They may also develop CHF or hypotension. *Electrical cardioversion* may be required in emergency circumstances (especially, when any PSVT is associated with angina, pulmonary edema, or severe hypotension and when initial therapy with vagal maneuvers and rapid-acting drugs fails). Electrical cardioversion is the use of a direct-current (DC) shock to treat certain tachyarrhythmias. The electrical shock transiently depolarizes the heart, interrupting a variety of abnormal rhythms and allowing the sinus node to "regain control" of the cardiac electrical cycle. The shock is administered with special paddles placed on the chest wall (see also Chapter 15

---

*Other drugs that may be used to prevent the reentrant mechanism in AVNRT are discussed in various texts cited in the Bibliography.

and Fig. 15-8). An *unsynchronized* DC shock is used to treat some arrhythmias (e.g., ventricular flutter or ventricular fibrillation). A *synchronized* DC shock must be used, however, to treat PSVT and other supraventricular arrhythmias (e.g., atrial fibrillation and atrial flutter). The shock is synchronized with the QRS complex so that it does not occur during the *vulnerable period* of ventricular repolarization (simultaneous with the apex of the T wave). Note that the DC shocks given to the heart during the vulnerable period may produce ventricular fibrillation. *Therefore, in treating PSVT, a synchronized DC shock must be given.*\*

For patients with recurrent episodes of AVNRT, *radiofrequency (RF) catheter ablation* may be curative. This special form of therapy involves delivering short pulses of RF current through an intracardiac catheter placed near the AV node during an electrophysiology procedure. The current produces a very small burn that effectively blocks part of the circuit that is supporting the reentrant-type wave.[†]

## ATRIOVENTRICULAR REENTRANT (BYPASS TRACT) TACHYCARDIA

A third common cause of PSVT has already been introduced in the discussion of preexcitation syndromes (see Chapter 12). As previously mentioned, the WPW syndrome is related to the presence of a so-called *bypass tract (accessory pathway),* an abnormal tract of cardiac muscle that connects the atria and ventricles, circumventing the AV node. Patients with this type of atrioventricular bypass tract may develop a tachycardia caused by a reentrant mechanism in which the impulse travels down the normal conduction system (AV node and His bundle) into the ventricles, recycles rapidly up into the atria via the bypass tract, and then goes down the AV node again. Repetition of this large reentrant circuit leads to atrioventricular reentrant (bypass tract) tachycardia (AVRT), a type of PSVT.

Of interest is the fact that in some patients the bypass tract is "concealed"; that is, it never becomes evident during sinus rhythm but can conduct in a retrograde direction, allowing a supraventricular tachycardia to occur.\* The ECG with a concealed-bypass-tract type of PSVT is very similar to the ECG findings described for AVNRT. One subtle difference is that the ECGs of some patients with tachycardia associated with a concealed bypass tract may show P waves occurring visibly after the QRS complexes in the ST segment (see Fig. 14-4D).

The therapy of PSVT resulting from a concealed bypass tract is quite similar to that of AVNRT. Drugs such as adenosine are used for acute episodes, and electrophysiologic testing is performed to evaluate the patient for possible RF catheter ablation of the bypass tract.

In summary, a PSVT should be suspected when a rhythm strip shows a rapid and typically very regular nonsinus rate at about 140 to 220 beats/min (range: 100 to 250 beats/min). The mechanism may be due to reentry in the AV node (AVNRT), atrioventricular reentrant (bypass tract) tachycardia (AVRT), or ectopic

---

\*For details on the use of electrical cardioversion to treat PSVT, see the appropriate texts cited in the Bibliography.
[†]AVNRT is due to the presence of so-called dual pathways located within the AV node area. These two pathways have different conduction and recovery (refractory) properties, allowing an impulse to travel down one path and loop back (reenter) along the other. In particular, there is a "fast" pathway that conducts relatively quickly but recovers slowly and a "slow" pathway that conducts more slowly but recovers more quickly. (See Bibliography for more details.)

---

\*To be evident during sinus rhythm, the bypass tract must conduct impulses rapidly from the atria to the ventricles, bypassing the AV node. This produces a short PR interval, a wide QRS complex, and a delta wave—the classic triad of WPW preexcitation (see Fig. 12-2). In some patients with a bypass tract, the pathway does not conduct antegrade effectively, but it can still conduct retrograde under certain conditions, thereby allowing an impulse to reenter the atria from the ventricles. Bypass tracts that conduct only in a retrograde direction, causing PSVT, are said to be "concealed."

AT. The differential diagnosis of PSVT and other supraventricular tachycardias is discussed further in Chapter 20.

## AV JUNCTIONAL RHYTHMS

With APBs, the ectopic pacemaker is located somewhere in the atria outside the SA node. Under certain circumstances, the AV junction may also function as an ectopic pacemaker, producing an AV junctional rhythm. In some discussions, the term *AV nodal* or *nodal* is used to refer to an AV junctional rhythm. The terms *AV junctional, junctional, AV nodal,* and *nodal* are, however, essentially synonymous.

Chapter 4 introduced the basic mechanism of AV junctional rhythms and the patterns seen with AV junctional beats. When the AV junction is the cardiac pacemaker, the atria are stimulated in a *retrograde* fashion, from bottom to top. An arrow representing the spread of atrial depolarization with junctional rhythm points upward, just opposite the direction of atrial depolarization when normal sinus rhythm is present (see Fig. 4-4). This retrograde stimulation of the atria produces a positive P wave in lead aV$_R$ and a negative P wave in lead II (see Fig. 4-5). With AV junctional rhythm, the ventricles are depolarized normally (unless a bundle branch block is present), resulting in a narrow QRS complex.

In some cases of AV junctional rhythm, the atria are stimulated just before the ventricles. In other cases the stimulus reaches the ventricles first. Finally, in many cases, the atria and the ventricles are stimulated simultaneously. If the atria are stimulated first, the P wave precedes the QRS complex. (A retrograde P wave preceding the QRS complex also occurs with some ectopic atrial beats from the lower part of either atrium. The distinction between such "low" ectopic atrial and AV junctional beats is usually not of clinical importance, however.) If the ventricles are first to be stimulated, the QRS complex precedes the P wave. If atrial and

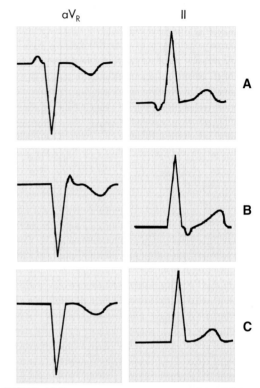

**FIGURE 14-8**  Atrioventricular junctional (nodal) beats produce P waves that point upward in lead aV$_R$ and downward in lead II; this is just the opposite of what is seen with sinus rhythm. The P wave may just precede the QRS complex (**A**), follow it (**B**), or occur simultaneously with it (**C**). In the last instance, no P wave is visible.

ventricular depolarizations are simultaneous, the P wave is hidden in the QRS and therefore is not seen.

In summary, AV junctional beats can be recognized on the ECG by one of the following patterns (Fig. 14-8):

- Retrograde P waves (positive in lead aV$_R$, negative in lead II) immediately preceding the QRS complexes

- Retrograde P waves immediately following the QRS complexes

- Absent P waves (buried in the QRS), so that the baseline between QRS complexes is flat

## AV JUNCTIONAL ESCAPE RHYTHMS

AV junctional escape beats were mentioned in the discussion of sinus arrest (see Chapter 13). An AV junctional escape beat (Fig. 14-9) is simply a beat that comes after a pause when the normal sinus pacemaker fails to function. The AV junctional escape beat is therefore a "safety beat." After this escape beat, the normal sinus pacemaker may resume function. If it does not, a slow AV junctional escape rhythm may continue. An AV junctional escape rhythm is a consecutive run of AV junctional beats. The heart rate is usually slow (30 to 50 beats/min).

Figure 14-10 shows an example of an AV junctional escape rhythm. Not surprisingly, the basic rate of the AV junction is slower than that of the SA node. If the AV junction had a faster inherent rate, it would compete with the SA node for control of the heartbeat.

AV junctional escape rhythms can be seen in a number of clinical settings, including the sick sinus syndrome (see Chapter 20), digitalis toxicity (see Chapter 18), excessive effects of beta blockers or calcium channel blockers (diltiazem and verapamil), acute myocardial infarction, hypoxemia, and hyperkalemia. The cause determines the treatment (e.g., stopping a toxic drug or oxygenating the patient). If the heart rate becomes excessively slow with an AV junctional rhythm, drugs such as atropine (a vagal blocker) or isoproterenol (a sympathomimetic stimulant) are sometimes used acutely. A pacemaker may be required.

## AV JUNCTIONAL TACHYCARDIAS

As is true of AV junctional escape rhythms, *AV junctional tachycardias* can arise in a number of settings. Probably the most common type is AVNRT (see Fig. 14-4C), an arrhythmia that results from a rapidly recirculating impulse in the nodal part of the AV junction. AV junctional tachycardias can also occur because of abnormally enhanced automaticity. This finding may, for example, occur with digitalis toxicity (see Chapter 18).*

---

*Additional information can be obtained from references cited in the Bibliography.

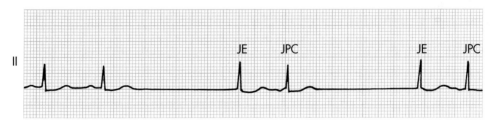

**FIGURE 14-9**   The junctional escape (JE) beat comes after a pause and is followed by a junctional premature complex (JPC). Notice the retrograde (inverted) P wave preceding the JPB in this lead II rhythm strip.

## Junctional Escape Rhythm

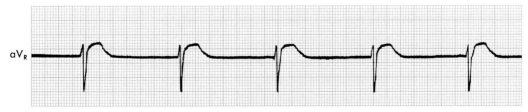

**FIGURE 14-10**   This rhythm strip shows a slow junctional escape rhythm at about 40 beats/min. No P waves are visible, and the baseline between QRS complexes is flat.

# REVIEW

Stimuli that pace the heart can arise not only in the sinoatrial (SA) node but also in other cardiac tissues, such as the atria, atrioventricular (AV) junction, or ventricles. The terms *ectopy, ectopic pacemaker, ectopic contraction,* and *ectopic beat* are used to describe these stimuli. Ectopic beats can be divided into two major categories:

1. *Premature beats* are extra beats that come before the next normal beat is expected. Examples include *atrial premature beats (APBs), junctional premature beats,* and *ventricular premature beats.* These beats originate in the atria, AV junction, and ventricles, respectively.

2. *Escape beats* are usually AV junctional or ventricular beats that are *not* premature but come after a pause in the normal rhythm.

APBs show the following ECG patterns:

1. Usually, the P wave has a different shape, and the PR interval is longer or shorter than in the preceding sinus complexes. Sometimes the P wave is hidden in the T wave of the preceding normal beat.

2. Not uncommonly, the atrial stimulus cannot penetrate the AV junction. In such cases of blocked APBs, the premature P wave is *not* followed by a QRS complex.

Paroxysmal ventricular tachycardia (PSVT) is a sudden run of three or more supraventricular beats. PSVT has three common types (see Fig. 14-4):

1. Atrial tachycardia (AT)

2. AV nodal reentrant tachycardia (AVNRT)

3. AV reentrant tachycardia (AVRT), which is associated with a bypass tract

AV junctional rhythms have the following features:

1. The P wave, when seen, is negative in lead II and positive in lead $aV_R$, which is just the reverse of the pattern seen with normal sinus rhythm. These are called *retrograde* P waves.

2. The retrograde P wave may immediately precede or follow the QRS complex.

3. In many cases, the retrograde P wave is buried within the QRS complex. When this occurs, the baseline between QRS complexes remains completely flat.

AV junctional rhythms are categorized as *junctional escape rhythms* and *junctional tachycardias.* An AV junctional escape rhythm is a run of AV junctional beats with a slow rate, generally between 30 and 50 beats/min. AV junctional tachycardia, by contrast, is a more rapid run of three or more consecutive beats originating in the AV junction. A common type is AVNRT. Other types are due to increased automaticity of AV junctional pacemaker cells.

# QUESTIONS

1. Based on the rhythm strip shown below, why might this patient complain of occasional palpitations?

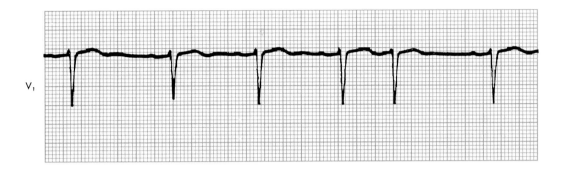

V₁

2. What is the beat marked $X$?

Monitor lead

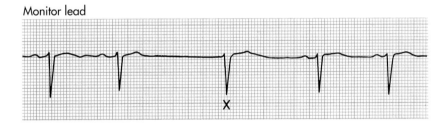

3. Examine the rhythm strip shown below and answer the questions on the next page:

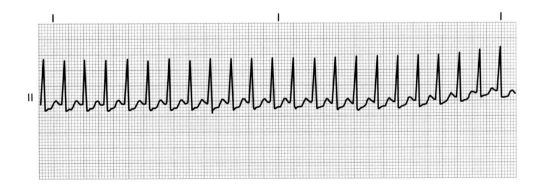

II

a. What is the heart rate?
b. What type of tachyarrhythmia is present?
   (1) Sinus tachycardia
   (2) Paroxysmal supraventricular tachy-cardia (PSVT)
   (3) Atrial flutter
   (4) Atrial fibrillation
   (5) Multifocal atrial tachycardia

4. *True or false:* Paroxysmal supraventricular tachycardia (PSVT) represents sinus tachycardia at a very rapid rate at rest (above 150/min).

## CHAPTER 15

# Supraventricular Arrhythmias Section II

## Atrial flutter and atrial fibrillation

**A**trial flutter and atrial fibrillation (AF) (Fig. 15-1) are two distinct but closely related tachyarrhythmias ("electrophysiologic cousins"). Like paroxysmal supraventricular tachycardia (PSVT), they are *ectopic* rhythms. In other words, with all three types of arrhythmias the atria are being stimulated *not* from the sinus node but from an ectopic site or sites. With PSVTs, the atria (or atrioventricular [AV] node) are stimulated at a rate generally between 140 and 250 cycles per minute. With atrial flutter, the atrial rate is even faster, generally 250 to 350 cycles/min. With AF, the atrial depolarization rate is typically between 350 and 600 cycles/min.*

With both atrial flutter and AF, no discrete P waves are seen on the ECG. Instead, characteristic *flutter* (F) waves and *fibrillation* (f) waves represent continuous atrial electrical activity. Notice the pronounced "sawtooth" shape of the F waves and the more rapid "tremulous" f waves in Figure 15-1. In some patients, atrial

fibrillation and atrial flutter can both occur, so that the ECG may show alternating patterns.

## ATRIAL FLUTTER

Atrial flutter, as introduced in Chapter 14, is an example of a *reentrant* type arrhythmia. Reentry is the term used to describe arrhythmias due to a traveling wave of excitation that circulates over a well-defined loop, "chasing its own tail." With typical atrial flutter, this wave originates in the right atrium, generally traveling in a counterclockwise direction from top to bottom to top (Fig. 15-2).

With atrial flutter, the atrial stimulation (depolarization) rate is about 300/min (Fig. 15-3). What happens to the ventricles during this rapid bombardment of the atria? The answer is that with atrial flutter (and atrial fibrillation) the ventricular (QRS) rate varies, depending on the ability of the atrioventricular (AV) junction to transmit stimuli from the atria to the ventricles. If the ventricles respond to each flutter wave, the ventricular rate is about 300 beats/min, a very unusual occurrence. Most commonly, the ventricular rate with atrial flutter is about 150, 100, or 75 beats/min. Atrial flutter with a

---

*The atrial depolarization rate with atrial flutter may be substantially less than 250 beats/min, especially in patients taking certain antiarrhythmic drugs such as flecainide, amiodarone, and quinidine.

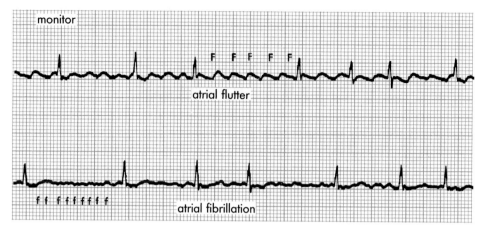

**FIGURE 15-1** Atrial flutter and fibrillation. Notice the "sawtooth" waves (F waves) with atrial flutter and the irregular fibrillatory waves (f waves) with atrial fibrillation.

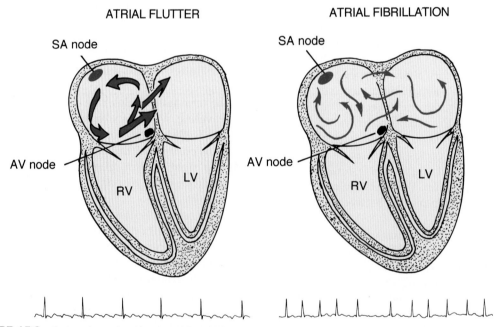

**FIGURE 15-2** Comparison of mechanisms of atrial flutter and atrial fibrillation (AF). Atrial flutter is typically due to a large reentrant wave originating in the right atrium. With typical atrial flutter, the wave spreads in counterclockwise direction. AF is attributed to either multiple reentrant wavelets and/or to multiple sites of atrial automaticity. AV, atrioventricular; LV, left ventricle; RV, right ventricle; SA, sinoatrial.

## Atrial Flutter

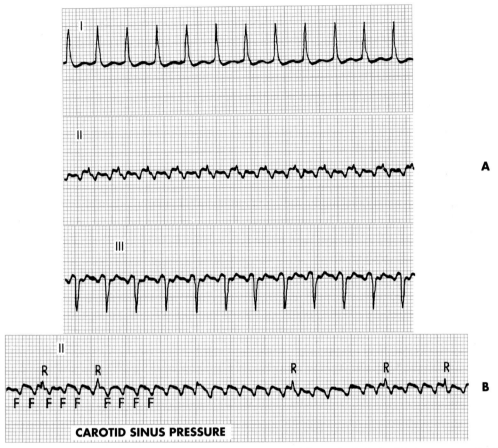

**FIGURE 15-3  A,** Notice the variable appearance of flutter waves in different leads. In lead I, the waves are barely apparent, whereas, in leads II and III, the classic "sawtooth" waves appear. The ventricular rate is about 160 beats/min, and the flutter rate is about 320 beats/min; thus 2:1 conduction is present. **B,** Carotid sinus massage produces marked slowing of the ventricular rate by increasing vagal tone.

ventricular response of about 150 beats/min is called 2:1 flutter because the ratio of the atrial rate (300) to the ventricular rate (150) is 2 to 1. Atrial flutter with a ventricular rate of about 100 beats/min is usually 3:1 flutter; with 75 beats/min, it is usually 4:1 flutter.

Characteristically, patients with atrial flutter increase or decrease their ventricular rate by stepwise fractions of the atrial rate (see Fig. 15-1). Thus a patient's ECG may change abruptly

from showing atrial flutter with a ventricular response of 75–100 beats/min to 150 beats/min. In some patients the ventricular response with atrial flutter is more variable.*

---

*The QRS pattern of "group beating" is not uncommon with atrial flutter and represents a Wenckebach-type variant associated with bombardment of the AV node by frequent atrial depolarization waves (e.g., at 300 cycles/min) (see Chapter 17).

## CLINICAL SIGNIFICANCE

Atrial flutter is rarely seen in people with normal hearts. This finding is in contrast to AF, which may occur in the absence of apparent organic heart disease. Atrial flutter, like atrial fibrillation, is not specific for any particular type of heart disease but occurs, for example, in patients with valvular (especially mitral) disease, chronic ischemic heart disease, cardiomyopathy, hypertensive heart disease, acute myocardial infarction (MI), chronic obstructive lung disease, and pulmonary emboli. Atrial flutter may also occur after cardiac surgery. Arial flutter and atrial fibrillation often occur in the same patient at different times.

Atrial flutter can lead to cardiac symptoms due to loss of normal atrial contraction and a fast or irregular heart rate. (Occasionally, an excessively slow ventricular response occurs with atrial flutter.) As a consequence, patients with atrial flutter (or atrial fibrillation) may complain of palpitations, light-headedness, or even syncope. They may also develop angina due to the rapid heart rate, especially in the presence of coronary disease, or symptoms of congestive heart failure, including shortness of breath and fatigue.

Atrial flutter is also clinically important because it may predispose to the formation of thrombi in the atria, leading to systemic embolization. This complication is most likely in patients who have both atrial fibrillation and atrial flutter and those with underlying rheumatic mitral valve disease or cardiomyopathy.

## TREATMENT CONSIDERATIONS

The treatment of atrial flutter depends on the clinical condition. In some patients, atrial flutter may revert spontaneously to normal sinus rhythm. In patients who are hypoxemic, oxygen therapy may help restore normal sinus rhythm.

Patients who have atrial flutter with a rapid ventricular response are usually treated initially with one drug or a combination of drugs (beta blockers, calcium channel blockers, digitalis) to slow impulse conduction through the AV node. Occasionally, the arrhythmia converts to normal sinus rhythm spontaneously in the course of this initial therapy. In some cases, an antiarrhythmic drug (e.g., ibutilide, dofetilide, amiodarone, procainamide) is used to help directly convert the flutter to normal sinus rhythm. Such drugs must be used with extreme care as they can cause life-threatening adverse effects, including cardiac arrest due to torsades de pointes (see Chapter 16).

Despite initial therapy, atrial flutter persists or recurs in many patients. Fortunately, it is one of the arrhythmias most easily treated with DC electrical cardioversion. As described in Chapter 14, a *synchronized* DC shock is given with the patient properly premedicated. Anticoagulation may also be indicated to decrease the risk of systemic embolization.

Another way of attempting to convert atrial flutter is with very rapid pacing of the atria by means of a temporary pacing wire. This therapy may be particularly useful shortly after cardiac surgery when electrical pacing wires are still in place.

In recent years, radiofrequency (RF) catheter ablation has emerged as a major modality to treat patients with atrial flutter. This method, briefly described in Chapter 14, is based on carefully burning out a small area of tissue involved in initiating or maintaining an arrhythmia. In treating atrial flutter, ablation therapy is usually directed to an area near the tricuspid valve, in the lower part of the right atrium.

In summary, atrial flutter is a tachyarrhythmia in which the atria are stimulated (depolarized) at a rate of usually 250 to 350 cycles/min, with a ventricular response that is often some fraction of the atrial rate (e.g., $\frac{1}{2}$, $\frac{1}{4}$). Atrial flutter may be treated with special drugs, synchronized DC shock, rapid atrial pacing, or RF ablation technology.

## ATRIAL FIBRILLATION

With atrial fibrillation (AF), one of the most common arrhythmias, the atria are stimulated (depolarized) at a very rapid rate, usually between 350 and 600 times/min. This fibrillatory activity produces a characteristically irregular wavy pattern in place of the normal P waves. The irregular waves are called *fibrillatory* or *f waves* (Fig. 15-4). In some cases, the f waves are relatively "coarse" (Fig. 15-5); in others, a faster "fine" pattern of fibrillation is seen (Fig. 15-6). Therefore AF is characterized by rapid depolarizations of the atria that produce irregular undulations of the ECG baseline without discrete (true) P waves.

The detailed electrophysiologic mechanism of AF is a subject of active study. Current analysis favors the view that the rapid atrial depolarization is related to multiple reentrant wavelets in the atria or to multiple foci of atrial automaticity. Figure 15-2 compares the atrial activation patterns in AF and atrial flutter.

Because of the rapid atrial depolarization rate, the AV junction in patients with AF is bombarded by innumerable stimuli from the atria. If every stimulus (each f wave) penetrated the AV junction, the ventricles would beat at a rate of up to 600 times per minute, with obvious catastrophic consequences. Fortunately, the AV junction is refractory to most of these impulses and allows only a fraction to reach the ventricles.

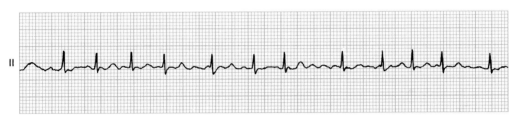

**FIGURE 15-4** Rapid oscillation of the baseline due to fibrillatory (f) waves. No true P waves are present, and the ventricular rate is irregular.

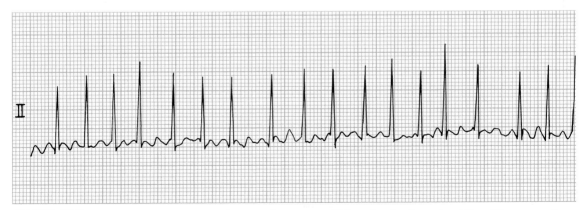

**FIGURE 15-5** Atrial fibrillation with a rapid ventricular response. This patient has hyperthyroidism. (The commonly used term *rapid atrial fibrillation* is actually a misnomer, because "rapid" is intended to refer to the ventricular rate rather than the atrial rate. The same is true for the term *slow atrial fibrillation*.) The atrial fibrillation waves here have a "coarse" appearance.

## Atrial Fibrillation

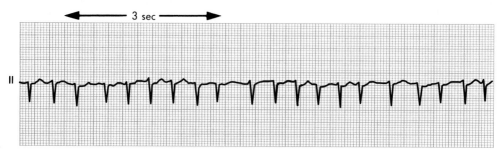

**FIGURE 15-6** Fibrillatory waves may be hard to find. In this tachyarrhythmia, no atrial waves are evident. The ventricular rate is about 140 beats/min and is irregular. No clear fibrillatory waves are visible; nevertheless, the rhythm is atrial fibrillation.

## Atrial Fibrillation

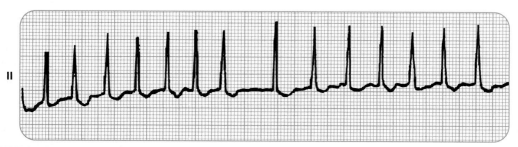

**FIGURE 15-7** Relatively subtle fibrillation waves give the baseline between irregularly spaced R waves a wrinkly appearance.

In patients with a normal AV junction in whom AF suddenly develops, the mean ventricular rate is generally between 110 and 180 beats/min. Figure 15-6 shows an example of AF with an average ventricular rate of about 140 beats/min. Characteristically, the ventricular rate with AF is haphazardly irregular because the AV junction is being stimulated in an apparently random fashion by the rapidly fibrillating atria.

In summary, AF has two ECG characteristics:

■ An irregular wavy baseline produced by the rapid f waves

■ A ventricular (QRS) rate that is usually quite irregular

When the ventricular rate is very fast (Fig. 15-7), the f waves may be difficult to distinguish. In such cases, the diagnosis of AF can usually be suspected by finding a very irregular ventricular rate in the absence of distinct P waves.

## GENERAL CLINICAL ASPECTS

AF is the most common arrhythmia causing hospital admissions. Over 2 million Americans have intermittent or chronic AF, and the incidence rises with age.

In some patients, AF occurs *paroxysmally* and may last only minutes, hours, or days. Some patients may experience only one episode or occasional episodes, whereas others have mul-

| BOX 15-1 | **Classification of Clinical Atrial Fibrillation (AF) Patterns** |
|---|---|

| Pattern | Features |
|---|---|
| Paroxysmal* | Stops spontaneously within 7 days and usually within 48 hours |
| Persistent* | Lasts for more than 7 days and usually requires cardioversion |
| Permanent (Established or Chronic) | Lasts indefinitely or fails to terminate (or recurs) even if cardioversion is attempted |

*Episodes are typically recurrent.
Note: AF of any pattern may be symptomatic (palpitations, chest discomfort, weakness, dyspnea, light-headedness) or asymptomatic.

tiple recurrences. In other patients, AF is more *persistent* and may become *permanent (chronic)*, lasting indefinitely, even if cardioversion is attempted (Box 15-1). With these fibrillatory episodes, some patients are quite symptomatic (typically complaining of palpitations, fatigue, dyspnea, light-headedness, and even syncope, or chest pain), whereas others have no specific complaints. In the asymptomatic patient, AF may first be discovered during a routine examination or when the patient presents with heart failure or stroke. AF can occur in people with no detectable heart disease and in patients with a variety of cardiac diseases (see Chapter 24). The term *lone atrial fibrillation* is sometimes used to describe recurrent or chronic AF in patients without other clinical evidence of heart disease. Paroxysmal AF may occur spontaneously, or it may be associated with excessive alcohol consumption in otherwise healthy individuals ("holiday heart syndrome"). In such cases, the arrhythmia often spontaneously reverts to normal sinus rhythm or is converted easily with pharmacologic therapy alone.

Changes in autonomic tone may provoke AF in susceptible individuals. Sometimes the arrhythmia is related to increased sympathetic tone (e.g., occurring during exercise or with emotional excitement). At other times, AF may occur in the context of high vagal tone (e.g., with sinus bradycardia during sleep).

AF is also one of the most frequently observed arrhythmias in patients with organic (structural) heart disease. The prevalence of this arrhythmia rises with advancing age. Common pathologic substrates include coronary artery disease, hypertensive heart disease, and valvular heart disease. Patients with coronary artery disease may experience AF for the first time during an acute MI or, more commonly, as a consequence of chronic ischemic myocardial disease, possibly because of associated atrial dilation or fibrosis. Hypertensive heart disease is often associated with left atrial enlargement. AF is also commonly caused by valvular heart disease, particularly when the mitral valve is involved. For example, severe mitral stenosis or mitral regurgitation produces atrial enlargement, which is a predisposing factor for atrial arrhythmias.

Numerous other conditions can also lead to AF. For example, patients with thyrotoxicosis (hyperthyroidism) may develop AF (see Fig. 15-6). AF (or atrial flutter) is quite common after cardiac surgery. It may also occur with pericardial disease (especially chronic disease), lung disease, obstructive sleep apnea, pulmonary emboli, cardiomyopathy, congenital heart disease (e.g., atrial septal defect), and other forms of heart disease. Often, patients have more than one predisposing factor for this arrhythmia.

Chapter 24 presents an "instant review" of the common substrates for AF.

## PATHOPHYSIOLOGY AND CLINICAL CONSEQUENCES

What happens physiologically when AF develops? After the P wave, the atria normally contract and pump blood into the ventricles. With AF, normal atrial depolarization is lost and the atria fibrillate (quiver) instead of contracting synchronously. In these circumstances, the normal atrial "kick" is lost, and the result is decreased cardiac output (since ventricular filling is decreased). Furthermore, the stagnation (stasis) of blood in the atria may lead to thromboembolic complications (discussion to follow).

### Decreased Cardiac Output

Hemodynamically the most significant effect of AF is decreased cardiac output, which is especially marked in patients with underlying cardiac impairment and in elderly people, who have stiffer cardiac musculature and are therefore more dependent on atrial contraction for filling of the ventricles. In addition, the amount of this decreased output depends importantly on the ventricular rate with AF. The faster the rate, the less time there is for adequate ventricular filling and the greater the decrease in cardiac output. Thus the patient with AF at a rate of 150 beats/min is more likely to be hypotensive or develop congestive heart failure (CHF) than is the patient with a rate of 100 beats/min. In patients with coronary artery disease, a rapid ventricular rate can also cause myocardial ischemia and even infarction, further reducing cardiac output (see Chapter 8).

### Atrial Thrombi and Embolization

The second significant effect of AF, resulting from the stagnation of blood, is a tendency in some patients for atrial thrombi to develop and dislodge into the arterial circulation, causing peripheral embolism. The thrombi can produce a cerebrovascular accident, occlusion of the blood supply to the legs, and other complications.

The risk of thrombus formation and embolization is highest in patients with chronic AF related to rheumatic mitral valve disease. Thrombi and embolization also occur, however, in patients with AF from other causes (so-called *nonrheumatic atrial fibrillation*). *Indeed, atrial fibrillation is a major substrate for embolic strokes, particularly in the elderly, as well as those with hypertension or heart failure.*

## TREATMENT APPROACHES

Rather than discussing the details of treating AF, this section focuses on the general clinical approach to patients with this arrhythmia. AF may convert to sinus rhythm in three principal ways. The first is spontaneous conversion in which the AF stops and sinus rhythm resumes without apparent reason. The second occurs with *pharmacologic* therapy. The third is with *electrical cardioversion* (as already described for PSVT and atrial flutter).

In approaching patients with AF, you need to address promptly three major clinical questions:

1. Is the arrhythmia acute and causing a life-threatening decrease in cardiac function, as indicated by severe myocardial ischemia, hypotension, or very severe CHF? As a general rule, patients with very recent–onset AF that is producing severe shock, severe myocardial ischemia, or pulmonary edema should be considered candidates for electrical cardioversion if they do not respond promptly to emergency drug therapy.

2. Is the AF likely of very recent onset (especially less than 48 hrs) or is it of longer duration?

3. Is there a specific cause (or causes) of the arrhythmia?

In most cases, acute AF does not require immediate electrical cardioversion. Drug therapy alone can be used initially to control the ventricular rate. Beta blockers, calcium channel blockers (verapamil, diltiazem), and digitalis all act by slowing conduction of stimuli through the AV node.*

---

*Digitalis glycosides act primarily by increasing vagal tone at the AV node. Beta blockers decrease sympathetic tone. Calcium channel blockers directly interfere with conduction by impairing the cellular entry of calcium ions, which play a major role in electrical impulse transmission in the AV node.

The usual sequence in treating AF pharmacologically is first to control the ventricular response with a beta blocker or a calcium channel blocker, and sometimes with digoxin. Always consider factors such as hypoxemia, severe anemia, fever, severe congestive heart failure, and hyperthyroidism, which can contribute to the rapid ventricular response and which, until addressed, will make rate control much more difficult.

If sinus rhythm is not spontaneously restored in association with rate slowing, the addition of a specific antiarrhythmic drug is often considered. Elective DC cardioversion (Fig. 15-8) is generally reserved for patients who fail to respond to an initial trial of drug therapy and who are felt to have a reasonable likelihood of maintaining sinus rhythm for an extended time. Sometimes, DC cardioversion is used without specific antiarrhythmic drug therapy.

*Attempts to convert AF to sinus rhythm with either pharmacologic therapy or DC cardioversion should not be made unless the patient has been sufficiently anticoagulated or atrial thrombus formation has been convincingly excluded (e.g., by transesophageal echocardiography).* The reason for this caveat is that restoration of normal atrial contractility during sinus rhythm may cause dislodgment of an atrial thrombus formed while the atria are fibrillating. The longer the duration of the fibrillation, the more likely thrombus formation becomes. Thrombus formation may also occur, however, with fibrillation of relatively short duration.

Not all patients with AF are candidates for pharmacologic or electrical cardioversion. Patients with persistent or recurrent AF who cannot be converted to or maintained in sinus rhythm are candidates for ventricular rate control along with long-term anticoagulation using warfarin or aspirin, depending on the circumstances. Antiarrhythmic drug therapy of AF has been disappointing because of the high failure rate and the toxicity of the agents, including the risk of potentially fatal ventricular arrhythmias *(proarrhythmia)* (see also Chapters 16 and 19).

Some patients with chronic AF who cannot be converted to sinus rhythm have an uncontrollably fast ventricular response despite maximal drug therapy. A useful approach to this problem is ablation of the AV node with RF current delivered by a special cardiac catheter (see Chapter 14). Because this therapy may result in complete heart block, a permanent pacemaker must also be implanted.

The limited efficacy and toxicities of drug therapies for preventing recurrence of atrial fibrillation has prompted major efforts to find new approaches to management. A number of nonpharmacologic therapies to treat recurrent atrial fibrillation are evolving. These include *atrial ablation* procedures and *atrial implanted defibrillators*. Atrial ablation therapy is based on the finding that many cases of AF originate with ectopic stimuli from the area around the pulmonary veins in the left atrium. Electrical "isolation" of the pulmonary veins using RF ablation techniques is being used as a new approach to therapy for carefully selected patients with drug-refractory, recurrent AF. Implanted atrial defibrillators may be useful in selected patients as well. These and other emerging approaches have exciting potential, but are not without serious risks. For example, atrial rupture and pulmonary vein thrombosis, among other serious complications, have occurred with ablation procedures. Atrial defibrillation from an implanted device can cause painful shocks, limiting the clinical use of this technology.

At the same time that you are starting to treat a patient with AF, you should be thinking of possible causes for this common arrhythmia. You should search for evidence of excessive chronic or acute alcohol use (holiday heart syndrome), hypertensive heart disease, cardiomyopathy, obstructive sleep apnea, valvular disease, coronary artery disease, or chronic pericardial disease, if indicated. A blood test for thyroid function should be performed in any

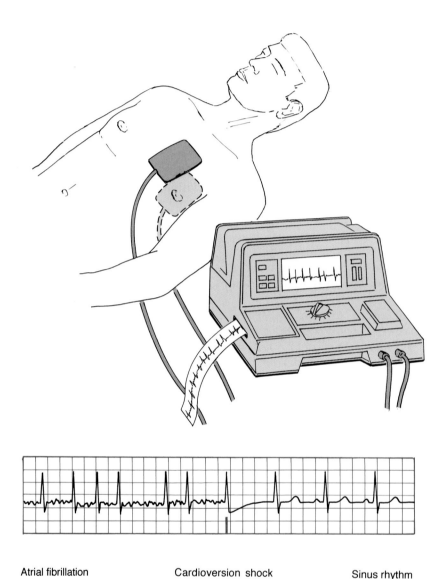

Atrial fibrillation        Cardioversion shock        Sinus rhythm

**FIGURE 15-8** Cardioversion of atrial fibrillation to sinus rhythm. With external direct-current (DC) cardioversion, an electric shock is administered to the heart via special electrode paddles placed on the chest wall. In the case depicted here, one electrode is placed on the anterior chest wall, to the left of the sternum, the other (indicated by *dashed lines*) is placed on the back, under the left scapula. The shock is synchronized with the peak of the QRS complex to avoid inducing ventricular fibrillation if the stimulus is delivered at the peak of the T wave.

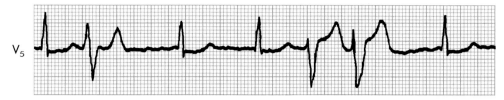

**FIGURE 15-9**   Atrial fibrillation with ventricular premature beats.

## Atrial Fibrillation with Complete Heart Block

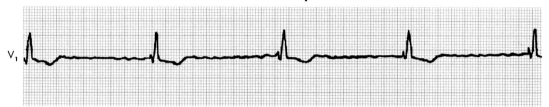

**FIGURE 15-10**   Atrial fibrillation with complete atrioventricular (AV) block. The ventricular rate is very slow and regular because of the block. (Notice the right bundle branch block morphology of the escape rhythm QRS complexes.)

patient with unexplained AF because thyro-toxicosis is an important treatable cause of this arrhythmia. The approach to the patient with AF in the setting of recent cardiac surgery is a subject of current interest and evolving strategies.

Patients with underlying AV nodal disease may develop persistent AF with a slow ventric-ular response in the absence of drug therapy. If the ventricular rate becomes exceedingly slow, a permanent (ventricular) pacemaker may be required. Atrial-based pacemaker therapy may be helpful in patients with sinus node dysfunc-tion ("sick sinus syndrome") who develop recurrent episodes of AF.

Guidelines for current therapy of AF are available at the websites of the American Heart Association and the American College of Car-diology (see Bibliography).

## ATRIAL FIBRILLATION AND OTHER ARRHYTHMIAS

Atrial fibrillation (or atrial flutter) may occur with other arrhythmias and conduction distur-bances, just as sinus rhythm can occur with ven-tricular premature beats (VPBs), AV heart block, and so on. An example of AF with VPBs is pre-sented in Figure 15-9. AF or atrial flutter can also occur with complete heart block (Fig. 15-10); in such cases, the ventricular response is very slow and regular. Possible digitalis toxic-ity should always be considered in the patient who has AF and a very slow or regularized ven-tricular rate (see Chapter 18).

The special case of AF with the Wolff-Parkinson-White (WPW) syndrome is dis-cussed in Chapter 20.

Occasionally, it can be difficult to decide whether AF or atrial flutter is present (see Chapter 23). The coarse atrial fibrillatory waves may resemble flutter waves (see Fig. 23-3). This arrhythmia, which is sometimes referred to as *fibrillation-flutter ("fib-flutter")*, usually has the same clinical significance and treatment as AF.

# REVIEW

With *atrial flutter,* the ECG shows the following features:

1. Characteristic "sawtooth" flutter waves instead of discrete P waves

2. A constant or variable ventricular rate (e.g., one QRS complex with every fourth flutter wave, 4:1 flutter; one QRS with every two flutter waves, 2:1 flutter, and the ventricular rate half the atrial rate; or the rare 1:1 flutter, in which the ventricles contract about 300 times a minute)

Atrial flutter rarely occurs in normal hearts but is most often seen in valvular heart disease, ischemic heart disease, lung disease, cardiomyopathy, or pulmonary emboli. It may also occur after cardiac surgery. Atrial flutter may be treated with a synchronized direct-current (DC) shock (cardioversion), rapid atrial pacing, radiofrequency catheter ablation, or drug therapy.

The ECG of a patient with *atrial fibrillation (AF)* shows the following:

1. Rapid irregular undulations of the baseline (fibrillatory waves) instead of P waves

2. A ventricular rate that is usually grossly irregular

In some patients, AF occurs permanently; in others, it is paroxysmal. Occasionally, AF is seen without evidence of underlying heart disease. Common factors predisposing to AF are coronary artery disease, hypertensive heart disease, and mitral valve disease. This arrhythmia may also occur in many other settings, such as with hyperthyroidism, cardiomyopathy, excessive alcohol use, cardiac surgery, pulmonary emboli, and chronic pericarditis. It may be seen with other arrhythmias (e.g., ventricular ectopy or complete heart block). With an extremely slow or regularized ventricular rate (50 beats/min or less), AF may signify digitalis toxicity. Sustained AF can sometimes be converted to normal sinus rhythm with DC cardioversion or pharmacologic therapy, or controlled with newer approaches using radiofrequency atrial ablation.

# QUESTIONS

1. Answer the following questions about the monitor lead rhythm strip below:

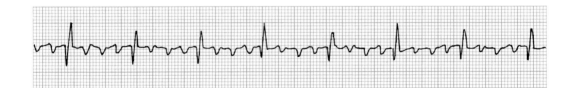

   a. What is the atrial rate?
   b. What is the ventricular rate?
   c. What is this arrhythmia?

2. Answer the following questions about this rhythm strip:

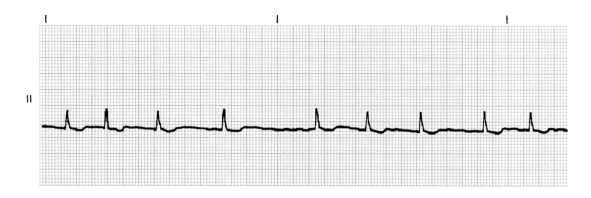

    a. What is the *average* heart rate?
    b. What is this arrhythmia?

3. The atrial rate with atrial flutter is *(faster, slower)* than the atrial rate with atrial fibrillation.

4. The atrial rate with atrial flutter is usually *(faster, slower)* than that with atrial tachycardia.

5. *True or false:* The ventricular rate with atrial fibrillation is always greater than 100 beats/min.

6. *True or false:* Systemic embolization causing stroke or vascular occlusion is not a risk with atrial flutter.

## CHAPTER 16

# Ventricular Arrhythmias

The three preceding chapters have focused on *supra*ventricular arrhythmias, which are rhythm disturbances arising in the sinus node, atria, or atrioventricular (AV) junction with normal ventricular depolarization. This chapter considers another major ECG topic—ventricular arrhythmias. Ectopic (nonsinus) beats frequently arise in the ventricles themselves, producing *premature ventricular beats (or complexes), ventricular tachycardia (VT)*, and sometimes *ventricular fibrillation (VF)* leading to cardiac arrest.

## VENTRICULAR PREMATURE BEATS

Ventricular premature beats (VPBs)* are premature depolarizations arising in the ventricles, analogous to atrial premature beats (APBs) and junctional premature beats (JPBs), which are supraventricular. Recall that, with APBs and JPBs, the QRS complex is usually of normal width because the stimulus spreads normally through the bundle branches to the ventricles. With VPBs, however, the premature depolarizations arise in either the right or left ventricle.

Therefore the ventricles are not stimulated simultaneously, and the stimulus spreads through the ventricles in an aberrant direction. Thus the QRS complexes are wide with VPBs, just as they are with the bundle branch block patterns. Examples of VPBs are shown in Figures 16-1 to 16-8.

VPBs have two major characteristics[†]:

1. They are premature and occur before the next normal beat is expected.

2. They are aberrant in appearance. The QRS complex is abnormally wide (usually 0.12 sec or more), and the T wave and QRS complex usually point in opposite directions.

VPBs usually precede a sinus P wave. Occasionally, they appear just after a sinus P wave but before the normal QRS complex (see Fig. 16-7). Sometimes they are followed by a nonsinus P wave (negative in lead II) that has arisen

---

*In the ECG literature, the terms *ventricular premature beat, ventricular premature depolarization, ventricular extrasystole,* and *premature ventricular complex* or *contraction (PVC)* are used interchangeably.

[†]The basic electrophysiologic mechanisms responsible for VPBs are a subject of active investigation. VPBs may arise by at least three mechanisms: *reentrant waves,* increased *spontaneous depolarizations* of ventricular cells (enhanced automaticity), and *triggered activity* or *afterdepolarizations* (i.e., premature firing of ventricular cells triggered by the previous depolarization).

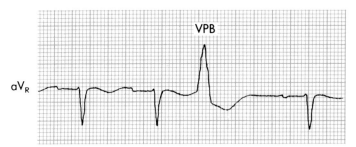

**FIGURE 16-1** A ventricular premature beat (VPB) is recognized because it comes before the next normal beat is expected and it has a wide aberrant shape. (Notice also the long PR interval in the normal sinus beats, indicating first-degree AV block.)

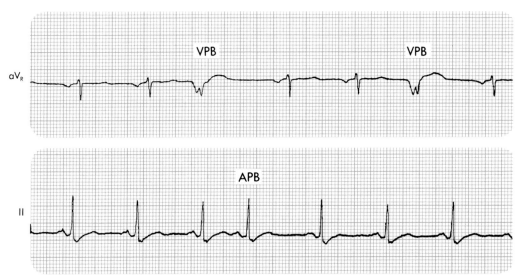

**FIGURE 16-2** Notice the wide aberrant shape of a ventricular premature beat (VPB) compared to the QRS complexes of an atrial premature beat (APB), which generally resembles the sinus QRS complexes.

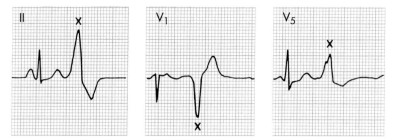

**FIGURE 16-3** Notice that the same ventricular premature beat (marked X) recorded simultaneously in three different leads has different shapes. By comparison, notice that the multiform ventricular premature beats shown in Figure 16-9 have different shapes in the *same* lead.

Monitor lead

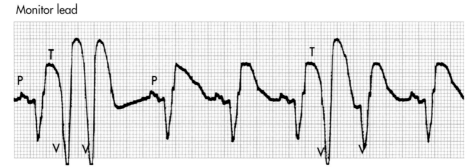

**FIGURE 16-4** Two ventricular premature beats (V) are referred to as a *pair* or a *couplet*. They also show the "R on T" phenomenon (see text and Fig. 16-10).

## Nonsustained Ventricular Tachycardia

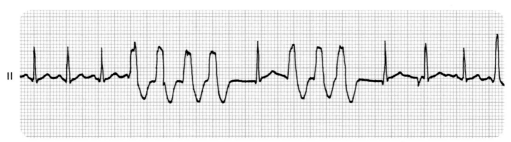

**FIGURE 16-5** Notice the two very short bursts of *nonsustained ventricular tachycardia* (VT). Compare this with the sustained VT shown in Fig. 16-12*A*.

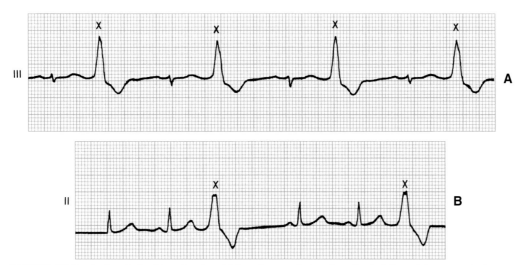

**FIGURE 16-6** **A,** Ventricular bigeminy, in which each normal sinus impulse is followed by a ventricular premature beat (marked *X*). **B,** Ventricular trigeminy, in which a ventricular premature beat occurs after every two sinus pulses.

because of retrograde stimulation of the atria by the VPB.

## FEATURES

Clinicians tend to comment on a number of features of VPBs that may have clinical relevance.

### Frequency

The frequency of VPBs refers to the number that is seen per minute or other unit of time. The VPB frequency may range from one or an occasional isolated premature depolarization to many.

VPBs may occur in various combinations. Two in a row (see Fig. 16-4) are referred to as a *pair* or *couplet*. Three or more in a row are, by definition, VT (see Fig. 16-5). Sometimes, as shown in Figure 16-6A, isolated VPBs occur so frequently that each normal beat is followed by a VPB. This produces a distinctive repetitive grouping of one normal beat and one VPB, which is called *ventricular bigeminy*. The sequence of two normal beats with a VPB is *ventricular trigeminy*.

### Morphology

As you might expect, the appearance of the VPBs will differ depending on the site(s) in the ventricles from which the VPBs originate. VPBs originating in the right ventricle generally have a left bundle branch block morphology, since the left ventricle is stimulated after the right ventricle. VPBs originating in the left ventricle generally have a right bundle branch block morphology. VPBs originating in the interventricular septum also often have a left bundle branch block morphology.

### Coupling Interval

The term *coupling interval* is applied to the interval between the VPB and the preceding normal beat. When multiple VPBs are present, *fixed coupling* often occurs, with the coupling interval approximately the same for each VPB (see Fig. 16-6A). At other times, VPBs may show a *variable coupling interval*.

**Fully Compensatory Pause**

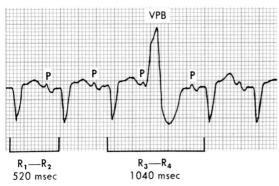

**FIGURE 16-7** Some ventricular premature beats (VPBs) cause a fully compensatory pause, with the interval between the two sinus beats that surround the VPB ($R_3$ and $R_4$, in this case) being two times the normal interval between sinus beats ($R_1$ and $R_2$). Notice that the P waves (P) come on time, except that the third P wave is interrupted by the VPB and therefore is not conducted through the AV junction, which is still refractory. The next (fourth) P wave also comes on time. The fact that the sinus node is continuing to pace despite the VPB results in the fully compensatory pause.

**Interpolated Ventricular Premature Beats**

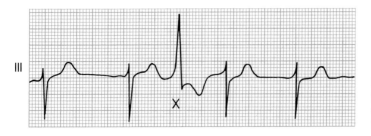

**FIGURE 16-8** Sometimes a ventricular premature beat (X) falls between two normal beats, in which case it is *interpolated*.

## Multiform Ventricular Premature Beats

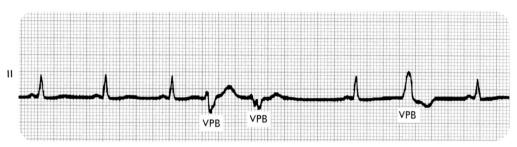

**FIGURE 16-9**  These multiform ventricular premature beats (VPBs) have different shapes in the same lead. (Compare this tracing with the one in Figure 16-6A.)

### Compensatory Pause

As you may have noticed, APBs and VPBs are usually followed by a pause before the next normal beat. The pause after a VPB is usually but not always longer than the pause after an APB. A fully compensatory pause indicates that the interval between the normal QRS complexes immediately before and immediately after the VPB is twice the basic RR interval (see Fig. 16-7). A fully compensatory pause is more characteristic of VPBs than APBs. Sometimes a VPB falls almost exactly between two normal beats; in such cases, the VPB is said to be *interpolated* (see Fig. 16-8).

### Uniform and Multiform VPBs

The terms *uniform* and *multiform* are used to describe the appearance of VPBs in any lead. Uniform VPBs have the same appearance in any lead and arise from the same anatomic site (focus) (see Fig. 16-6). (Of course, they have different shapes in different leads, just as normal beats do.) By contrast, multiform VPBs have different morphologies in the same lead (Fig. 16-9). Multiform VPBs often but not always arise from different foci. Uniform VPBs are uni*focal*, but multiform VPBs are not necessarily multi*focal*. Uniform VPBs may occur in normal hearts and hearts with underlying organic heart disease. Frequent multiform VPBs often indicate that organic heart disease is present.

### R on T Phenomenon

The *R on T* or *VPB on T phenomenon* refers to VPBs that are timed so that they fall at the peak* of the T wave of the preceding normal beat (see Figs. 16-10 and 16-16). Those falling on the T wave are noteworthy in that they may precipitate VT or VF, particularly in the course of an acute myocardial infarction (MI) or myocardial ischemia or with very long QT intervals (discussed later in this chapter). Recall from the discussion of synchronized direct-current (DC) cardioversion that the peak of the T wave is a time during which an external stimulus is especially likely to produce VF (see Chapter 15). VT and VF most commonly occur, however, without a preceding "R on T" beat, and most "R on T" beats do not precipitate a sustained ventricular tachyarrhythmia.

### CLINICAL SIGNIFICANCE

VPBs are among the most common arrhythmias. They may occur in normal hearts and with serious organic heart disease. Individuals with VPBs may be asymptomatic, or they may complain of palpitations (i.e., sensations of a "skipped" or "extra" beat). VPBs may be a stable and benign finding, or they may be a

---

*Equivalently, the VPBs may fall at the nadir of a negative T wave.

Monitor lead

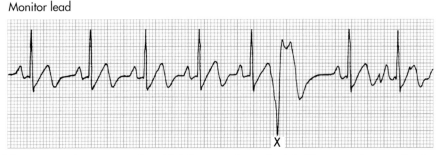

**FIGURE 16-10**  A ventricular premature beat (X) falling near the peak of the T wave of the preceding beat may be a predisposing factor for ventricular tachycardia or ventricular fibrillation, particularly when this "R on T" phenomenon occurs in the setting of acute myocardial ischemia or infarction or with long QT(U) intervals.

marker of severe organic heart disease associated with an increased risk of cardiac arrest and sudden death from VF. Clearly, clinicians need certain ground rules to help decide when VPBs are of concern. A few general principles are discussed here.

As mentioned, VPBs are not uncommon in normal adults of all ages although they occur more frequently with advancing age. Young adults, for example, may have VPBs because of anxiety or excessive caffeine intake. Certain drugs used in asthmatics (e.g., epinephrine, isoproterenol, and aminophylline) can provoke VPBs in normal hearts. Nevertheless, if a patient has frequent VPBs, you should search carefully for underlying cardiac disease (heart murmurs, abnormal echocardiographic findings, and so on) and also obtain a careful drug history. Occasional or even frequent isolated VPBs in an otherwise healthy person without organic heart disease are not usually a source of concern. VPBs are also common with mitral valve prolapse, and they may be seen with virtually any type of heart disease. For example, a patient with valvular, hypertensive, or ischemic heart disease with or without MI may have them. VPBs are the most common arrhythmia seen with acute MI.

As noted, VPBs can be caused by the effects on the heart of numerous drugs, including epinephrine, isoproterenol, and aminophylline, which are cardiac stimulants. Ventricular ectopy is also an important sign of digitalis toxicity (see Chapter 18). VPBs may be seen in patients with electrolyte disturbances such as hypokalemia or hypomagnesemia and in patients with lung disease or hypoxemia from any cause.

## DRUG THERAPY

As mentioned, VPBs are common in healthy people. Even in patients with underlying heart disease, the suppression of frequent isolated VPBs or even short runs of VT with antiarrhythmic drugs has not been shown to improve survival. In fact, the drugs used to treat ventricular ectopy (e.g., quinidine, procainamide, disopyramide, mexiletine, propafenone, moricizine, amiodarone, and flecainide) all have serious and sometimes life-threatening side effects. Furthermore, antiarrhythmic drugs may actually make the situation worse by increasing the severity of the ectopy (*proarrhythmic effect*). Indeed, treating a patient with so-called antiarrhythmic drugs may sometimes provoke a potentially fatal, sustained ventricular tachyarrhythmia.

For patients with frequent VPBs associated with very bothersome palpitations, beta-blocker therapy is sometimes used. Beta blockers may also be helpful in patients who have ventricular ectopy associated with coronary artery disease and in patients who have certain types of cardiomyopathy.

These complex and sometimes controversial therapeutic issues are discussed more completely in texts cited in the Bibliography. Again, *whenever you see a patient with frequent VPBs, you must search for potentially reversible causes and contributors, particularly hypokalemia, hypomagnesemia, and certain stimulant drugs.* Underlying structural heart disease should be assessed by history and physical examination, and by noninvasive techniques such as echocardiography and exercise testing where specifically indicated.

## VENTRICULAR TACHYCARDIA

VT is, by definition, simply a run of three or more consecutive VPBs. Examples are shown in Figures 16-5, 16-11, and 16-12. VT is usefully classified by duration (nonsustained and sustained) and by morphology (monomorphic and polymorphic) (Box 16-1).

Sustained VT (typically lasting longer than 30 sec) is usually a life-threatening arrhythmia for two major reasons:

1. Most patients are not able to maintain an adequate blood pressure at very rapid ventricular rates and eventually become hypotensive.

2. The condition may degenerate into VF (Fig. 16-13), causing immediate cardiac arrest.

VT, whether sustained or not, can also be characterized as *monomorphic* (see Fig. 16-12*A*)

## Paroxysmal Nonsustained Ventricular Tachycardia

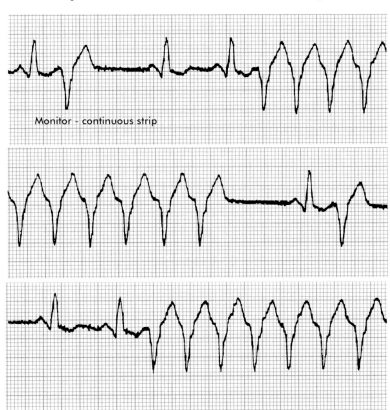

Monitor - continuous strip

**FIGURE 16-11** The monitor lead shows short bursts of ventricular tachycardia.

**Sustained, Monomorphic Ventricular Tachycardia Terminated by Direct-Current Shock**

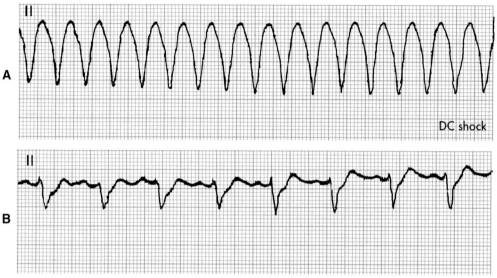

**FIGURE 16-12**   **A,** Long run of monomorphic ventricular tachycardia. **B,** Normal sinus rhythm restored after direct-current (DC) cardioversion.

---

<table>
<tr><td>

**BOX 16-1**   **Classification of Ventricular Tachycardia**

**Duration**

Nonsustained (lasting three beats to 30 sec)
Sustained (lasting 30 sec or more, or somewhat shorter runs if associated with symptoms of syncope or near-syncope)

**Morphology**

Monomorphic
Polymorphic
   With long QT(U) syndrome: torsades de pointes
   Without long QT(U) syndrome: for example, polymorphic ventricular tachycardia with acute ischemia

</td></tr>
</table>

or *polymorphic* (see Fig. 16-16), depending on whether consecutive VPBs have the same or a variable appearance in a single lead.

Very rapid VT with a sine-wave appearance is sometimes referred to as *ventricular flutter.*

This arrhythmia often leads to cardiac arrest with VF (Fig. 16-14).

## SUSTAINED MONOMORPHIC VENTRICULAR TACHYCARDIA: CAUSES AND THERAPIES

Sustained VT, which may lead to syncope or sudden death, rarely occurs in patients without underlying structural heart disease.* Most patients with this type of high-grade ventricular ectopy (i.e., long runs of ventricular tachycardia) have some basic structural cardiac abnormality, such as prior MI, cardiomyopathy or valvular disease associated with fibrosis (scarring), or ventricular enlargement. The most common cause of sustained, recurrent monomorphic VT in American adults is coronary artery disease with prior MI.

Despite pharmacologic therapy, some patients are at high risk for life-threatening

---

*See also references cited in the Bibliography for discussion of the types of VT that may occur *without* structural heart disease.

## Ventricular Fibrillation

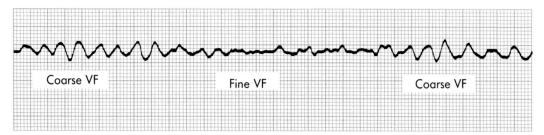

**FIGURE 16-13**   Ventricular fibrillation (VF) may produce both coarse and fine waves. Immediate defibrillation should be performed.

## Cardiac Arrest

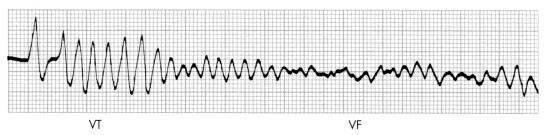

**FIGURE 16-14**   Ventricular tachycardia (VT) and ventricular fibrillation (VF) recorded during the onset of cardiac arrest. The rapid sine-wave type of VT seen here is sometimes referred to as *ventricular flutter.*

recurrences of sustained VT or VF. For these patients, a special device called an *implantable cardioverter defibrillator (ICD)* has been developed to deliver an internal electric shock directly to the heart during a life-threatening tachycardia (Chapter 21).

## ACCELERATED IDIOVENTRICULAR RHYTHM

Figures 16-15 and 16-16 present a distinctive arrhythmia that has been called *accelerated idioventricular rhythm (AIVR)* or *slow ventricular tachycardia.* Recall that, with typical VT, the heart rate is faster than 100 beats/min. With AIVR, the heart rate is usually between 50 and 100 beats/min, and the ECG shows wide QRS complexes without associated sinus P waves.

AIVR is particularly common with acute MI, and it may be a sign of *reperfusion* after the use of thrombolytic agents or after interventional coronary artery procedures. This arrhythmia is generally short lived, lasting minutes or less, and usually requires no specific therapy.

In many cases (see Fig. 16-15), AIVR appears to be a benign "escape" rhythm that competes with the underlying sinus mechanism. When the sinus rate slows, AIVR appears; when the sinus rate speeds up, the arrhythmia disappears. In other cases (see Fig. 16-16), AIVR is initiated by premature beats rather than escape beats. This latter type is more likely to be associated with actual VT.

## Accelerated Idioventricular Rhythm

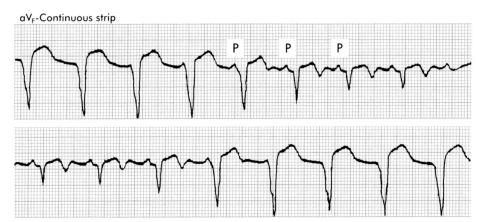

**FIGURE 16-15**   Accelerated idioventricular rhythm (AIVR) in a patient with an acute inferior wall infarction. The first four beats show the typical pattern, followed by a return of sinus rhythm, then the reappearance of the AIVR. Notice that the fifth, sixth, twelfth, and thirteenth QRS complexes are "fusion beats" because of the nearly simultaneous occurrence of a sinus beat and a ventricular beat.

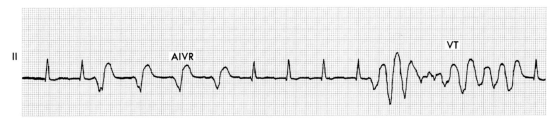

**FIGURE 16-16**   Accelerated idioventricular rhythm (AIVR) and nonsustained polymorphic ventricular tachycardia (VT) occurring together. Notice the "VPB on T" beats that initiate both the AIVR and the VT episodes.

## TORSADES DE POINTES: A SPECIFIC FORM OF POLYMORPHIC VENTRICULAR TACHYCARDIA

A distinct type of polymorphic VT is called *torsades de pointes* (a French term meaning "twisting of the points"). Figures 16-17 and 16-18 show examples of this tachycardia. Notice how the direction of the QRS complexes appears to rotate cyclically, pointing downward for several beats and then twisting and pointing upward in the same lead.

Torsades de pointes is important because of its diagnostic and therapeutic implications. As shown in Figure 16-17, torsades de pointes

occurs in the setting of delayed ventricular repolarization, evidenced by prolongation of the QT intervals or the presence of prominent U waves. It is often initiated by a VPB that occurs near or on the T or U wave of the preceding beat. Reported causes and contributors include the following (also see Chapter 24 for a more complete list):

■ Drugs, particularly quinidine (see Chapter 10 and Fig. 19-7) and related antiarrhythmic agents (disopyramide and procainamide), as well as ibutilide, dofetilide, sotalol, amiodarone (less commonly), psychotropic agents (phenothiazines and tricyclic antidepres-

### Torsades de Pointes: Nonsustained

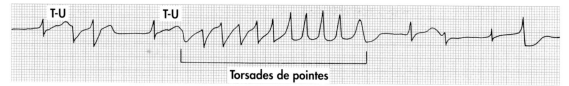

**FIGURE 16-17**  Notice the shifting polarity and amplitude of the QRS complexes during an episode of nonsustained torsades de pointes. QT(U) prolongation (0.52 sec) is also present in the normal sinus beats.

### Torsades de Pointes: Sustained

Monitor lead

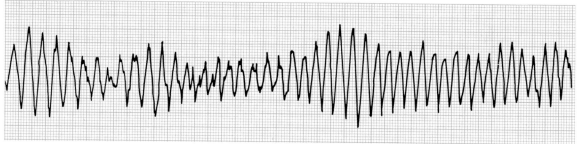

**FIGURE 16-18**  Classic pattern of the sustained torsades de pointes type of ventricular tachycardia. Notice the pattern of depolarization in which the QRS axis appears to rotate or turn in a systematic way. Figure 16-17 shows a short, nonsustained run of the same arrhythmia, which typically occurs in the setting of QT(U) prolongation.

sants), and other noncardiac drugs (e.g., probucol, cisapride, pentamidine, and erythromycin and related antibiotics)

■ Electrolyte imbalances, especially hypokalemia and hypomagnesemia, and, less commonly, hypocalcemia, which prolong repolarization

■ Severe bradyarrhythmias (e.g., complete heart block)

■ Miscellaneous factors, such as liquid protein diets

■ Hereditary long QT syndromes (see Fig. 19-8)

Recognition of torsades de pointes is critical because this type of potentially lethal ventricular tachycardia is often caused by drugs conventionally recommended for the treatment of arrhythmias. Therefore the therapy of torsades de pointes must include removing or correcting causative factors such as drug effects, electrolyte imbalance, or underlying bradycardia. In emergency settings, a temporary pacemaker may be inserted to accomplish "overdrive" suppression of the arrhythmia by increasing the underlying heart rate and shortening of the QT interval, thereby decreasing ventricular repolarization time and inhomogeneity. Intravenous magnesium sulfate has proved useful for suppressing this arrhythmia. Drug therapy with isoproterenol has been used in selected cases. Sustained episodes of torsades de pointes associated with cardiac arrest require attempted cardioversion. The arrhythmia usually recurs, however, unless causative factors are corrected.*

Polymorphic VT may also occur without QT prolongation (see Fig. 16-16), for example, in the setting of acute myocardial ischemia.

## VENTRICULAR FIBRILLATION

With VF (see Figs. 16-13 and 16-14), the ventricles do not beat in any coordinated fashion but instead fibrillate or quiver asynchronously and ineffectively. No cardiac output occurs, and the patient becomes unconscious immediately. VF is one of the three major ECG patterns seen with cardiac arrest. The other two are *brady-asystolic*

*patterns* and *pulseless electrical activity* (see Chapter 19).

The ECG in VF shows characteristic fibrillatory waves with an irregular pattern that may be either coarse or fine (see Fig. 16-13).

VF requires immediate defibrillation with an unsynchronized DC shock. Patients who have just been resuscitated from an episode of VF are generally given an immediate dose of an intravenous antiarrhythmic drug in an attempt to suppress further ventricular ectopy.

This lethal tachyarrhythmia can occur in patients with heart disease of any type. It may be preceded by a warning arrhythmia (e.g., VPBs or VT), or it may occur spontaneously. VF is the most common cause of *sudden cardiac death* (see Chapter 19) in patients with acute MI, although it may also occur in normal hearts, sometimes because of drugs (e.g., epinephrine, cocaine).

---

*Consult texts cited in the Bibliography for further discussions of torsades de pointes.

## REVIEW

Ventricular premature beats (VPBs) may occur normally or with organic heart disease. VPBs have the following characteristics:

1. They are premature, occurring before the next normal beat is expected.

2. They have an aberrant shape. The QRS complex is abnormally wide, usually 0.12 second or more in duration, and the T wave and QRS complex usually point in opposite directions.

VPBs may occur with varying frequency. Two in a row are called a *couplet*. Three or more in a row constitute *ventricular tachycardia (VT)*. When a VPB occurs regularly after each normal beat, the grouping is called *ventricular bigeminy*. When the rhythm is two normal beats followed

by a VPB, this grouping is termed *ventricular trigeminy.*

A VPB is often followed by a compensatory pause before the next beat. *Uniform* VPBs have the same shape in a single lead. *Multiform* VPBs have different shapes in the same lead.

A VPB occurring simultaneously with the apex of the T wave of the preceding beat is called an *R on T phenomenon*. It may be the precursor of VT or ventricular fibrillation (VF), particularly in the setting of acute myocardial infarction or long QT syndromes.

VT is a run of three or more VPBs. Short runs of VT are called *nonsustained*. In *sustained* VT, episodes last longer than 30 seconds and may lead to syncope or even cardiac arrest. VT may be classified as *monomorphic* or *polymorphic*. *Torsades de pointes* is a particular type of polymorphic VT associated with prolonged repolarization syndromes such as long QT(U) syndrome.

*Accelerated idioventricular rhythm (AIVR)* is a ventricular arrhythmia that resembles a slow VT with a rate between 50 and 100 beats/min. It is commonly seen with MI and is usually self-limited.

*Torsades de pointes* is a form of VT in which the QRS complexes in the same lead appear to twist periodically and turn in the opposite direction. It is generally seen in the setting of delayed ventricular repolarization (increased QT interval or prominent U waves) caused by drugs (quinidine, procainamide, disopyramide, dofetilide, ibutilide), electrolyte abnormalities (hypokalemia, hypomagnesemia), or other factors summarized in Chapter 24.

VF occurs when the ventricles stop beating and, instead, fibrillate or twitch in an ineffective fashion. It is one of the three major ECG patterns seen with cardiac arrest; the other two are *brady-asystole* and *pulseless electrical activity* (see Chapter 19).

## QUESTIONS

1. What is the arrhythmia shown below?

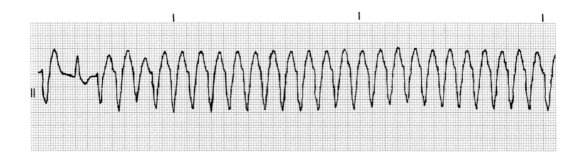

2. Which arrhythmia does this rhythm strip show?

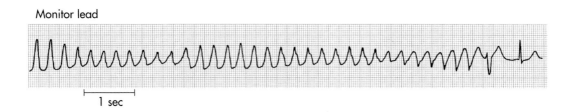

3. Name three potentially treatable causes of ventricular premature beats.

## 4. What is the arrhythmia here?

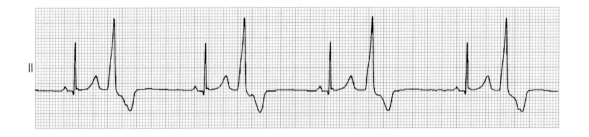

## CHAPTER 17

# Atrioventricular (AV) Heart Block

**H**eart block is the general term for atrioventricular (AV) conduction disturbances. Normally, the AV junction (AV node and His bundle area) acts as a bridge between the atria and ventricles. As mentioned in Chapter 2, the PR interval is primarily a measure of the lag in AV conduction between initial stimulation of the atria and initial stimulation of the ventricles. The normal PR interval in adults is between 0.12 and 0.2 second.

Heart block occurs when transmission through the AV junction is impaired either transiently or permanently (Table 17-1). The mildest form is called *first-degree heart block*. The term *first-degree AV block* is actually a misnomer, however, because the impulse is not blocked but delayed. Therefore a preferable term is *prolonged PR interval*. With first-degree heart block, the PR interval is uniformly prolonged beyond 0.2 second. *Second-degree heart block* is an intermediate grade of AV conduction disturbance in which impulse transmission between the atria and ventricles fails *intermittently.* The most extreme form is *third-degree* or *complete heart block.* In this case, the AV junction does not conduct any stimuli between the atria and ventricles. The present chapter describes these three degrees of heart block, along with the related topic *AV dissociation.*

## PROLONGED PR INTERVAL (FIRST-DEGREE AV BLOCK)

With first-degree heart block, the PR interval is prolonged beyond 0.2 second and is relatively constant from beat to beat (Fig. 17-1). A moderately prolonged PR interval does not produce symptoms or significant change in cardiac function. The PR interval may become prolonged for many reasons. Most factors that produce PR prolongation can also produce second- and third-degree block. For example, digitalis, which has a vagal effect on the AV junction, can produce any degree of heart block. Other drugs such as amiodarone, beta blockers, and calcium channel blockers (e.g., verapamil and diltiazem) can also severely depress AV conduction.

Patients with ischemic heart disease may have heart block of any degree. This finding may occur with chronic myocardial ischemia over a long time or with acute myocardial infarction (MI). Varying degrees of heart block are particularly common with inferior wall infarction because the right coronary artery, which generally supplies the inferior wall of the heart, also usually supplies the AV node. In addition, acute inferior MI is often associated with increased vagal tone. Heart block during inferior wall infarction tends to be transient.

| TABLE 17-1 | Classification of AV Heart Blocks |
| --- | --- |
| **Degree** | **AV Conduction Pattern** |
| First-degree block | Uniformly prolonged PR interval |
| Second-degree block* | Intermittent conduction failure* Mobitz type I (Wenckebach): progressive PR prolongation Mobitz type II: sudden conduction failure |
| Third-degree block | No atrioventricular conduction |

*Two special types are also designated: 2:1 AV block and advanced AV block (3:1, 4:1, and so on.)

Hyperkalemia may cause prolonged AV conduction. Other signs of hyperkalemia include peaking of the T waves and widening of the QRS complexes (see Chapter 10). Prolonged PR intervals may also occur with acute rheumatic fever. Not uncommonly, mild PR interval prolongation is seen as a normal variant, especially with physiologic sinus bradycardia during rest or sleep.

## SECOND-DEGREE AV BLOCK

Second-degree AV block is somewhat more complicated because it has two major types: *Mobitz type I block* (also called *Wenckebach block*) and *Mobitz type II block*.

### MOBITZ TYPE I (WENCKEBACH) AV BLOCK

With Mobitz type I or Wenckebach pattern, each stimulus from the atria to the ventricles appears to have a more difficult time passing through the AV junction. Finally the stimulus is not conducted at all. This *blocked beat* is followed by relative recovery of the AV junction, and the whole cycle starts again.

The characteristic ECG picture of Wenckebach block is progressive lengthening of the PR interval from beat to beat until a beat is "dropped." The dropped beat is a P wave that is not followed by a QRS complex, indicating failure of the AV junction to conduct the stimulus from the atria to the ventricles. Importantly, the PR interval after the nonconducted P wave is shorter than the PR interval of the beat just before the nonconducted P wave. Figure 17-2 diagrammatically depicts the Wenckebach phenomenon, and Figure 17-3 shows an actual example of this pattern. The number of P waves occurring before a QRS complex is "dropped" may vary. In many cases, just two or three conducted P waves are seen. In other cases, longer cycles are seen.

*What characterizes the classic Wenckebach pattern is (1) the sequence of a progressive lengthening of the PR interval followed by a nonconducted P wave, and then (2) shortening of the PR interval in the beat immediately after the nonconducted one.* (Not all cases of type I AV block, however, show the classic pattern of progressive PR prolongation before the nonconducted beat. In some cases, for example, the PR interval may not

### First-Degree AV Block

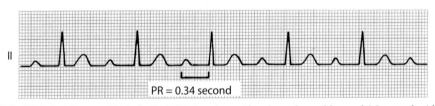

**FIGURE 17-1**  With first-degree AV block, the PR interval is uniformly prolonged beyond 0.2 second with each beat.

### Mobitz Type I (Wenckebach) Second-Degree AV Block

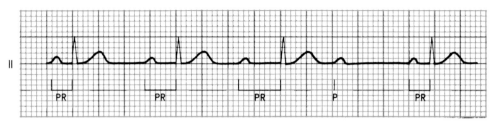

II

**FIGURE 17-2**  The PR interval lengthens progressively with successive beats until one sinus P wave is not conducted at all. Then the cycle repeats itself. Notice that the PR interval after the nonconducted P wave is shorter than the PR interval of the beat just before it.

### Mobitz Type I (Wenckebach) Second-Degree AV Block

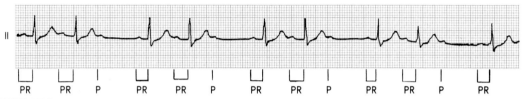

II

**FIGURE 17-3**  Notice the progressive increase in PR intervals, with the third sinus P wave in each sequence not followed by a QRS complex. Mobitz type I (Wenckebach) block produces a characteristically syncopated rhythm with grouping of the QRS complexes (group beating).

prolong noticeably. Even in such atypical cases, however, the PR interval after the nonconducted beat will always be shorter than the PR interval before it.)

As you can see from the examples, the Wenckebach cycle also produces a distinct clustering of QRS complexes separated by a pause that results from the dropped beat. Any time you encounter an ECG with this type of *group beating*, you should suspect a Wenckebach block and look for the diagnostic pattern of lengthening PR intervals.

Clinically, patients with the Wenckebach type of AV block are usually without symptoms unless the ventricular rate is very slow. The pulse rate is irregular.

Common causes of Wenckebach block include drugs such as beta blockers, calcium channel blockers (diltiazem and verapamil),

and digoxin. Wenckebach block is not uncommon with acute inferior wall MI. In such cases, it is usually transient and generally does not require any treatment except observation. Occasionally, these patients may progress into complete heart block. Of note, a physiologic increase in vagal tone may cause Wenckebach AV block in endurance athletes at rest or in young individuals during sleep.

## MOBITZ TYPE II SECOND-DEGREE AV BLOCK

Mobitz type II AV block is a rarer and more serious form of second-degree heart block. Its characteristic feature is the sudden appearance of a single, nonconducted sinus P wave without (1) the progressive prolongation of PR intervals seen in classic Mobitz type I (Wenckebach) AV block, and (2) shortening of the PR interval in

| TABLE 17-2 | Mobitz Type I and Mobitz Type II AV Blocks | |
|---|---|---|
| **Characteristic** | **Mobitz Type I** | **Mobitz Type II** |
| | 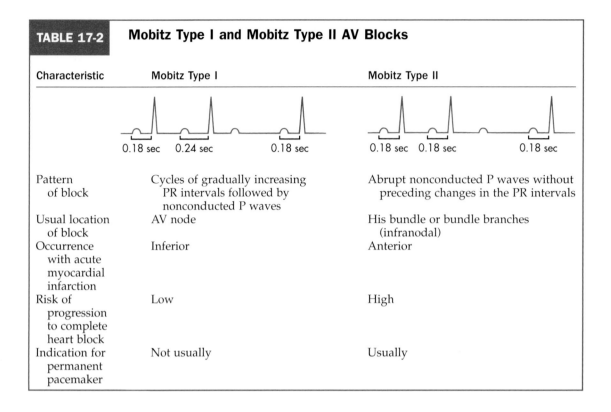 | |
| Pattern of block | Cycles of gradually increasing PR intervals followed by nonconducted P waves | Abrupt nonconducted P waves without preceding changes in the PR intervals |
| Usual location of block | AV node | His bundle or bundle branches (infranodal) |
| Occurrence with acute myocardial infarction | Inferior | Anterior |
| Risk of progression to complete heart block | Low | High |
| Indication for permanent pacemaker | Not usually | Usually |

the beat after the nonconducted P wave as seen with type I block.*

Mobitz type II block is generally a sign of severe conduction system disease involving the region below the AV node (i.e., the His-Purkinje system). Because Mobitz type II block often progresses into complete heart block, cardiologists generally consider it an indication for a pacemaker. Unlike Wenckebach AV block, Mobitz type II block is *not* usually caused by beta-blocker therapy, digitalis excess, or inferior wall MI. Mobitz type II block may be seen, however, with anterior wall MI, and these patients often progress into complete heart block. Therefore cardiologists generally treat patients with anterior wall MI and Mobitz type II AV block by inserting a pacemaker.

Mobitz I and Mobitz II AV blocks are compared in Table 17-2.

## ADVANCED SECOND-DEGREE AV BLOCK

The term *advanced second-degree AV block* refers to the distinct ECG finding of two or more consecutive nonconducted sinus P waves (Fig. 17-4). For example, with sinus rhythm and 3:1

*For clarification of a point of common confusion, it should be noted that 2:1 AV block per se does not necessarily indicate a Mobitz type II block. Not uncommonly, 2:1 AV block is due to a type I mechanism in which the block in the AV node occurs after every other P wave. In such cases a careful search of a long rhythm strip often reveals 3:2, 4:3, and other types of classic Wenckebach block in addition to the 2:1 periods. Furthermore, in most (but not all) cases of Wenckebach AV block, the QRS complex is of normal duration. By contrast, when 2:1 block is due to a type II mechanism, the His-Purkinje system (not just the AV node) is involved and the QRS duration is often prolonged. Thus 2:1 block with a narrow QRS complex most likely represents a type I mechanism. However, 2:1 block with a wide QRS complex may be due to either mechanism. Definitive assessment in any case of 2:1 block may require an intracardiac electrophysiologic study. Therefore pure 2:1 block should be labeled as such without specifying a type I or type II mechanism.

**Advanced Second-Degree AV Block**

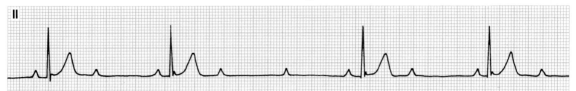

**FIGURE 17-4** Lead II recorded during a Holter monitor ECG in a patient with intermittent light-headedness. The recording shows sinus rhythm with 2:1 block alternating with 3:1 block (i.e., two consecutive nonconducted P waves followed by a conducted one). The term *advanced second-degree atrioventricular block* is applied when the ECG shows two or more nonconducted P waves in a row.

block, every third P wave is conducted; with 4:1 block, every fourth P wave is conducted, and so forth. This type of advanced block does not necessarily indicate a Mobitz II mechanism. However, unless advanced second-degree AV block has a reversible cause (e.g., drug toxicity or hyperkalemia), a permanent pacemaker is usually required.

## THIRD-DEGREE (COMPLETE) HEART BLOCK

First- and second-degree heart blocks are examples of *incomplete* block because the AV junction conducts at least some stimuli to the ventricles. With complete heart block, no stimuli are transmitted from the atria to the ventricles. Instead, the atria and ventricles are paced independently. The atria generally continue to be paced by the sinus node, or sinoatrial (SA) node. The

ventricles, however, are paced by an escape pacemaker located somewhere below the point of block in the AV junction. The resting ventricular rate with complete heart block may be lower than 30 beats/min or as high as 50 to 60 beats/min. The atrial rate is generally faster than the ventricular rate.

Examples of complete heart block are shown in Figures 17-5 and 17-6. The ECG with sinus rhythm and complete heart block has the following three characteristics:

- P waves are present, with a regular atrial rate faster than the ventricular rate.

- QRS complexes are present, with a slow (usually fixed) ventricular rate.

- The P waves bear no relation to the QRS complexes, and the PR intervals are completely variable because the atria and ventricles are electrically disconnected.

**Third-Degree (Complete) AV Block**

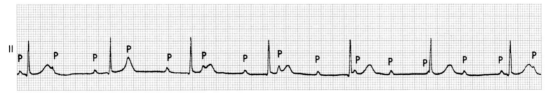

**FIGURE 17-5** Complete heart block with underlying sinus rhythm is characterized by independent atrial (P) and ventricular (QRS complex) activity. The atrial rate is almost always faster than the ventricular rate. The PR intervals are completely variable. Some sinus P waves fall on the T wave, distorting its shape. Others may fall in the QRS complex and be "lost." Notice that the QRS complexes are of normal width, indicating that the ventricles are being paced from the atrioventricular junction. Compare this example with Fig. 17-6, which shows complete heart block with wide, very slow QRS complexes because the ventricles are most likely being paced from below the atrioventricular junction (idioventricular pacemaker).

## Third-Degree (Complete) Heart Block

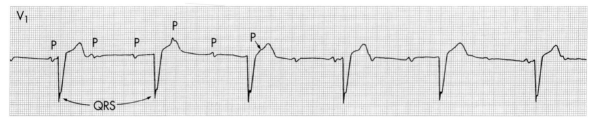

**FIGURE 17-6** This example of complete heart block shows a very slow idioventricular rhythm and a faster independent atrial (sinus) rhythm.

Complete heart block may also occur in patients whose basic atrial rhythm is flutter or fibrillation. In these cases, the ventricular rate is very slow and almost completely regular (see Fig. 15-10).

With complete heart block, the QRS complexes may be either of normal width (see Fig. 17-5) or abnormally wide (see Fig. 17-6) with the appearance of a bundle branch block pattern. The width of the QRS complexes depends in part on the location of the block in the AV junction. If the block is in the first part (the AV node), the ventricles are stimulated normally by a junctional pacemaker and the QRS complexes are narrow (see Fig. 17-5) unless the patient has an underlying bundle branch block. If the block is within, or particularly below, the bundle of His, the ventricles are paced by an *idioventricular pacemaker,** producing wide QRS complexes (see Fig. 17-6). As a general clinical rule, complete heart block with wide QRS complexes tends to be less stable than complete heart block with narrow QRS complexes because the ventricular escape pacemaker is usually slower and less consistent.

Complete heart block can occur for a number of reasons. It is most commonly seen in older patients who have chronic degenerative changes (sclerosis or fibrosis) in their conduction systems *not* related to MI. Digitalis intoxication, which can cause second-degree heart

block, may also lead to complete heart block (see Chapter 18). Varying degrees of AV block, including some cases of complete block, have been reported with Lyme disease. Complete heart block may occur abruptly after open heart surgery, particularly with aortic valve replacement. Complete heart block occurring with bacterial endocarditis is an ominous finding that suggests a perivalvular abscess involving the conduction system.

Complete heart block may also be seen acutely as a complication of MI. The course and therapy of complete heart block with MI depend to a large extent on whether the infarct is anterior or inferior. Transient AV conduction disturbances are commonly seen with acute inferior wall MI because of the common blood supply to the AV node and inferior wall (via the right coronary artery). Occlusion of the right coronary artery with inferior MI also often leads to temporary ischemia of the AV node, sometimes resulting in complete heart block. (In addition, acute inferior MI may cause an increase in vagal tone.) Complete heart block occurring with inferior wall MI is often a transient and reversible complication that does not usually require a temporary pacemaker unless the patient is hypotensive or is having concomitant episodes of tachyarrhythmia.

With acute anterior MI and complete heart block, the situation is more serious. Patients with anterior wall infarcts and complete heart block generally have extensive myocardial damage. The *idioventricular escape rhythm* that

---

*An idioventricular pacemaker may be located in the His-Purkinje system or the ventricular myocardium.

develops is usually slow and unstable. Therefore if complete heart block occurs with an acute anterior MI, cardiologists insert a temporary pacemaker (and subsequently a permanent one).

Regardless of its cause, complete heart block is a serious and potentially life-threatening arrhythmia. If the ventricular rate becomes too slow, the cardiac output drops and the patient may faint. Fainting spells associated with complete heart block (or other types of bradycardia) are referred to as *Stokes-Adams attacks*. In some patients, complete heart block is a chronic and persistent finding. In others, the block may occur transiently and may be recognized only with more prolonged monitoring.

## BIFASCICULAR BLOCK, TRIFASCICULAR BLOCK, AND COMPLETE HEART BLOCK

Cardiologists have been interested in developing criteria to predict which patients with acute MI (particularly, anterior wall infarcts) will develop life-threatening complete heart block. Current information suggests that certain high-risk patients can be identified, although precise predictions are not possible. Specifically, patients with acute anterior wall MI and complete heart block often have other conduction disturbances before the onset of complete heart block. These conduction disturbances are referred to as *bifascicular blocks*.

Recall from Chapter 7 that the ventricular conduction system is *trifascicular*, consisting of the right bundle branch and the left bundle branch, the latter further dividing into left anterior and left posterior fascicles. Blockage of just the left anterior fascicle produces left anterior fascicular block (hemiblock) with left axis deviation (LAD). Blockage of just the left posterior fascicle produces left posterior fascicular block (hemiblock) with right axis deviation (RAD). Bifascicular block indicates blockage of any two of the three fascicles. For example, right bundle branch block (RBBB) with left anterior fascicu-

lar block produces an RBBB pattern with marked LAD (see Figs. 8-20 and 17-7); RBBB with left posterior fascicular block (Fig. 17-8) produces an RBBB pattern with RAD (provided other causes of RAD, especially right ventricular hypertrophy and lateral MI, are excluded). Similarly, a complete LBBB may indicate blockage of both the anterior and posterior fascicles.

Bifascicular blocks are potentially significant because they make ventricular conduction dependent on the single remaining fascicle. Additional damage to this third remaining fascicle may completely block AV conduction, producing complete heart block *(trifascicular block)*. Therefore the acute development of new bifascicular block (especially with a prolonged PR interval) during an acute anterior wall MI is an important warning signal of possible impending complete heart block.

An important distinction must be made between *acute* bifascicular blocks occurring with anterior wall MI (see Fig. 8-20) and *chronic* bifascicular blocks (Figs. 17-7 and 17-8). Many asymptomatic people have ECGs resembling the one in Figure 17-7 showing RBBB with left axis deviation due to left anterior fascicular block. Patients with chronic bifascicular block of this kind do not generally require a permanent pacemaker unless they develop second- or third-degree AV block (Fig. 17-9). The risk of complete heart block in asymptomatic patients with *chronic* bifascicular block is relatively low. By contrast, patients with acute anterior MI in whom bifascicular block suddenly occurs have a poor prognosis because of underlying extensive myocardial necrosis, and they are also at higher risk of abruptly developing complete heart block.

## AV DISSOCIATION

Cardiologists use the term *AV dissociation* in two related though not identical ways. This classification continues to cause considerable (and understandable) confusion among students and clinicians.

## Bifascicular Block: Right Bundle Branch Block with Left Anterior Fascicular Block

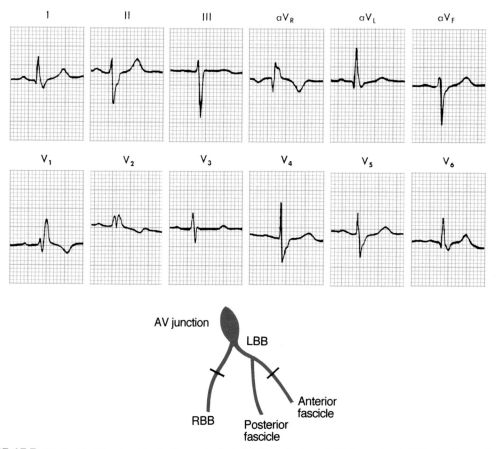

**FIGURE 17-7** Notice that the chest leads show a typical right bundle branch block pattern (rSR' in lead $V_1$ and qRS in lead $V_6$). The limb leads show marked left axis deviation (mean QRS axis about $-60°$), consistent with left anterior hemiblock. Thus a bifascicular block involving the right bundle branch (RBB) and the anterior fascicle of the left bundle branch (LBB) system is present (as shown in the diagram). AV, atrioventricular.

AV dissociation is widely used as a *general* term for any arrhythmia in which the atria and ventricles are controlled by independent pacemakers. The definition includes complete heart block, as well as some instances of ventricular tachycardia in which the atria remain in sinus rhythm (see Chapter 16).

AV dissociation is also used as a more *specific* term to describe a particular family of arrhythmias that are often mistaken for complete heart block. With this type of AV dissociation, the SA node and AV junction appear to be "out of synch"; thus the SA node loses its normal control of the ventricular rate. As a result, the atria and ventricles are paced independently—the atria from the SA node, the ventricles from the AV junction. This situation is similar to what occurs with complete heart block. *With AV dissociation, however, the ventricular rate is the same as or slightly faster than the atrial rate.* When the

## Bifascicular Block: Right Bundle Branch Block with Left Posterior Fascicular Block

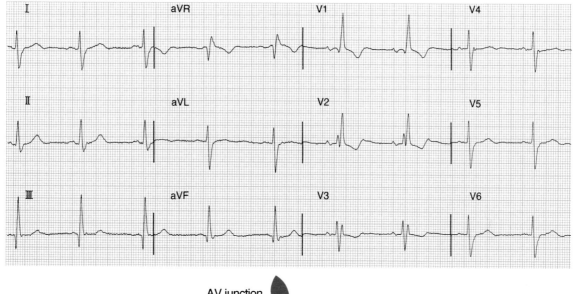

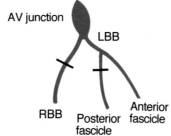

**FIGURE 17-8** Notice that the chest leads, as in Fig. 17-7, show a typical right bundle branch block (RBBB) pattern. The limb leads show prominent right axis deviation (RAD). The combination of these two findings (in the absence of other more common causes of RAD such as right ventricular hypertrophy or lateral MI) is consistent with chronic bifascicular block due to left posterior fascicular block in concert with the RBBB. This elderly patient had severe coronary artery disease. The Q waves in leads III and aVF are consistent with prior inferior MI. Left atrial abnormality is also present.

atrial and ventricular rates are almost the same, the term *isorhythmic AV dissociation* is used. (*Iso* is the Greek root for "same.")

The critical difference between AV dissociation (resulting from "desynchronization" of the SA and AV nodes) and actual complete heart block (resulting from true conduction failure) is as follows: with AV dissociation (e.g., isorhythmic) a properly timed P wave can be conducted through the AV node, whereas with complete heart block no P wave reaches the ventricles.

AV dissociation (Fig. 17-10) therefore can be regarded as a "competition" between the SA node and the AV node for control of the heartbeat. It may occur either when the SA node slows down (e.g., because of the effects of beta blockers or calcium channel blockers or with increased vagal tone) or when the AV node is accelerated (e.g., by ischemia or digitalis toxicity). Not uncommonly, isorhythmic AV dissociation is seen in healthy young individuals, particularly when they are sleeping.

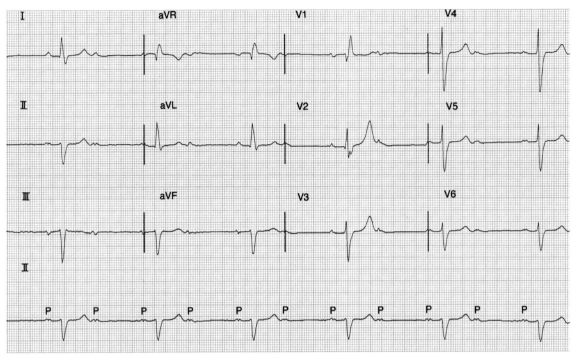

**FIGURE 17-9** This elderly patient with chronic bifascicular block (RBBB and left anterior fascicular block) developed 2:1 heart block, probably due to a block below the AV node (infranodal block). A dual chamber pacemaker was implanted. (The broad notched P waves here indicate left atrial abnormality.)

## Isorhythmic AV Dissociation

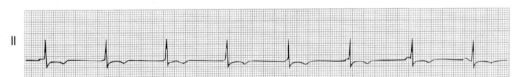

**FIGURE 17-10** This common type of AV dissociation is characterized by transient desynchronization of the sinus and AV node pacemakers such that they beat at nearly the same rate. Because they are "out of synch" with each other, the P waves (representing the sinus node pacemaker) appear to "slide" in and out of the QRS (representing the AV junction pacemaker). This type of AV dissociation, a minor arrhythmia due to desynchronization of SA and AV nodes, must be distinguished from actual complete AV block, a life-threatening conduction problem (compare with Figs. 17-5 and 17-6).

Figure 17-10 presents an example of isorhythmic AV dissociation. Notice the P waves with a variable PR interval because the ventricular (QRS) rate is nearly the same as the atrial rate. At times, the P waves may merge with the QRS complexes and become imperceptible for several beats. If the sinus rate speeds up sufficiently (or the AV junctional rate slows), the stimulus may be able to penetrate the AV junction, reestablishing sinus rhythm.

# REVIEW

Three types of atrioventricular (AV) heart block may occur:

1. With PR interval prolongation, or *first-degree block*, the PR interval is uniformly prolonged beyond 0.2 second.

2. *Second-degree* heart block has two major types, with two specific subtypes designated:
   a. In *Mobitz type I (Wenckebach) block*, the PR interval becomes increasingly prolonged until a P wave is blocked and not followed by a QRS complex; this produces a distinctive clustering of QRS complexes separated by a pause resulting from the nonconducted beat (known as *group beating*). Further, the PR interval just after the nonconducted P wave is shorter than the PR interval just before it.
   b. In *Mobitz type II block*, a single nonconducted sinus P wave appears suddenly without prolongation of the preceding PR interval; in addition, the PR interval after the nonconducted P wave is the same as the one before it.
   c. Two special subtypes have been designated: *2:1 AV block*, which may be due to a nodal or infranodal block, and *advanced second-degree atrioventricular block*, in which two or more nonconducted P waves are present (i.e., 3:1 or 4:1 block).

3. Third-degree (complete) block shows the following:

   a. Atria and ventricles that beat independently because stimuli cannot pass through the AV junction
   b. An atrial rate that is almost always faster than the ventricular rate
   c. A PR interval that is constantly changing

Complete heart block with acute anterior wall myocardial infarction (MI) is sometimes preceded by the sudden appearance of *bifascicular block* (right bundle branch block with left anterior or posterior fascicular block or a new complete left bundle branch block). Patients with *chronic* bifascicular block who have no symptoms, however, usually do not require any special therapy.

The significance of complete heart block with acute MI depends on the location of the infarct. Complete heart block occurring with acute inferior wall MI is usually transient and can sometimes be managed without a pacemaker. By contrast, complete heart block with acute anterior wall MI is usually associated with a very poor prognosis and requires a pacemaker.

Complete heart block must be distinguished from other forms of *AV dissociation*. With *isorhythmic* AV dissociation, the atria and ventricles beat independently; however, the ventricular rate is about the same as the atrial rate. AV dissociation of this type is a minor, usually transient arrhythmia.

Current guidelines for pacemaker therapy of AV heart block syndromes are given on the websites of the American Heart Association and the American College of Cardiology.

# QUESTIONS

1. The rhythm strip below shows sinus rhythm with which of the following?

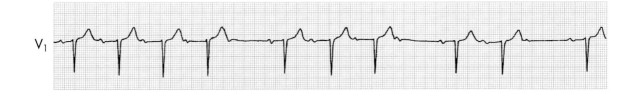

    a. Wenckebach-type second-degree atrioventricular (AV) block
    b. Complete heart block
    c. 3:1 AV block
    d. AV dissociation
    e. Blocked premature atrial beats

2. Based on the rhythm strip below, answer the following questions:

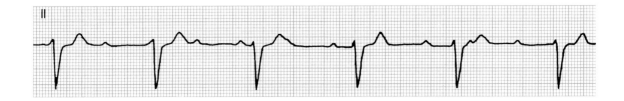

    a. What is the approximate atrial (P wave) rate?
    b. What is the approximate ventricular (QRS) rate?
    c. Is the PR interval constant?
    d. What is the ECG abnormality shown?

3. *True or false:* Complete heart block may occur with underlying atrial fibrillation.

## CHAPTER 18

# Digitalis Toxicity

This chapter focuses on the arrhythmias and conduction disturbances caused by digitalis toxicity. This subject is included in an introductory textbook for several reasons. The most important is that digitalis glycosides (mainly digoxin) are still frequently prescribed and digitalis toxicity remains an important clinical problem. Furthermore, digitalis toxicity can cause fatal arrhythmias. Therefore, all clinicians should strive to prevent and recognize digitalis toxicity early. Finally, because digitalis toxicity can produce a wide variety of arrhythmias and all degrees of heart block, this topic provides a convenient review of material presented in previous chapters.

## BASIC AND CLINICAL BACKGROUND

*Digitalis* refers to a class of cardioactive drugs called glycosides that have specific effects on the mechanical and electrical function of the heart. The most commonly used digitalis preparation in current practice is digoxin.

Digitalis is used in clinical practice for two major reasons. First, in selected patients with dilated hearts and congestive heart failure (CHF), it increases the strength of myocardial contractions. This effect is its *mechanical* action. Second, it affects the conductivity of certain heart tissues. This is its *electrical* action. Thus digitalis is useful for treating selected arrhythmias. Its antiarrhythmic action results primarily from its slowing of conduction through the atri-

oventricular (AV) junction (node) as the result of an increase in vagal tone. Consequently, digitalis is used for controlling the ventricular response in atrial fibrillation (AF) and atrial flutter, which are characterized by the excessive transmission of stimuli from the atria to the ventricles through the AV junction. In addition, it is sometimes still used in the treatment of certain reentrant types of paroxysmal supraventricular tachycardia (PSVT).

Although digitalis has continued indications in the treatment of heart failure and selected supraventricular arrhythmias, it also has a relatively low margin of safety. The difference between therapeutic and toxic concentrations is narrow.

The basic mechanisms involved in digitalis-related arrhythmias are complex and incompletely understood. Bradyarrhythmias may be due to excessive increases in vagal tone caused by digitalis. Increased automaticity and tachycardias may be due at least in part to activating effects of toxic doses of digitalis on the sympathetic nervous system. The automaticity of certain cardiac cells may also be directly increased by the calcium loading effects of digitalis.

## SIGNS OF DIGITALIS TOXICITY

Digitalis toxicity can produce general systemic symptoms as well as specific cardiac arrhythmias and conduction disturbances. Common

---

| **BOX 18-1** | **Arrhythmias and Conduction Disturbances Caused by Digitalis Toxicity** |

**Bradycardias**

Sinus bradycardia (including sinoatrial block)
Junctional (nodal) escape rhythms*
Atrioventricular (AV) heart block, including
   Mobitz type I (Wenckebach) AV block and
   complete heart block*

**Tachycardias**

Accelerated or junctional rhythm such as
   nonparoxysmal or junctional tachycardia*
Atrial tachycardia with block
Ventricular ectopy, including ventricular
   premature beats, monomorphic ventricular
   tachycardia, bidirectional ventricular
   tachycardia, and ventricular fibrillation

---

*These arrhythmias and conduction disturbances may occur with underlying atrial fibrillation leading to slow or regularized ventricular response. AV dissociation without complete heart block may also occur.

extracardiac symptoms include weakness, anorexia, nausea, and vomiting. Visual effects (altered color perception) and mental changes may occur. This section of the chapter concentrates on the arrhythmias and conduction disturbances produced by digitalis excess.

As a general clinical rule, *virtually any arrhythmia and all degrees of AV heart block can be produced by digitalis intoxication.* Of all the arrhythmias discussed in this book, AF and atrial flutter with a rapid ventricular response are the *least* likely to be caused by digitalis toxicity. A number of other arrhythmias and conduction disturbances, however, are commonly seen with digitalis toxicity (Box 18-1).

## VENTRICULAR ARRHYTHMIAS

Ventricular premature beats (VPBs) are often the first sign of digitalis toxicity. Isolated VPBs may occur at first. Ventricular bigeminy (Fig. 18-1), with each normal beat followed by a VPB, is common. Ventricular tachycardia (VT) and

fatal ventricular fibrillation (VF) may occur if digitalis toxicity is not recognized and treated (see Chapter 16).

## BIDIRECTIONAL VENTRICULAR TACHYCARDIA

*Bidirectional* VT (Fig. 18-2) is a special type of VT in which each successive beat in any lead alternates in direction. This distinctive tachyarrhythmia should always raise the question of digitalis intoxication.

## AV JUNCTIONAL (NODAL) RHYTHMS

AV junctional rhythms are frequently a sign of digitalis toxicity.* Most AV junctional rhythms resulting from excessive digitalis have a rate of less than 130 beats/min.

## SINUS BRADYCARDIA AND SINOATRIAL BLOCK

Sinus bradycardia may be one of the earliest signs of digitalis excess. Sinoatrial (SA) block with sinus arrest may also occur.

## ATRIAL TACHYCARDIA WITH AV BLOCK

Atrial tachycardia (AT) with AV block is another tachyarrhythmia that has not been discussed in earlier chapters (an example appears in Figure 18-3). This arrhythmia is usually characterized by regular, rapid P waves occurring at a rate between 150 and 250 beats/min and, because of the AV block, a slower ventricular rate. Not uncommonly, 2:1 AV block is present so that the ventricular rate is half the atrial rate. Mobitz type I (Wenckebach) AV block is also common. Digitalis toxicity is an important but not the only cause of these arrhythmias. Superficially, AT with block may resemble atrial flutter; however, in AT with block, the baseline between P waves is isoelectric. Furthermore, when atrial

---

*Two classes of junctional (nodal) rhythms may occur: (1) a typical junctional escape rhythm with a rate of 60 beats/min or less, and (2) an accelerated junctional rhythm (also called nonparoxysmal junctional tachycardia) at a rate of about 60 to 130 beats/min.

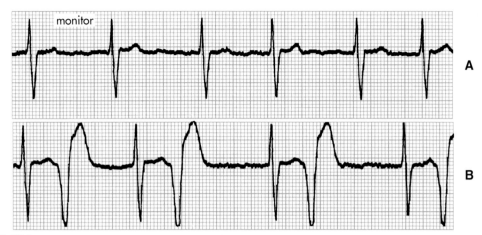

**FIGURE 18-1**   Ventricular bigeminy caused by digitalis toxicity. Ventricular ectopy is one of the most common signs of digitalis toxicity. **A,** The underlying rhythm is atrial fibrillation. **B,** Each normal QRS complex is followed by a ventricular premature beat.

## Bidirectional Ventricular Tachycardia

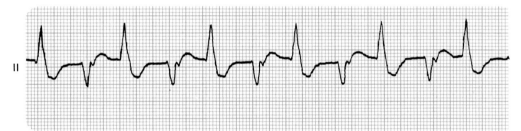

**FIGURE 18-2**   This digitalis-toxic arrhythmia is a special type of ventricular tachycardia with QRS complexes that alternate in direction from beat to beat. No P waves are present.

## Atrial Tachycardia with Block

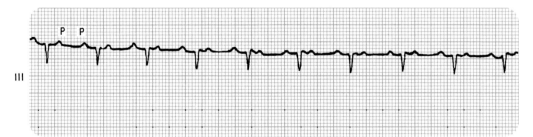

**FIGURE 18-3**   This rhythm strip shows atrial tachycardia (about 200 beats/min) with 2:1 block, producing a ventricular rate of about 100 beats/min.

flutter is present, the atrial rate is faster (usually 250 to 350 beats/min).

## AV HEART BLOCK AND AV DISSOCIATION

Because digitalis slows conduction through the AV junction, it is not surprising that toxic doses can result in any degree of AV heart block.

### First-Degree Block

With first-degree AV block, PR intervals are uniformly prolonged beyond 0.2 second. Some degree of PR lengthening may be expected with digitalis therapy. More marked widening of the PR interval suggests early digitalis toxicity.

### Second-Degree Block

With higher doses of digitalis, PR prolongation may progress to second-degree block of the Mobitz type I (Wenckebach) variety.

### Complete Heart Block

Third-degree, or complete, heart block may also occur with digitalis toxicity.

Digitalis toxicity can cause other types of AV dissociation as well (see Chapter 17).

## ATRIAL FIBRILLATION OR FLUTTER WITH SLOW VENTRICULAR RATE

Rarely, digitalis causes AF and atrial flutter with a rapid ventricular response. In such cases, the toxicity is often shown by marked slowing of the ventricular rate to less than 50 beats/min (Fig. 18-4) and/or the appearance of VPBs. In some cases, the earliest sign of digitalis toxicity

in a patient with AF may be a subtle *regularization* of the ventricular rate. The need for potentially toxic doses of digoxin to control the ventricular rate in AF has been obviated by the availability of other drugs (beta blockers and calcium channel blockers) and AV nodal ablation procedures (see Chapter 15).

In summary, digitalis toxicity causes a number of important arrhythmias and conduction disturbances. Therefore, because of the frequency and potential lethality of digitalis toxicity, you should suspect this problem in any patient taking a digitalis preparation who has an unexplained arrhythmia, until you can prove otherwise.

## FACTORS PREDISPOSING TO DIGITALIS TOXICITY

A number of factors significantly increase the hazard of digitalis intoxication (Box 18-2). For example, a low serum potassium concentration increases the likelihood of certain digitalis-induced arrhythmias, particularly ventricular ectopy and AT with block. Hypokalemia is not uncommon in patients who are taking digitalis because these patients frequently receive diuretics for the treatment of heart failure and edema. The serum potassium concentration must be checked periodically in any patient taking digitalis and in every patient suspected of having digitalis toxicity.

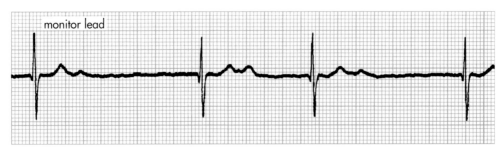

**FIGURE 18-4** Atrial fibrillation with an excessively slow ventricular rate because of digitalis toxicity. Atrial fibrillation with a rapid ventricular rate is rarely caused by digitalis toxicity. In patients with underlying atrial fibrillation, however, digitalis toxicity is sometimes manifested by excessive slowing or regularization of the QRS rate.

**Predisposing Factors for Digitalis Toxicity**

Cardiac amyloidosis
Chronic lung disease
Hypercalcemia
Hypertrophic cardiomyopathy (an inherited
　　heart condition associated with excessive
　　cardiac contractility)
Hypokalemia
Hypomagnesemia
Hypothyroidism
Hypoxemia
Myocardial infarction
Old age
Renal insufficiency
Wolff-Parkinson-White syndrome and atrial
　　fibrillation

Hypomagnesemia occurs in a variety of settings, including alcoholism, intestinal malabsorption, and diuretic therapy. Hypercalcemia is seen with hyperparathyroidism and certain tumors, among other conditions. Both hypomagnesemia and hypercalcemia can be predisposing factors for digitalis toxicity.

Hypoxemia and chronic lung disease may also increase the risk of digitalis toxicity, probably because they are associated with increased sympathetic tone. Patients with acute myocardial infarction (MI) or ischemia appear to be more sensitive to digitalis. Patients with hypothyroidism appear to be more sensitive to the effects of digitalis.

Digoxin, the most widely used preparation of digitalis, is excreted primarily in the urine. Therefore, any degree of renal insufficiency, as measured by increased blood urea nitrogen (BUN) and creatinine concentrations, requires a lower maintenance dose of digoxin. Thus elderly patients may be more susceptible to digitalis toxicity, in part because of decreased renal excretion of the drug.

Even therapeutic levels of digoxin can be dangerous in certain special clinical settings.

For example, digitalis may worsen the symptoms of patients with hypertrophic cardiomyopathy, an inherited heart condition associated with excessive cardiac contractility. Patients with heart failure due to amyloidosis are also extremely sensitive to digitalis. In patients with the Wolff-Parkinson-White syndrome and AF (see Chapter 20), digitalis may facilitate extremely rapid transmission of impulses down the atrioventricular bypass tract, leading to a potentially lethal tachycardia (see Fig. 20-10A).

## TREATMENT OF DIGITALIS TOXICITY

The first step in treatment is prevention. Before any patient is started on digoxin or a related drug, the indications should be carefully reviewed. Some patients continue to receive digoxin or related drugs for inappropriate reasons. The patient should have a baseline ECG, serum electrolytes, and BUN and creatinine measurements. Serum magnesium blood levels should also be considered, particularly if indicated by diuretic therapy and other factors. Additional considerations include the patient's age and pulmonary status, as well as whether the patient is having an acute MI. Early signs of digitalis toxicity (e.g., VPBs, sinus bradycardia, or increasing AV block) should be carefully checked. Furthermore, concomitant administration of a number of different drugs (including amiodarone, propafenone, quinidine, and verapamil) increases the digoxin level.

Definitive treatment of digitalis toxicity depends on the particular arrhythmia. With minor arrhythmias (e.g., isolated VPBs, sinus bradycardia, prolonged PR interval, Wenckebach AV block or AV junctional rhythms), discontinuation of digitalis and careful observation are usually adequate. More serious arrhythmias (e.g., prolonged VT) may require suppression with an intravenous drug such as lidocaine. For tachycardias with hypokalemia, potassium supplements should be given to raise the serum potassium level to well within normal limits.

Patients with complete heart block from digitalis toxicity may require a temporary pacemaker while the effect of the digitalis dissipates, particularly if they have symptoms of syncope, hypotension, or CHF. In other cases, complete heart block can be managed conservatively while the digitalis wears off.

Occasionally, patients present with a large overdose of digitalis taken inadvertently or in a suicide attempt. In such cases, the serum digoxin level is markedly elevated, and severe brady- or tachyarrhythmias may develop. In addition, massive digitalis toxicity may cause life-threatening *hyperkalemia* because the drug blocks the cell membrane mechanism that pumps potassium into the cells in exchange for sodium. Patients with a potentially lethal overdose of digitalis can be treated with a special digitalis-binding antibody given intravenously (digoxin immune Fab [antigen-binding fragment; Digibind]).

Finally, *direct-current electrical cardioversion of arrhythmias in patients who have digitalis toxicity is extremely hazardous and may precipitate fatal ventricular tachycardia and fibrillation.* Therefore, you should not electrically cardiovert any patient who has atrial tachycardia with block, AF, or atrial flutter and is suspected of having digitalis toxicity.

## SERUM DIGOXIN LEVELS

The concentration of digoxin in the serum can be measured by means of radioimmunoassay. "Therapeutic concentrations" are reported to range from about 0.5 to 2 ng/mL in most laboratories. Concentrations exceeding 2 ng/mL are associated with a very high incidence of digitalis toxicity. In ordering a test of digoxin level in a patient, you must be aware that "therapeutic levels" do not rule out the possibility of digitalis toxicity. As previously mentioned, some patients are more sensitive to digitalis and may show signs of toxicity with "therapeutic" levels. For most patients being treated for systolic heart failure or atrial fibrillation, it is safest to keep the digoxin levels at the low end of the therapeutic range.

In other patients, factors such as hypokalemia or hypomagnesemia may potentiate digitalis toxicity despite a therapeutic serum level. Although a "high" digoxin level does not necessarily indicate overt digitalis toxicity, these patients should be examined for early evidence of digitalis excess, including extracardiac symptoms (e.g., gastrointestinal symptoms) and all cardiac effects that have been discussed. Efforts should be made to keep the digoxin level well within therapeutic bounds; lower levels appear to be as efficacious as (and safer than) higher ones in the treatment of heart failure. (A spuriously high digoxin level may be obtained if blood is drawn within a few hours of the administration of digoxin.)

## DIGITALIS TOXICITY VS. DIGITALIS EFFECT

*Digitalis toxicity*, which refers to the arrhythmias and conduction disturbances produced by this drug, should not be confused with digitalis effect. *Digitalis effect* (see Fig. 10-1) refers to the distinct scooping of the ST-T complex (associated with shortening of the QT) typically seen in patients taking digitalis glycosides. The presence of digitalis effect by itself does not imply digitalis toxicity and may be seen at therapeutic doses.

# REVIEW

Digitalis toxicity can produce almost any arrhythmia and all degrees of AV heart block.

Atrial fibrillation or atrial flutter with a rapid ventricular response rarely occurs as a result of digitalis toxicity. Furthermore, digitalis toxicity does not produce bundle branch blocks.

Factors such as renal failure, hypokalemia, hypercalcemia, hypomagnesemia, hypoxemia, old age, and acute myocardial infarction are predisposing factors for digitalis toxicity. The concomitant administration of certain drugs (e.g., quinidine, verapamil, amiodarone, propafenone) also increases serum digoxin levels.

Digitalis toxicity should not be confused with digitalis effect. *Digitalis effect* refers to the shortening of the QT interval and scooping of the ST-T complex produced by *therapeutic* doses of digitalis.

# QUESTIONS

1. Name three factors that can potentiate digitalis toxicity.

   *True or false* (2 to 7):
2. Ventricular premature beats are a frequent manifestation of digitalis toxicity.

3. Atrial fibrillation with a rapid ventricular response is a common manifestation of digitalis toxicity.

4. Left bundle branch block may result from digitalis toxicity.

5. Mobitz type I (Wenckebach) AV block may be caused by digitalis toxicity.

6. A therapeutic digoxin level indicates that digitalis toxicity is not present.

7. DC cardioversion is very hazardous in the presence of digitalis toxicity and may lead to ventricular fibrillation.

## CHAPTER 19

# Cardiac Arrest and Sudden Cardiac Death

The preceding chapters systematically discussed the major disorders of heart rhythm and atrioventricular (AV) conduction. Instead of considering entirely new ECG patterns, this chapter reviews some earlier topics, placing them in a special clinical perspective. The subject of this chapter is the recognition of life-threatening arrhythmias that cause cardiac arrest. By definition, *cardiac arrest occurs when the heart stops contracting effectively and ceases to pump blood.* The important and closely related topic of *sudden cardiac death* is also introduced.

## CLINICAL ASPECTS OF CARDIAC ARREST

The patient in cardiac arrest loses consciousness within seconds and may even have a seizure as a result of inadequate blood flow to the brain. Irreversible brain damage usually occurs within 4 minutes and sometimes sooner. Furthermore, shortly after the heart stops pumping, spontaneous breathing also ceases *(cardiopulmonary arrest)*. Respiration sometimes stops first (primary respiratory arrest) and cardiac activity stops shortly thereafter.

*The diagnosis of cardiac arrest should be made clinically even before the patient is connected to an ECG machine.* Laypeople should immediately recognize cardiac arrest in any unresponsive person who is not breathing. Trained clinicians should examine the patient very quickly by trying to feel for pulses in the carotid arteries. The patient in cardiac arrest becomes cyanotic (bluish gray) from lack of oxygenated blood. No heart tones are audible with a stethoscope placed on the chest, and the blood pressure is, of course, unobtainable. The arms and legs become cool. If the brain becomes severely hypoxic, the pupils are fixed and dilated. Seizure activity may occur. However, *the absence of pulses in an unresponsive individual is the major diagnostic sign of cardiac arrest.*

When cardiac arrest is recognized, *cardiopulmonary resuscitation* (CPR) must be started without delay. In capsule form, the initial basic life support treatment of any cardiac arrest consists of the following four (*A, B, C, D*) steps:

- Establish an *Airway*.
- *Breathe* for the patient, either by mouth-to-mouth or mouth-to-mask methods or by

manually compressing a bag-valve device, forcing air into the patient's nose or mouth.

- Maintain Circulation by external cardiac compression.

- Defibrillate the heart.

The specific details of CPR and advanced cardiac life support, including intubation, drug dosages, the use of automatic emergency defibrillators (AEDs) and standard defibrillators, along with other matters related to definitive diagnosis and treatment, lie outside the scope of this book but are discussed in selected references cited in the Bibliography. This chapter concentrates on the particular ECG patterns seen during cardiac arrest and the clinical implications of these major abnormalities.

*Initial treatment with ventilation and external cardiac compression should never be delayed while the patient in cardiac arrest is being connected to an ECG recorder.*

## BASIC ECG PATTERNS IN CARDIAC ARREST

The three basic ECG patterns seen with cardiac arrest were mentioned in earlier chapters.

Cardiac arrest may be associated with the following:

- Ventricular tachyarrhythmia, including ventricular fibrillation (VF) or a sustained type of pulseless ventricular tachycardia (VT)

- Ventricular asystole or a brady-asystolic rhythm with an extremely slow rate

- Pulseless electrical activity (PEA), also referred to as *electromechanical dissociation (EMD)*

The ECG patterns seen in cardiac arrest are briefly reviewed in the following sections, with emphasis placed on their clinical implications (Figs. 19-1 to 19-6).

## VENTRICULAR TACHYARRHYTHMIA (VF OR PULSELESS VT)

With VF, the ventricles do not contract but instead twitch rapidly in a completely ineffective way. No cardiac output occurs, and the patient loses consciousness within seconds. The characteristic ECG pattern, with its unmistakable fast oscillatory waves, is illustrated in Figure 19-1.

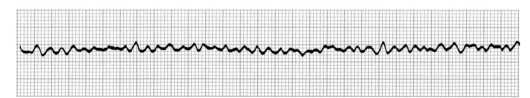

**FIGURE 19-1** Ventricular fibrillation causing cardiac arrest.

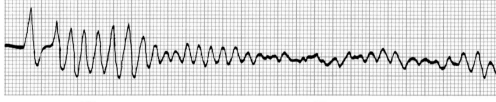

VT                                    VF

**FIGURE 19-2** Ventricular tachycardia (VT) and ventricular fibrillation (VF) recorded during cardiac arrest (monitor leads). The rapid sine-wave type of ventricular tachycardia seen here is sometimes referred to as *ventricular flutter*.

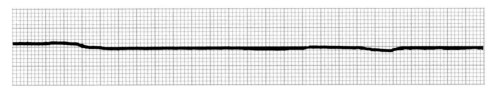

**FIGURE 19-3**  Complete ventricular standstill (asystole) producing a straight-line pattern during cardiac arrest.

## Cardiac Arrest: Brady-Asystolic Patterns

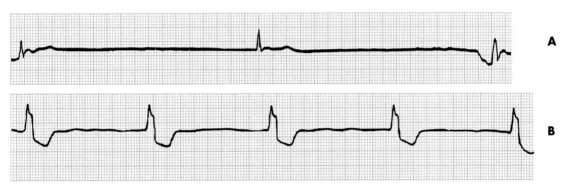

A

B

**FIGURE 19-4**  Escape rhythms with underlying ventricular standstill (monitor leads). **A,** Junctional escape rhythm with narrow QRS complexes. **B,** Idioventricular escape rhythm with wide QRS complexes. Treatment should include the use of intravenous atropine and, if needed, sympathomimetic drugs in an attempt to speed up these bradycardias, which cannot support the circulation. If hyperkalemia is present, it should be treated.

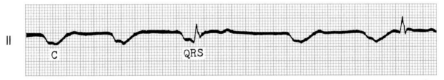

**FIGURE 19-5**  External cardiac compression artifact. External cardiac compression during resuscitation produces artifactual ECG complexes (C), which may be mistaken for *QRS* complexes.

Of the three basic ECG patterns seen with cardiac arrest, VF is the most common one encountered initially. It may appear spontaneously, although as noted in Chapter 16, it often is preceded by another ventricular arrhythmia (usually VT or premature ventricular beats). Figure 19-2 shows a run of VT degenerating into VF during cardiac arrest.

The treatment of VF was described in Chapter 16. The patient should be immediately defibrillated, with a *defibrillator (cardioverter)* used to administer a direct-current electric shock to the heart by means of paddles placed on the chest wall. An example of successful defibrillation is presented in Figure 19-6*D.*

Success in defibrillating any patient depends on a number of factors. *The single most important factor in treating ventricular fibrillation is haste: the less delay in defibrillation, the greater the chance of succeeding.*

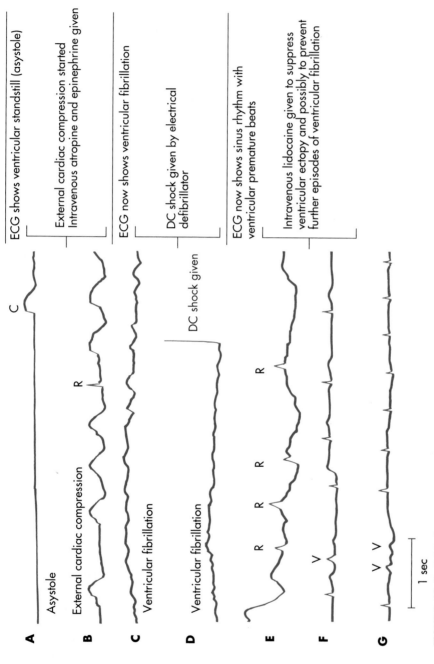

**A** Asystole

**B** External cardiac compression

R

**C** Ventricular fibrillation

**D** Ventricular fibrillation

DC shock given

**E**   R   R   R

**F**   V   R

**G**   V   V

1 sec

ECG shows ventricular standstill (asystole)

External cardiac compression started
Intravenous atropine and epinephrine given

ECG now shows ventricular fibrillation

DC shock given by electrical defibrillator

ECG now shows sinus rhythm with ventricular premature beats

Intravenous lidocaine given to suppress ventricular ectopy and possibly to prevent further episodes of ventricular fibrillation

**FIGURE 19-6**   ECG "history" of cardiac arrest and successful resuscitation. The left panel shows the ECG sequence during an actual cardiac arrest. The right panel shows sequential therapy used in this case for the different ECG patterns. **A** and **B**, Initially, the ECG showed ventricular asystole with a straight-line pattern, which was treated by external cardiac compression, along with intravenous medications. Intravenous vasopressin may also be used here. **C** and **D**, Next ventricular fibrillation was seen. Intravenous amiodarone and other medications may also be used in this setting (see text and references). **E** to **G**, Sinus rhythm appeared after defibrillation with a direct-current electric shock. C, external cardiac compression artifact; DC, direct current; R, R wave from the spontaneous QRS complex; V, ventricular premature beat.

Sometimes repeated shocks must be administered before the patient is successfully defibrillated. In other cases, all attempts fail. Finally, external cardiac compression *must* be continued between attempts at defibrillation.

In cases where VF or pulseless VT persists or recurs despite initial defibrillation attempts, additional measures are indicated, including drugs to support the circulation (epinephrine or vasopressin), intravenous antiarrhythmic agents such as amiodarone or lidocaine, and magnesium sulfate (if hypomagnesemia is suspected).

## VENTRICULAR ASYSTOLE AND BRADY-ASYSTOLIC RHYTHMS

Ventricular standstill and slow escape rhythms are described in Chapter 13. The normal pacemaker of the heart is the sinus node, which is located in the right atrium. Failure of the sinus node to function (sinus arrest) leads to ventricular standstill (asystole) if no other subsidiary pacemaker (e.g., in the atria, AV junction, or ventricles) takes over. In such cases, the ECG records a *straight-line pattern* (see Fig. 19-3), indicating asystole. Whenever you encounter a straight-line pattern, you need to confirm this finding in at least two leads and check to see that all electrodes are connected to the patient. Electrodes often become disconnected during a cardiac arrest, leading to the mistaken diagnosis of asystole. Very low–amplitude VF may also mimic a straight-line pattern.

The treatment of ventricular standstill also requires continued external cardiac compression. Sometimes spontaneous cardiac electrical activity resumes. Drugs such as vasopressin or epinephrine may help support the circulation or stimulate cardiac electrical activity. Patients with refractory ventricular standstill require a *temporary pacemaker,* which may be inserted at the bedside in an emergency situation. As described in Chapter 21, the temporary *transvenous* pacemaker is a special catheter wire electrode that is usually inserted through a vein into the right ventricle and connected to a battery outside the body. A type of *external* temporary pacemaker that does not require intravenous insertion is also commercially available. This noninvasive *(transcutaneous)* pacemaker uses special electrodes that are pasted on the chest wall. Transcutaneous pacing may not always be effective, however, and it can be quite painful in conscious patients.

Hyperkalemia should always be excluded in cases of brady-asystolic rhythms.

Not uncommonly with ventricular standstill, you also see occasional QRS complexes appearing at infrequent intervals against the background of the basic straight-line rhythm. These are *escape beats* and represent the attempt of intrinsic cardiac pacemakers to restart the heart's beat (see Chapter 13). Examples of escape rhythms with underlying ventricular standstill are shown in Figure 19-4. In some cases, the escape beats are narrow, indicating their origin from either the atria or the AV junction (see Fig. 19-4A). In others, they come from a lower focus in the ventricles, producing a slow *idioventricular* rhythm with wide QRS complexes (see Fig. 19-4B). The term *brady-asystolic pattern* is used to describe this type of cardiac arrest ECG.

Escape beats should not be confused with *artifacts* produced by external cardiac compression. Artifacts are large wide deflections that occur with each compression (see Fig. 19-5). Their size varies with the strength of the compression, and their direction varies with the lead in which they appear (i.e., usually negative in leads II, III, and aV$_F$, positive in leads aV$_R$ and aV$_L$).

## PULSELESS ELECTRICAL ACTIVITY (ELECTROMECHANICAL DISSOCIATION)

In the large majority of patients with cardiac arrest, the ECG shows either a sustained ventricular tachyarrhythmia (VF or VT) or a brady-asystolic pattern. Occasionally, however, the ECG of patients in cardiac arrest surprisingly continues to show identifiable, narrow QRS complexes at a relatively physiologic rate. The actual heart rhythm in such cases may be a sinus rhythm, AV junctional (nodal) rhythm, AF, or other supraventricular mechanism. Despite the presence of recurring QRS complexes and even P waves on the ECG, however, the patient is unconscious and does not have a palpable pulse or blood pressure detectable by usual clinical methods. In other words, the patient has cardiac electrical activity but insufficient mechanical heart contractions to pump blood effectively. The term *pulseless electrical activity* (PEA) or *electromechanical dissociation* (EMD) is used in such cases.

PEA with a physiologic rate can arise in a number of settings. When assessing a patient with PEA, you must consider potentially *reversible* causes first. These include *severe hypovolemia, hypoxemia,* and *acidosis.* Another important reversible cause of EMD is *pericardial (cardiac) tamponade,* in which pericardial effu-

sion decreases cardiac output and ultimately causes cardiac arrest. Pericardial tamponade can be treated by removing some of the fluid from the pericardial sac with a special needle inserted through the chest wall *(pericardiocentesis).* Because the disease process is primarily extracardiac (i.e., involving the pericardium), the ECG generally shows relatively normal electrical activity, despite the impaired mechanical function of the heart. Low voltage with sinus tachycardia is often present. Electrical alternans may be seen (see Chapter 11). *Tension pneumothorax* and *massive pulmonary embolism* are two other potentially reversible causes of EMD (Table 19-1).

One of the most common settings in which EMD occurs is when the myocardium has sustained severe generalized injury that may not be reversible, such as with myocardial infarction (MI). In such cases, even though the heart's con-

| TABLE 19-1 | Some Conditions That Cause Pulseless Electrical Activity |
| --- | --- |

| Condition | Clues |
| --- | --- |
| Hypovolemia | History of blood or fluid loss, flat neck veins |
| Hypoxia | Cyanosis, abnormal blood gases, airway problems |
| Cardiac (pericardial) tamponade | History of trauma, renal failure, or thoracic malignancy; no pulse with cardiopulmonary resuscitation, neck vein distension, impending tamponade (tachycardia, hypotension, low pulse pressure) changing to sudden bradycardia as the terminal event |
| Tension pneumothorax | History of asthma, ventilator use, chronic obstructive pulmonary disease, or trauma; no pulse with cardiopulmonary resuscitation, absent breath sounds, neck vein distension, tracheal deviation |
| Hypothermia | History of exposure to cold; low central body temperature |
| Massive pulmonary embolism | Relevant history, no pulse felt with cardiopulmonary resuscitation, distended neck veins |
| Drug overdose (tricyclic antidepressants, digoxin, beta blockers, calcium channel blockers) | Bradycardia, history of drug ingestion, empty medication bottles at the scene, neurologic examination |
| Hyperkalemia | ECG showing wide QRS complexes without P waves and then asystole; history of renal failure, diabetes, dialysis, or selected medications |
| Severe acidosis | History of preexisting acidosis, renal failure, diabetes mellitus |
| Acute, massive myocardial infarction | Relevant history, ECG, cardiac enzymes |

Modified from Cummins RO (ed): Textbook of Advanced Cardiac Life Support, Dallas, TX, American Heart Association, 1997.

duction system may be intact enough to generate a relatively normal rhythm, the amount of functional ventricular muscle is insufficient to respond to this electrical signal with an adequate contraction. Sometimes the myocardial depression is temporary and reversible ("stunned myocardium"), and the patient may respond to resuscitative efforts.

In summary, the three basic ECG patterns seen with cardiac arrest are a sustained ventricular tachyarrhythmia, ventricular asystole (or brady-asystolic patterns), and pulseless electrical activity. During the course of resuscitating any patient, you may see two or even all three of these ECG patterns at different times during the arrest. Figure 19-6 shows the "ECG history" of a cardiac arrest.

## CLINICAL CAUSES OF CARDIAC ARREST

Cardiac arrest associated with any of the three electrical mechanisms—ventricular tachyarrhythmia, ventricular asystole, or PEA—may occur in numerous settings. It can be due to any type of organic heart disease. For example, a patient with an acute MI may have cardiac arrest for several reasons. Myocardial ischemia and increased ventricular electrical instability may precipitate VF. Damage to the conduction system may result in ventricular standstill. Finally, EMD may occur with extensive myocardial injury. Occasionally, actual rupture of the infarcted ventricular wall occurs, leading to fatal pericardial tamponade. Cardiac arrest also occurs when electrical instability is associated with *chronic* heart disease resulting from previous infarction, valvular abnormalities, hypertension, or cardiomyopathy.

A lightning strike or an electric shock may produce cardiac arrest in the normal heart. Cardiac arrest may also occur during surgical procedures, particularly in patients with underlying heart disease. Drugs such as epinephrine can produce VF. Quinidine, disopyramide, procainamide, ibutilide, dofetilide, and related drugs may lead to torsades de pointes (see Chapter 16). Excessive digitalis can also lead to fatal ventricular arrhythmias (see Chapter 18). Hypokalemia and hypomagnesemia may potentiate arrhythmias associated with a variety of antiarrhythmic drugs and with digitalis glycosides. Other cardiac drugs can also precipitate sustained ventricular tachyarrhythmias through their so-called *proarrhythmic effects* (see Chapter 16). The recreational use of *cocaine* may also induce fatal arrhythmias.

Brady-asystolic cardiac arrest may occur with intrinsic conduction disease resulting from sick sinus syndrome (see Chapters 13 and 20) or with high-degree AV block (see Chapter 17). You need to exclude very important reversible causes of brady-asystolic arrest such as hyperkalemia (see Chapter 10) and drug toxicity (e.g., digitalis, tricyclic antidepressant overdose, beta blockers, calcium channel blockers). Systemic hypothermia may be associated with severe bradycardia. Conditions that may directly cause or contribute to pulseless electrical activity (including brady-asystolic patterns or actual EMD) are summarized in Table 19-1.

During and after successful resuscitation of the patient in cardiac arrest, an intensive search for the cause must be started. Serial 12-lead ECGs and serum cardiac enzyme levels are helpful in diagnosing MI. A complete blood count, serum electrolyte concentrations, and arterial blood gas measurements should be obtained. A portable chest x-ray unit and, if needed, an echocardiograph machine can be brought to the bedside. In addition, a pertinent medical history should be obtained from every available source, with particular attention to drug use (e.g., digitalis, antiarrhythmics, psychotropics, "recreational" drugs) and previous cardiac problems.

## SUDDEN CARDIAC DEATH

The term *sudden cardiac death* is used to describe the situation in which an individual who sustains an unexpected cardiac arrest and is not

### Quinidine-Induced Long QT and Torsades de Pointes

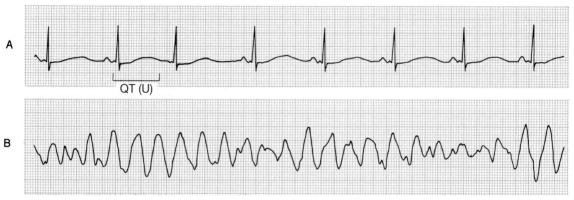

**FIGURE 19-7**  Patient on quinidine (monitor lead) developed marked prolongation of repolarization with low amplitude T-U waves **(A)** followed by cardiac arrest with torsades de pointes ventricular tachycardia **(B)**. (Note that the third beat in panel A is a premature atrial complex.)

resuscitated dies instantly or within an hour or so of the development of acute symptoms. More than 400,000 such deaths occur each year in the United States, striking individuals both with and without known cardiovascular disease. Unexpected sudden cardiac death is most often initiated by a sustained ventricular tachyarrhythmia, less commonly by a brady-asystolic mechanism or EMD.

Most individuals with unexpected cardiac arrest have underlying structural heart disease. An estimated 20% of patients with acute MI die suddenly before reaching the hospital. Another important substrate for sudden death is severe left ventricular scarring from previous (chronic) MI. Other patients with sudden cardiac death have structural heart disease with valvular abnormalities or myocardial disease associated, for example, with severe aortic stenosis, dilated or hypertrophic cardiomyopathy, acute or chronic myocarditis, arrhythmogenic right ventricular dysplasia, or anomalous origin of a coronary artery.

Some individuals with sudden cardiac death do not have mechanical cardiac dysfunction, but they may have intrinsic electrical instability

as a result of the long QT syndromes (predisposing to torsades de pointes), Wolff-Parkinson-White (WPW) preexcitation syndrome (particularly when associated with atrial fibrillation precipitating ventricular fibrillation), the Brugada syndrome, or severe SA or AV conduction system disease causing prolonged sinus arrest or high grade heart block, respectively.

QT prolongation, a marker of risk for torsades de pointes type of ventricular tachycardia, was discussed in Chapters 10 and 16. QT prolongation syndromes may be divided into acquired and hereditary (congenital) subsets. The major acquired causes include drugs, electrolyte abnormalities, and bradyarrhythmias. Figure 19-7 shows an example of marked QT prolongation due to quinidine that was followed by torsades de pointes and cardiac arrest. Hereditary long QT syndromes (Fig. 19-8) are due to a number of different abnormalities of cardiac ion channel function ("channelopathies"). A detailed list of clinical factors causing long QT is given in Chapter 24.

The Brugada syndrome refers to the association of a characteristic ECG pattern with risk

## Hereditary Long QT Syndrome

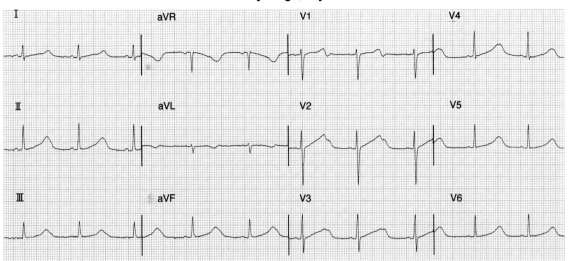

**FIGURE 19-8** Hereditary long QT syndrome. ECG from 21-year-old woman with history of recurrent syncope, initially mistaken for a seizure disorder. The ECG demonstrates a prolonged QT interval of 0.6 second. Note the broad T waves with notching (or possibly U waves) in the precordial leads. Syncope, with risk of sudden cardiac death, is due to episodes of torsades de pointes type of ventricular tachycardia.

of ventricular tachyarrhythmias. The Brugada pattern consists of distinctive ST elevations in the right chest leads ($V_1$ to $V_3$) with a QRS pattern somewhat resembling a right bundle branch block (Fig. 19-9). The basis of the Brugada pattern and associated arrhythmias is a topic of active study. Abnormal repolarization of right ventricular muscle related to sodium channel dysfunction appears to play an important role.

As noted, "recreational" drugs such as cocaine or cardiac antiarrhythmic agents may induce lethal arrhythmias. Finally, a small subset of individuals sustain cardiac arrest without having any demonstrable structural or currently identifiable electrophysiologic abnormality.

The term *commotio cordis* (Latin for "cardiac concussion") refers to the syndrome of sudden cardiac arrest in healthy individuals who sustain nonpenetrating chest trauma, triggering ventricular fibrillation. This syndrome has been most frequently reported after chest wall impact during sports such as baseball or softball, football or rugby, boxing, ice hockey, karate, and lacrosse, but may occur in other settings, such as car or motorcycle accidents.

The identification and management of patients at high risk for sudden death are central areas of investigation in cardiology today. The important role of *implantable cardioverter-defibrillator (ICD)* devices in preventing sudden death in carefully selected high-risk patients is discussed in Chapter 21.

## Brugada Pattern

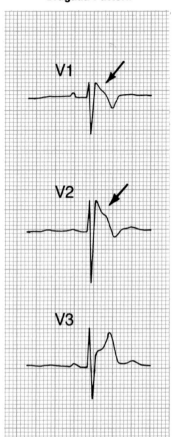

**FIGURE 19-9** Brugada pattern showing characteristic ST elevations in the right chest leads. The ECG superficially resembles a right bundle branch block (RBBB) pattern. Typical RBBB, however, produces an rSR' pattern in right precordial leads and is not associated with ST elevation in this distribution. The Brugada pattern appears to be a marker of abnormal right ventricular repolarization and in some individuals is associated with an increased risk of life-threatening ventricular arrhythmias.

# REVIEW

Cardiac arrest occurs when the heart stops pumping blood. The diagnosis should be made clinically even before the patient is connected to an electrocardiograph. The major clinical sign of cardiac arrest is the absence of pulses in an unconscious patient.

Cardiac arrest may be associated with one or more of the following ECG patterns:

1. *Ventricular tachyarrhythmias,* including ventricular fibrillation, sustained typical ventricular tachycardia, torsades de pointes, or ventricular flutter

2. *Ventricular standstill (asystole)* or *brady-asystolic pattern,* which is a straight-line pattern, sometimes with interruptions by junctional or ventricular escape beats

3. *Pulseless electrical activity (PEA)/Electro-mechanical dissociation (EMD),* in which recurring QRS complexes and sometimes

even P waves are not associated with a palpable pulse or blood pressure. EMD is usually caused by diffuse myocardial injury, although it may be due to pericardial tamponade, tension pneumothorax, or massive pulmonary embolism, among other causes.

Any or all of these patterns may be seen during the resuscitation of a patient in cardiac arrest.

With cardiac arrest, the ECG may show distinctive *artifacts* caused by external cardiac compression. These large wide deflections should not be mistaken for the intrinsic electrical activity of the heart.

The term *sudden cardiac death* is used in reference to individuals who sustain an unexpected cardiac arrest and, unless resuscitated, die instantly or within an hour or so of the development of acute symptoms.

# QUESTIONS

1. Would a pacemaker be of any value in treating a patient with cardiac arrest and electromechanical dissociation (EMD)?

2. The rhythm strip shown below was obtained from a patient during the course of a cardiac arrest and attempted resuscitation. Answer the following questions:

Monitor lead

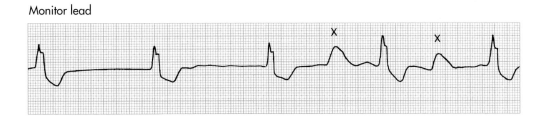

   a. What is the basic rhythm?
   b. What is the likely cause of the complexes marked *X*?

3. Name four drugs that can produce cardiac arrest associated with a sustained ventricular tachyarrhythmia (i.e., ventricular fibrillation, monomorphic ventricular tachycardia, torsades de pointes, or ventricular flutter).

# Bradycardias and Tachycardias

## Review and differential diagnosis

The preceding chapters described the major arrhythmias and atrioventricular (AV) conduction disturbances. These abnormalities can be classified in numerous ways. This "review and overview" chapter simply divides them into two major clinical groups—bradycardias and tachycardias—and discusses the differential diagnosis of each group (Box 20-1).

## BRADYCARDIAS (BRADYARRHYTHMIAS)

A number of arrhythmias and conduction disturbances associated with a slow heart rate have been described. The term *bradycardia* (or *bradyarrhythmia*) refers to arrhythmias and conduction abnormalities that produce a heart rate of less than 60 beats per minute. Fortunately, the differential diagnosis of a slow pulse is relatively simple in that only a few causes must be considered. Bradyarrhythmias fall into five general classes (Box 20-2).

### SINUS BRADYCARDIA

Sinus bradycardia is sinus rhythm with a rate less than 60 beats/min (Fig. 20-1).* Each QRS complex is preceded by a P wave; the P wave is negative in lead $aV_R$ and positive in lead II, indicating that the sinoatrial (SA) node is the pacemaker. Some patients may have a sinus bradycardia of 40 beats/min or less.

Sinus bradycardia may be related to a decreased firing rate of the sinus node pacemaker cells or to actual SA block.† The most extreme example is SA node arrest (see Chapter 13).

### AV JUNCTIONAL (NODAL) ESCAPE RHYTHM

With a slow AV junctional escape rhythm (Fig. 20-2), either the P waves (seen immediately before or just after the QRS complexes) are *retrograde* (inverted in lead II and upright in lead $aV_R$), or no P waves are apparent if the atria and ventricles are stimulated simultaneously.

### AV HEART BLOCK (SECOND OR THIRD DEGREE) OR AV DISSOCIATION

A slow ventricular rate of 60 beats/min or less (even as low as 20 beats/min) is the rule with complete heart block because of the slow intrinsic rate of the junctional or idioventricular pacemaker (Fig. 20-3). In addition, patients with second-degree AV block (either Mobitz type I

---

*Some cardiologists reserve the term *sinus bradycardia* for rates less than 50 beats/min.

†*SA block* refers to situations in which impulses formed in the sinus node fail to depolarize the atria.

---

### BOX 20-1 Major Tachyarrhythmias: Simplified Classification

| Narrow QRS Complexes | Wide QRS Complexes |
|---|---|
| Sinus tachycardia | Ventricular tachycardia |
| Paroxysmal supraventricular tachycardias (PSVTs)* | Supraventricular tachycardia with aberration caused by a bundle branch block–type or Wolff-Parkinson-White pattern |
| Atrial flutter | |
| Atrial fibrillation preexcitation syndrome | |

*The three most common types of PSVTs are AV nodal reentrant tachycardias (AVNRT), atrioventricular reentrant tachycardia (AVRT) involving a bypass tract, and atrial tachycardia (AT) including unifocal and multifocal atrial tachycardia, as discussed in Chapter 14. Other *non*paroxysmal supraventricular tachycardias may also occur, including types of so-called *incessant* atrial, junctional, and bypass-tract tachycardias. (For further details of this advanced topic, see selected references cited in the Bibliography.)

---

### BOX 20-2 Bradycardias: Simplified Classification

Sinus bradycardia, including sinoatrial block
Atrioventricular (AV) junctional (nodal) escape rhythm
AV heart block (second or third degree) or AV dissociation
Atrial fibrillation or flutter with a slow ventricular response
Idioventricular escape rhythm

---

## ATRIAL FIBRILLATION OR FLUTTER WITH A SLOW VENTRICULAR RATE

Paroxysmal atrial fibrillation (AF), prior to treatment, is generally associated with a rapid ventricular rate. The rate may become excessively slow (less than 50 to 60 beats/min), however, because of drug effects or toxicity (beta blockers, calcium channel blockers, digitalis) or because of underlying disease of the AV junction (Fig. 20-4). In such cases, the ECG shows the characteristic atrial fibrillatory (f) waves with a slow ventricular (QRS) rate. The f waves may be very fine and easily overlooked. (A very slow, regularized ventricular response in AF suggests the presence of underlying complete AV heart block; see Chapter 17.)

## IDIOVENTRICULAR ESCAPE RHYTHM

When the SA nodal and AV junctional escape pacemakers fail to function, a very slow pace-

[Wenckebach] or Mobitz type II) sometimes have a bradycardia because of the dropped beats (see Fig. 17-3 and Table 17-1).

Isorhythmic AV dissociation, which may be confused with complete heart block, is also frequently associated with a heart rate of less than 60 beats/min (see Chapter 17).

---

**Sinus Bradycardia**

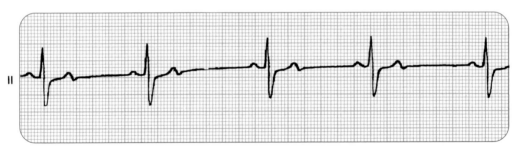

**FIGURE 20-1** Sinus bradycardia with a slight sinus arrhythmia.

## AV Junctional Escape Rhythm

Monitor lead

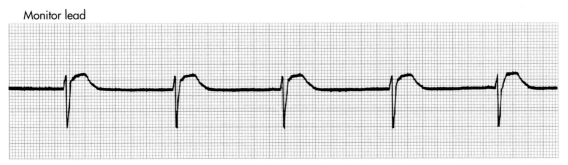

**FIGURE 20-2**   The heart rate is about 43 beats/min. The baseline between the QRS complexes is perfectly flat (i.e., no P waves are evident).

## Complete Heart Block

II

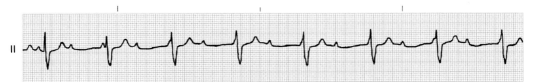

**FIGURE 20-3**   The atrial (P wave) rate is about 80 beats/min. The ventricular (QRS) rate is about 43 beats/min. Because the atria and ventricles are beating independently, the PR intervals are variable. The QRS complex is wide because the ventricles are being paced by an idioventricular pacemaker.

## Atrial Fibrillation with a Slow, Regularized Ventricular Rate

Monitor lead

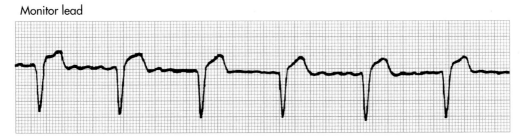

**FIGURE 20-4**   Regularization and excessive slowing of the ventricular rate with atrial fibrillation are usually a sign of drug toxicity (especially digitalis) or intrinsic AV node disease (see Chapter 18).

maker in the ventricular conduction (His-Purkinje) system may take over. This rhythm is referred to as an *idioventricular escape rhythm.* The rate is usually very slow (less than 45 beats/min), and the QRS complexes are wide without any preceding P wave (see Fig. 17-6).

*In such cases, hyperkalemia should always be excluded.*

## CLINICAL SIGNIFICANCE

With the exception of sinus bradycardia, which is a common normal variant, the other bradycardias are often abnormal.* The possible causes of AV junctional rhythms, heart block, and AF were described in earlier chapters.

Digitalis excess or other drug toxicity (e.g., beta blockers, calcium channel blockers, lithium carbonate) must always be considered in any patient with a bradycardia. Hyperkalemia is another important, reversible, life-threatening cause of bradyarrhythmias (see Chapter 10). Prominent intermittent sinus bradycardia and sinus pauses at night may occur with obstructive sleep apnea syndrome.

Patients with any of the bradycardias just discussed may have no symptoms, or they may complain of light-headedness or fainting because of decreased cardiac output. The treatment depends on the particular arrhythmia and the clinical setting.

In summary, most patients with an ECG heart rate of less than 60 beats/min have one of the five following classes of arrhythmia: sinus bradycardia (including SA block), AV junctional escape rhythm, AV heart block (or AV dissociation), AF or atrial flutter with a very slow ventricular rate, or idioventricular escape rhythm.[†]

## TACHYCARDIAS (TACHYARRHYTHMIAS)

At the opposite end of the spectrum from bradyarrhythmias are the tachycardias. These rhythm disturbances produce a heart rate faster than 100 beats/min. The tachyarrhythmias can be usefully divided into two general groups: those with a "narrow" (normal) QRS duration and those with a "wide" QRS duration. Narrow-complex tachycardias are almost invariably *supra*ventricular (i.e., the focus of stimulation is within or *above* the AV junction). Wide-complex tachycardias, by contrast, are either ventricular or supraventricular with aberrant ventricular conduction (supraventricular tachycardia [SVT] with aberrancy).

The four major classes of supraventricular tachyarrhythmia[‡] are sinus tachycardia, paroxysmal supraventricular tachycardia (PSVT), atrial flutter, and AF. With each class, cardiac activation occurs at one or more sites in the atria or AV junction (node), above the ventricles (hence *supra*ventricular). This is in contrast to ventricular tachycardia (VT), in which the stimulus starts in the ventricles themselves. VT is defined as a rapid run of three or more consecutive premature ventricular depolarizations (see Fig. 16-5). The QRS complexes are always wide because the ventricles are not being stimulated simultaneously. The rate of VT is usually between 100 and 200 beats/min. By contrast, with supraventricular arrhythmias, the ventricles are stimulated normally (simultaneously), and the QRS complexes are therefore narrow (unless a bundle branch block–type pattern is also present).

The first step in analyzing a tachyarrhythmia is to look at the width of the QRS complex in all 12 leads if possible. If the QRS complex is narrow (0.1 sec or less), you are dealing with some type of supraventricular arrhythmia and not VT. If the QRS complex is very wide (particularly if greater than 0.14 sec), you should

---

*Normal persons (in particular, athletes with increased vagal tone at rest) occasionally show a slow junctional rhythm or even Wenckebach AV block.
[†]Bradycardia can also be due to a wandering atrial pacemaker (see Fig. 20-15) or isorhythmic AV dissociation (see Fig. 17-10).

[‡]Be aware of possible confusion in terminology. Cardiologists use the term *supraventricular tachycardia (SVT)* in two related, but different ways. First, SVT refers most generally to any arrhythmia originating in area of the AV junction, atria, or SA node, above the ventricular conduction system (hence *supra*ventricular). Second, SVT is also used more specifically to refer to a class of paroxysmal supraventricular tachycardias (PSVTs) originating in the region of the atria or AV junction (node) or involving an atrioventricular bypass tract. These PSVTs, caused by reentry or automaticity, are distinct from sinus tachycardia, AF, or atrial flutter (see Chapters 14 and 15).

consider the rhythm to be VT unless it can be proved otherwise.

## DIFFERENTIAL DIAGNOSIS OF NARROW-COMPLEX TACHYARRHYTHMIAS

The characteristics of sinus tachycardia, PSVTs, AF, and atrial flutter have been described in previous chapters. *Sinus tachycardia* in adults generally produces a heart rate between 100 and 180 beats/min, with the higher rates (150 to 180 beats/min) generally occurring in association with exercise. If you find a narrow-complex tachycardia with a rate of 150 beats/min or more in a resting adult, you are most likely dealing with one of the other three types of (nonsinus) arrhythmias mentioned previously.

PSVT and AF can generally be distinguished on the basis of their regularity. PSVT resulting from AV nodal reentry or a concealed bypass tract is usually an almost perfectly regular tachycardia with a ventricular rate between 140 and 250 beats/min (see Chapter 14). AF, on the other hand, is distinguished by its irregularity. Remember that with rapid AF (Fig. 20-5) the f waves may not be clearly visible, but the diagnosis can be made in almost every case by noting the absence of P waves and the haphazardly irregular QRS complexes.

*Atrial flutter* is characterized by "sawtooth" flutter (F) waves between QRS complexes (Fig. 20-6). When atrial flutter is present with 2:1 block (e.g., the atrial rate is 300 beats/min and the ventricular response is 150 beats/min), however, the F waves are often hidden. Therefore atrial flutter at 150 beats/min can be confused with sinus tachycardia, PSVT, or AF (Fig.

### Atrial Fibrillation with a Rapid Ventricular Rate

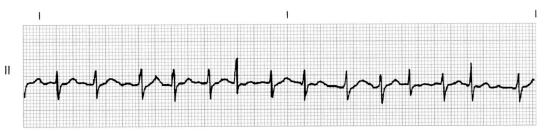

**FIGURE 20-5**  The ventricular rate is about 130 beats/min (13 QRS cycles in 6 sec). Notice the characteristic haphazardly irregular rhythm.

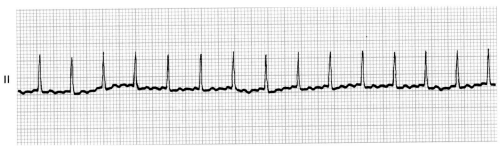

**FIGURE 20-6**  Atrial flutter with 2:1 conduction.

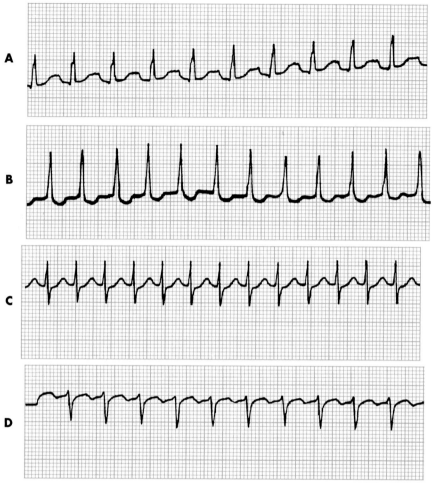

**FIGURE 20-7** Four "look-alike" narrow-complex tachyarrhythmias (lead II). **A,** Sinus tachycardia. **B,** Atrial fibrillation. **C,** Paroxysmal supraventricular tachycardia (PSVT) resulting from AV nodal reentrant tachycardia (AVNRT). **D,** Atrial flutter with 2:1 block. When the ventricular rate is about 150 beats/min, these four arrhythmias may be difficult if not impossible to tell apart on the standard ECG, particularly from a single lead. In the example of sinus tachycardia, the P waves can barely be seen in this case. Next, notice that the irregularity of the atrial fibrillation here is very subtle. In the example of PSVT, the rate is quite regular without evident P waves. In the strip illustrating atrial flutter, the flutter waves cannot be seen clearly in this lead.

20-7). AF can be excluded because atrial flutter with 2:1 conduction is generally very regular.

Nevertheless, the differential diagnosis of sinus tachycardia, PSVT with a ventricular rate of about 150 beats/min, AF, and atrial flutter can be a problem (see Fig. 20-7). One measure often used to help separate these arrhythmias is

*carotid sinus massage* (CSM).* Pressure on the carotid sinus produces a reflex increase in vagal

---

*CSM is not without risks, particularly in elderly patients. Consult texts cited in the Bibliography for details on this maneuver and the use of adenosine in the differential diagnosis of tachycardias.

## Multifocal Atrial Tachycardia

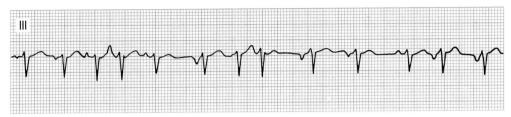

**FIGURE 20-8**   Note the rapidly occurring P waves showing variable shapes, variable PR intervals, or both.

tone. The effects of CSM on sinus tachycardia, reentrant-types of PSVT, and atrial flutter are described next.

### Sinus Tachycardia

Sinus tachycardia generally slows slightly with CSM. No abrupt change in heart rate usually occurs, however. Slowing of sinus tachycardia may make the P waves more evident. Sinus tachycardia generally begins and ends gradually, not abruptly.

### Paroxysmal Supraventricular Tachycardias

PSVT resulting from AV nodal reentry (AVNRT) or atrioventricular reentry (AVRT) involving a concealed bypass tract usually has an *all-or-none* response to CSM. In successful cases, it breaks suddenly, and sinus rhythm resumes during the CSM (see Fig. 14-7). At other times, CSM has no effect, and the tachycardia continues at the same rate. In cases of PSVT caused by atrial tachycardia (AT), CSM may have no effect or may increase the degree of block, resulting in a rapid sequence of one or more nonconducted P waves.

### Atrial Flutter

CSM often increases the degree of block in atrial flutter, converting flutter with a 2:1 response to 3:1 or 4:1 flutter with a ventricular rate of 100 or 75 beats/min. Slowing of the ventricular rate unmasks the characteristic F waves (see Fig. 15-2).

## MULTIFOCAL ATRIAL TACHYCARDIA

Another variant of PSVT that has not yet been specifically discussed is *multifocal atrial tachycardia (MAT)*. An example is shown in Figure 20-8. This tachyarrhythmia is characterized by multiple ectopic foci stimulating the atria. The diagnosis of MAT requires the presence of three or more (nonsinus) P waves with different shapes at a rate of 100 or more per minute. The PR intervals often vary. MAT is usually seen in patients with chronic lung disease. Because the ventricular rate is irregular and rapid, this arrhythmia is most likely to be mistaken for AF. MAT is caused by multiple atrial pacemakers firing in an unpredictable fashion. This is in contrast to classic (unifocal) atrial tachycardia, which typically involves only a single ectopic pacemaker in the atrium (see Chapter 14).

## DIFFERENTIAL DIAGNOSIS OF VENTRICULAR TACHYCARDIA

Tachycardias are divided into SVTs and ventricular tachycardia (VT). This section briefly describes the differential diagnosis of VT. A tachycardia with widened (broad) QRS complexes indicates two possible diagnostic considerations. The first and more important is VT, a potentially life-threatening arrhythmia.* As

---

*Most cases of VT are associated with a very wide QRS complex. More rarely, VT may occur with a QRS complex that is only mildly prolonged, particularly if the arrhythmia originates in the upper part of the ventricular septum or in the proximal part of the fascicles.

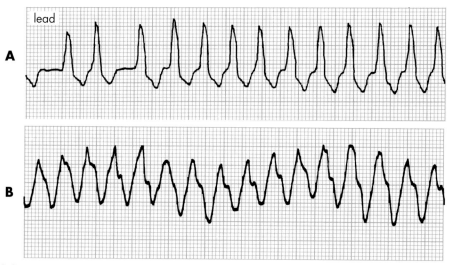

**FIGURE 20-9    A,** Atrial fibrillation with a left bundle branch block pattern. **B,** Ventricular tachycardia. Based on the ECG appearance, differentiating supraventricular tachycardia with bundle branch block from actual ventricular tachycardia may be difficult and sometimes impossible.

noted, VT is a consecutive run of three or more ventricular premature beats at a rate generally between 100 and 200 or more beats/min. It is usually very regular. The second possible cause of a tachycardia with widened QRS complexes is so-called *SVT with aberration*. The term *aberration* simply means that some abnormality in ventricular activation is present, causing widened QRS complexes.

## DIFFERENTIATION OF SVT WITH ABERRANCY AND VENTRICULAR TACHYCARDIA

Aberrancy with an SVT has two major mechanisms: bundle branch block and, much more rarely, Wolff-Parkinson-White (WPW) preexcitation.

### Supraventricular Tachycardia with Bundle Branch Block

If any of the SVTs just discussed occurs in association with a bundle branch block (or related pattern), the ECG shows a wide-complex tachycardia that may be mistaken for VT. For example, a patient with sinus tachycardia, AF, atrial flutter, or PSVT and concomitant right bundle branch block (RBBB) or left bundle branch block (LBBB) has a wide-complex tachycardia.

Figure 20-9*A* shows AF with a rapid ventricular response occurring in conjunction with LBBB. Figure 20-9*B* shows an example of VT. Because the arrhythmias look so similar, it can be difficult to tell them apart. The major distinguishing feature is the irregularity of the AF as opposed to the regularity of the VT. VT can sometimes be irregular, however.

You need to remember that in some cases of SVT with aberration, the bundle branch block is seen only during the episodes of tachycardia. Such rate-related bundle branch blocks are said to be *tachycardia (or acceleration) dependent*.

### Supraventricular Tachycardias with Wolff-Parkinson-White Preexcitation

The second mechanism responsible for a wide-complex tachycardia is SVT with a Wolff-Parkinson-White (WPW) pattern. As noted, patients with WPW preexcitation have an accessory pathway connecting the atria and ventricles, thus bypassing the AV node. Such patients are especially prone to a reentrant type of PSVT with narrow (normal) QRS complexes. Some-

## Atrial Fibrillation and Wolff-Parkinson-White Syndrome

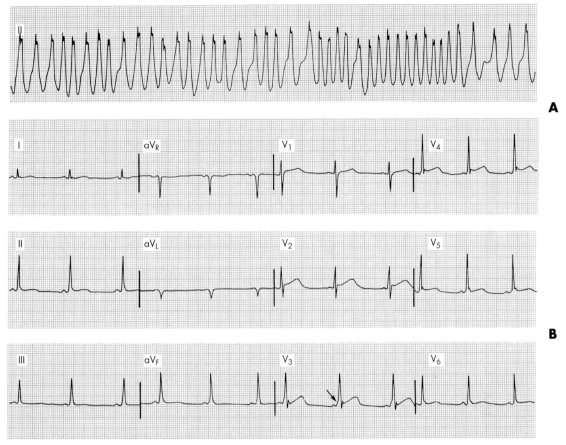

**FIGURE 20-10** **A,** Atrial fibrillation with the Wolff-Parkinson-White preexcitation syndrome may lead to a wide-complex tachycardia that has a very rapid rate. Notice that some of the RR intervals are less than 0.20 sec. Irregularity is due to the underlying atrial fibrillation. **B,** After the arrhythmia has been converted to sinus rhythm, the classic triad of the Wolff-Parkinson-White syndrome is visible but subtle: relatively short PR interval, wide QRS complex, and delta wave (*arrow* in lead V₃).

times, however, particularly if AF or atrial flutter develops, a wide-complex tachycardia may result from conduction down the bypass tract at very high rates. This kind of wide-complex tachycardia obviously mimics VT. An example of WPW with AF is shown in Figure 20-10.*

*WPW with AF should be strongly suspected if you encounter a wide-complex tachycardia that is (1) irregular, and (2) has a very high rate (very short RR intervals).* In particular, RR intervals of 0.20 second or less are rarely seen with conventional AF, and very rapid VT is usually quite regular. These very short RR intervals are related to the ability of the bypass tract (in contrast to the AV node) to conduct impulses in extremely rapid succession (see Fig. 20-10*A*).

The recognition of WPW with AF is of considerable clinical importance because digitalis may paradoxically enhance conduction down the bypass tract. As a result, the ventricular response may increase, leading to possible

## Ventricular Tachycardia: AV Dissociation

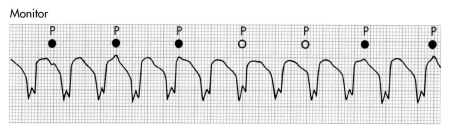

Monitor

**FIGURE 20-11** Sustained monomorphic ventricular tachycardia with atrioventricular (AV) dissociation. Note the independence of the atrial (sinus) rate (75 beats/min) and ventricular (QRS) rate (140 beats/min). The visible sinus P waves are indicated by ●, and the hidden P waves are indicated by ○.

## Ventricular Tachycardia: Fusion and Capture Beats

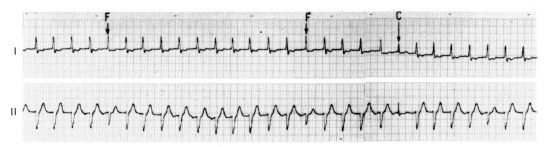

**FIGURE 20-12** Sustained monomorphic ventricular tachycardia with atrioventricular dissociation producing fusion (F) and capture (C) beats. Leads I and II were recorded simultaneously.

myocardial ischemia and, in some cases, to ventricular fibrillation. A similar hazardous effect has been reported with intravenous verapamil.

### VT vs. SVT: Diagnostic Clues

Differentiating VT from SVT (e.g., PSVT, atrial flutter, or atrial fibrillation) with bundle branch block–type aberrancy can be very challenging. Three clues may be especially helpful in favoring VT.

1. *AV dissociation* is an important clue that may be helpful in differentiating SVT with aberrancy from VT. Recall from Chapter 17 that, with AV dissociation, the atria and ventricles are paced from separate sites. Some patients with VT also have AV dissociation; in other words, the ventricles are stimulated from an *ectopic* site at a rapid rate, while the atria continue to be paced independently by the SA

node. In such cases, you may be able to see P waves occurring at a slower rate than the rapid wide QRS complexes, as shown in Figure 20-11. Some of the P waves may be buried in the QRS complexes and therefore difficult to discern.

Unfortunately, only a minority of patients with VT clearly show ECG evidence of AV dissociation. Therefore the absence of AV dissociation does not exclude VT. The presence of AV dissociation in a patient with wide QRS complexes at a rapid rate, however, is virtually diagnostic of VT. Furthermore, in some cases of VT with AV dissociation, the SA node may transiently "capture" the ventricles, producing a *capture beat*, which has a normal QRS duration, or a *fusion beat*, in which the sinus and ventricular beats coincide to produce a hybrid complex. Figure 20-12 illustrates capture and fusion beats occurring with VT.

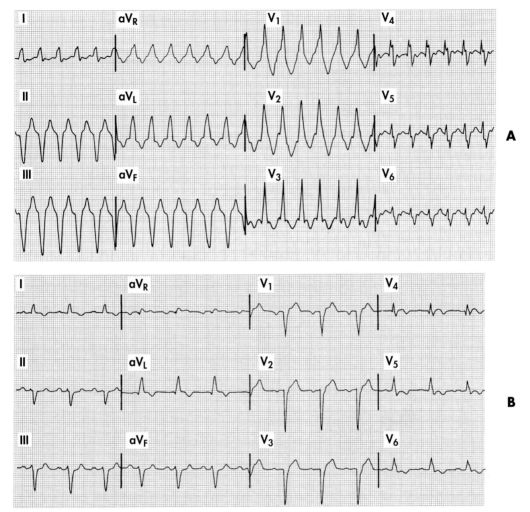

**FIGURE 20-13**   **A,** Sustained monomorphic ventricular tachycardia at a rate of about 200 beats/min. Notice the wide QRS complexes with a right bundle branch block morphology. The QRS complex in leads $V_1$ and $V_2$ shows a broad R wave. **B,** Following conversion to sinus rhythm, the pattern of an underlying anterior wall myocardial infarction and possible ventricular aneurysm becomes evident. Q waves and ST elevations are seen in leads in $V_1$, $V_2$, and $V_3$; ischemic T wave inversions are present in leads $V_4$, $V_5$, and $V_6$. Note also that the QRS complex is wide (0.12 sec) because of an intraventricular conduction delay (IVCD) with left axis deviation (left anterior fascicular block). The prominent negative P waves in lead $V_1$ are due to left atrial abnormality.

2. *The shape of the QRS in $V_1/V_2$ and $V_6$.* When the QRS shape resembles an RBBB pattern, a typical rSR' shape in lead $V_1$ suggests SVT and a single broad R wave or a qR, QR, or RS complex in that lead strongly suggests VT (Fig. 20-13). When the QRS shape resembles an LBBB pattern, a broad (0.04 sec or longer) initial R wave in lead $V_1$ or $V_2$ or a QR complex in lead $V_6$ strongly suggests VT.

3. *The QRS duration.* A QRS width of greater than 0.14 sec with an RBBB morphology or greater than 0.16 sec with an LBBB morphology

---

| **BOX 20-3** | **Wide Complex Tachycardia: Selected Criteria Favoring Ventricular Tachycardia** |

1. AV dissociation
2. QRS width: >0.14 s with RBBB configuration*
   >0.16 s with LBBB configuration*
3. Shape of the QRS complex
   RBBB: Mono- or biphasic complex in $V_1$

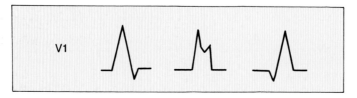

   LBBB: Broad R waves in $V_1$ or $V_2 \geq 0.04$ s
   Onset of QRS to tip of S wave in $V_1$ or $V_2 \geq 0.07$ s
   QR complex in $V_6$

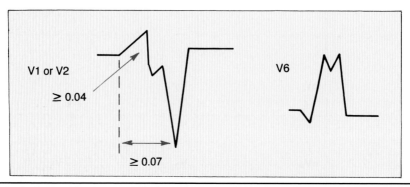

*QRS duration may also be increased in supraventricular tachycardias in presence of drugs that prolong QRS derivation or with hyperkalemia.
Modified from: Josephson ME, Zimetbaum P: The tachyarrhythmias. In Kasper DL, Braunwald E, Fauci A, et al (eds): Harrison's Principles of Internal Medicine, 16th ed. New York, McGraw-Hill, 2004.

---

suggests VT. (This criterion is not reliable if the patient is on a drug that widens the QRS, or in the presence of hyperkalemia.)

Box 20-3 summarizes some of the major findings that favor VT over SVT with bundle branch block aberrancy. For more detailed discussion, consult the Bibliography.

At times, you may find it impossible to distinguish reliably between VT and SVT with aberration from the 12-lead ECG. In such cases,

clinical judgment must be used. For example, if the patient is hypotensive, the tachycardia is generally treated as VT (see Box 20-1). On the other hand, remember that not all patients with VT are hypotensive. Indeed, occasional patients may have minimal symptoms at rest when they are in sustained VT.

Remember that *intravenously administered verapamil should not be used in undiagnosed wide-complex tachycardias*. This drug may cause hemodynamic collapse in patients with VT or AF with WPW preexcitation syndrome that may simulate VT.

## CLINICAL SIGNIFICANCE

As mentioned previously, the first question to ask in looking at any tachyarrhythmia is whether the rhythm is VT. If sustained VT is present, emergency treatment is required (see Chapter 16).

The treatment of narrow-complex tachycardias depends on the clinical setting. In patients with sinus tachycardia (see Chapter 13), treatment is directed at the underlying cause (e.g., fever, sepsis, congestive heart failure, or hyperthyroidism). Similarly, the treatment of MAT should be directed at the underlying problem (usually decompensated chronic pulmonary disease). Direct-current electrical cardioversion should *not* be used with MAT because it is unlikely to be helpful and it may induce serious ventricular arrhythmias. A calcium channel blocker (verapamil or diltiazem) can be used to slow the ventricular response in MAT.

In assessing any patient with a narrow-complex tachycardia, you should ask the following three key questions about the effects of the tachycardia on the heart and circulation:

1. Is the patient's blood pressure abnormally low? In particular, is the patient severely hypotensive or actually in shock?

2. Is the patient having an acute myocardial infarction or severe ischemia?

3. Is the patient in severe congestive heart failure (pulmonary edema)?

Patients in any one of these categories who have AF or atrial flutter with a rapid ventricular response or a PSVT require emergency therapy. If they do not respond promptly to initial drug therapy, electrical cardioversion should be considered.

Another major question to ask about any patient with a tachyarrhythmia (or any arrhythmia, for that matter) is whether digitalis or other drugs are part of the therapeutic regimen. Some arrhythmias (e.g., AT with block) may be digitalis-toxic rhythms, disturbances for which electrical cardioversion is contraindicated (see Chapter 18). Drug-induced QT prolongation is an important substrate for *torsades de pointes* type VT as discussed in Chapter 16.

## SICK SINUS SYNDROME AND THE BRADY-TACHY SYNDROME

An interesting group of patients has bradyarrhythmia sometimes alternating with episodes of tachyarrhythmia. The term *sick sinus syndrome* was coined to describe patients with SA node dysfunction that causes marked sinus bradycardia or sinus arrest, sometimes with junctional escape rhythms, which may lead to symptoms of light-headedness and even syncope.

In some patients with sick sinus syndrome, bradycardia episodes are interspersed with paroxysms of tachycardia (usually AF, atrial flutter, or some type of PSVT). Sometimes the bradycardia occurs immediately after spontaneous termination of the tachycardia. The term *brady-tachy syndrome* has been used to describe patients with sick sinus syndrome who have both tachyarrhythmias and bradyarrhythmias (Fig. 20-14).

The diagnosis of sick sinus syndrome and, in particular, the brady-tachy variant often requires monitoring the patient's heartbeat over several hours or even days. A single ECG strip may be normal or may reveal only the bradycardia or tachycardia episode. Treatment generally requires a permanent pacemaker to prevent sinus arrest and radiofrequency ablation therapy or antiarrhythmic drugs to control the tachycardias after the pacemaker has been inserted.

## WANDERING ATRIAL PACEMAKER

Wandering atrial pacemaker (sometimes abbreviated as WAP) is an arrhythmia that is some-

## Brady-Tachy Syndrome

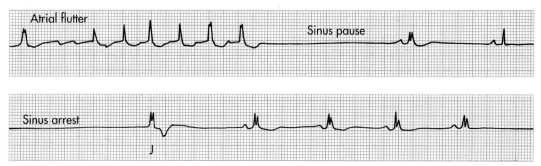

**FIGURE 20-14**   Brady-tachy (sick sinus) syndrome. This rhythm strip shows a narrow-complex tachycardia (probably atrial flutter) followed by a prominent sinus pause, two sinus beats, an atrioventricular junctional escape beat (J), and then sinus rhythm again.

## Wandering Atrial Pacemaker

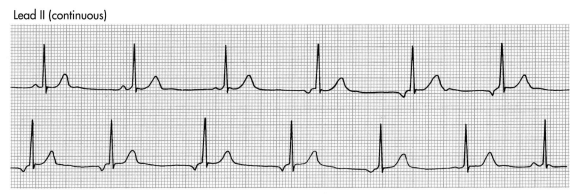

**FIGURE 20-15**   The variability of the P wave configuration in this lead II rhythm strip is caused by shifting of the pacemaker site between the sinus node and ectopic atrial locations.

what difficult to classify. As shown in Figure 20-15, this rhythm is characterized by multiple P waves of varying configuration with a relatively normal or slow heart rate. This pattern reflects rapid shifting of the pacemaker between the sinus node and different ectopic atrial sites, and sometimes the AV junction. Wandering atrial pacemaker may be seen in a variety of settings. Occasionally, it develops in normal persons (particularly during sleep). It may also occur with digitalis excess or certain other drug toxicity, sick sinus syndrome, and different types of organic heart disease.

Wandering atrial pacemaker is quite distinct from MAT, another arrhythmia with multiple different P waves. In wandering atrial pacemaker, the rate is normal or slow. In MAT, it is rapid.

# REVIEW

Arrhythmias can be grouped into *bradycardias* (heart rate *slower* than 60 beats/min) and *tachycardias* (heart rate *faster* than 100 beats/min).

Bradycardias include five major classes of arrhythmias or conduction disturbances:

1. Sinus bradycardia

2. Atrioventricular (AV) junctional (nodal) escape rhythm

3. Second- or third-degree heart block or AV dissociation

4. Atrial fibrillation or flutter with a slow ventricular rate

5. Idioventricular escape rhythm.

Digitalis or other drug toxicity, or hyperkalemia, may be responsible for any of these arrhythmias.

Tachycardias can be subdivided into those with *narrow* QRS complexes and those with *wide* QRS complexes. The narrow-complex QRS tachycardias are almost always *supraventricular* in origin and include the following:

1. Sinus tachycardia

2. Paroxysmal supraventricular tachycardias (PSVTs), including atrial tachycardia (AT),

AV nodal reentrant tachycardia (AVNRT), and AV reentrant tachycardia (AVRT) (see Chapter 14)

3. Atrial fibrillation

4. Atrial flutter

Carotid sinus massage is sometimes helpful in differentiating these arrhythmias at the bedside. Tachycardias with wide QRS complexes may be either *ventricular* or any of the supraventricular tachycardias associated with a *bundle branch block* or *Wolff-Parkinson-White* preexcitation mechanism.

The term *sick sinus syndrome* describes patients with sinoatrial node dysfunction who have a marked sinus bradycardia, sometimes with sinus arrest or slow junctional rhythms that causes light-headedness or syncope. Some patients with sick sinus syndrome have periods of tachycardia alternating with the bradycardia *(brady-tachy syndrome)*.

*Wandering atrial pacemaker* is an arrhythmia characterized by multiple P waves of varying configuration, usually with a relatively normal or slow heart rate.

## QUESTIONS

1. Answer the following questions about the rhythm strip below:

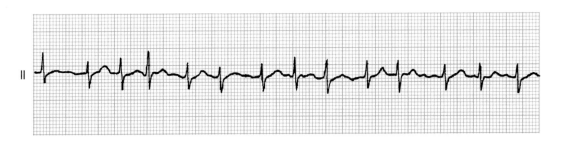

   a. Is the rate regular or irregular?
   b. Are discrete P waves present?
   c. What is this arrhythmia?

2. What is the most likely diagnosis for the wide complex tachycardia arrhythmia shown below?

Monitor lead

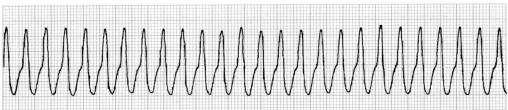

3. A 40-year-old woman complaining of occasional palpitations with a fast heartbeat is found to have runs of narrow QRS complex tachycardia at a rate of 200 beats/min without evident P waves on her Holter monitor tracing. The rhythm is very regular. What is the most likely diagnosis?

4. What is the cause of the bradycardia in the rhythm strip shown below?

V1

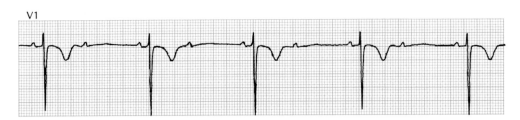

5. Name five reversible pharmacologic or metabolic causes of bradycardia.

# Pacemakers and Implantable Cardioverter-Defibrillators

A brief introduction

This chapter provides a brief overview of an important aspect of clinical electro-cardiography—electronic cardiac devices, including pacemakers and implantable cardioverter-defibrillator (ICD) devices. Particular emphasis is placed on introducing the different types of pacemakers, major indications for pacemaking, recognition of pacemaker malfunction, and the functions and uses of ICD devices.

## PACEMAKERS

*A pacemaker is a battery-powered device designed to stimulate the heart electrically.* This device is used primarily when a patient's own heart rate is excessively slow (see Chapter 20 for discussion of bradycardias). A pacemaker has two major components: a battery that serves as the power source and wire electrodes that are attached to the heart chamber(s) being stimulated.

Pacemakers are either *temporary* or *permanent (implanted)*. With temporary pacemakers, the pacing wire is connected to a battery outside the body. With long-term implanted pacemakers, the battery is inserted subcutaneously, usually under the chest wall. With both types, the pacemaker wire is usually threaded through a vein into the right ventricular cavity so that the pacemaker electrode can stimulate the endocardium of the right ventricle (Fig. 21-1). Occasionally, an *epicardial* pacemaker wire is used. This wire is sewn directly into the epicardium of the left or right ventricle, and the battery is implanted under the skin of the abdomen. Atrial pacing can also be performed. Many patients benefit from a *dual-chamber* pacemaker therapy in which electrodes are placed in both the right atrium and right ventricle.

As described later, pacemakers have two additional specialized uses: (1) treating certain types of tachycardias, and (2) improving

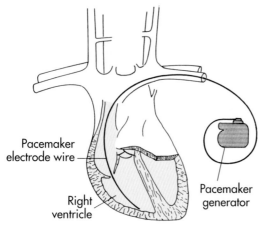

**FIGURE 21-1** Implanted pacemaker generator (battery) with a wire electrode inserted through the left subclavian vein into the right ventricle.

ventricular function in selected patients with congestive heart failure as part of *cardiac resynchronization therapy* using *biventricular pacing.*

## PACEMAKER ECG PATTERNS

When a ventricular pacemaker fires, it produces a sharp vertical deflection (pacemaker spike) followed by a QRS complex (representing depolarization of the ventricle). Can you predict what the ECG shows with a functioning right ventricular pacemaker? The ECG should show a left bundle branch block (LBBB) pattern (see Fig. 7-8). Recall that the pacemaker is initially stimulating the right ventricle and therefore left ventricular depolarization is delayed.

Typical pacemaker tracings are shown in Figures 7-8 and 21-2. The vertical line preceding each QRS complex is the pacemaker spike. This sharp deflection is followed by a wide QRS complex with LBBB morphology (QS in lead $V_1$ and wide R wave in lead $V_6$). What pattern would you predict with an epicardial pacemaker stimulating the left ventricle? It would be a right bundle branch block pattern.

An atrial pacemaker produces a spike followed by a P wave (Fig. 21-3).

Pacemaker patterns seen with biventricular pacing as part of cardiac resynchronization therapy are described later in this chapter.

## PACEMAKER BATTERIES

A variety of battery units can be used to power implanted pacemakers. Early pacemaker batteries used mercury-zinc cells. Because of their relatively short life span, however, these units were supplanted by lithium batteries, which

### Ventricular (VVI) Pacemaker

Lead II

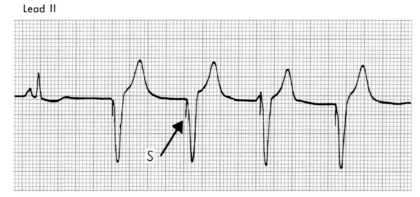

**FIGURE 21-2** Pacemaker beats. The first P-QRS cycle is from a normal sinus beat. It is followed by four pacemaker beats. Notice the pacemaker spike (S) preceding each paced beat. Pacemaker beats are wide and resemble bundle branch block beats. Because this type of pacemaker senses and paces only in the right ventricle and is inhibited by the intrinsic QRS complexes, it is termed a *VVI unit.* (See Appendix at the end of this chapter.)

## Atrial Pacemaker

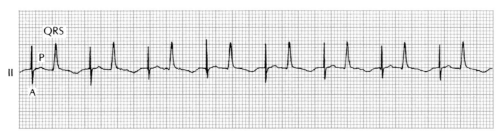

**FIGURE 21-3** With the pacemaker electrode placed in the right atrium, a pacemaker spike (A) is seen before each P wave. The QRS complex is normal because the ventricle is not being electronically paced.

may last 5 or more years. As the power cell of a conventional pacemaker wears out, the pacemaker rate usually starts to slow.

### VENTRICULAR PACING: FIXED-RATE AND DEMAND PACEMAKERS

The two modes of pacemaker function are *fixed rate* and *demand*. A fixed-rate pacemaker is one that fires at a specific preset rate, regardless of the patient's own heart rate. The earliest pacemakers were fixed-rate devices. Contemporary pacemakers are demand units. A demand pacemaker literally functions "on demand," that is, only when the patient's heart rate falls below a preset value. Therefore a demand pacemaker incorporates two distinct features: (1) a *sensing* mechanism designed so that the pacemaker is inhibited when the patient's own heart rate is adequate, and (2) a *pacing* mechanism designed to trigger the pacemaker when no intrinsic QRS complexes occur within a predetermined period. By contrast, fixed-rate pacemakers lack a sensing mechanism.

Demand units can be temporarily converted to fixed-rate mode by placing a special magnet on the chest wall over the battery. The magnet test is routinely performed when the pacemaker rate is being checked. Present-day demand-type pacemakers are also "programmable." This means that the pacing rate can be adjusted once a pacemaker is implanted. Adjustment of rate is accomplished by placing a special telemetry device on the chest wall to allow communication with the pacemaker.

Demand ventricular pacemakers usually are QRS (R wave) inhibited. They emit pulses only when the spontaneous heart rate falls below the escape rate of the pacemaker (e.g., 70 beats/min) (Fig. 21-4). They do not emit pulses when the patient's spontaneous heart rate is faster than the escape rate of the pacemaker. Each time a QRS-inhibited pacemaker senses a spontaneous QRS complex, formation of a pacemaker pulse is inhibited. Therefore these pacemakers show pacemaker spikes only when the spontaneous heart rate is slower than the escape

**FIGURE 21-4** A ventricular demand (QRS-inhibited) pacemaker emits an electronic pulse only when the intrinsic heart rate falls below the escape rate of the pacemaker.

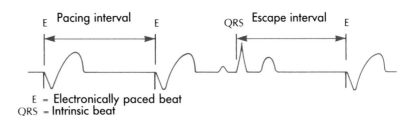

E = Electronically paced beat
QRS = Intrinsic beat

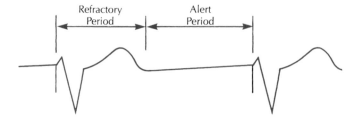

**FIGURE 21-5** During the refractory period a ventricular demand pacemaker does not sense any electrical activity. The refractory period is followed by the alert period. If no QRS complex is sensed by the end of the alert period, the pacemaker emits an escape pulse.

rate of the pacemaker. The spikes appear before each QRS complex.

The QRS-inhibited pacemaker also has a *refractory* period (e.g., 0.4 sec) that begins whenever the pacemaker senses a QRS complex or emits a pulse (Fig. 21-5). During the refractory period, the pacemaker cannot sense another R wave. If spontaneous ventricular beats or ventricular premature complexes occur during the refractory period, however, they are not inhibited but appear on the ECG.

The refractory period is followed by an *alert* period, during which the pacemaker can sense an R wave. If no QRS complex is sensed by the end of the alert period, the pacemaker emits another pulse (see Fig. 21-5). If a spontaneous QRS complex occurs, however, the pacemaker is recycled into another refractory period and then into another alert period.

### DUAL-CHAMBER PACING

In dual-chamber pacemakers, electrodes are inserted into both the right atrium and right ventricle. With most models in use today, the circuitry permits sensing and pacing in both chambers. Thus the atrial lead is able to sense the patient's intrinsic P waves and stimulates the atrium when the atrial rate becomes too slow. The circuitry is designed to allow for a physiologic delay between atrial and ventricular stimulation. This *atrioventricular (AV) delay* (interval between the atrial and ventricular pacemaker spikes) is analogous to the PR interval seen in physiologic conduction.

With the type of dual-chamber pacemaker that allows for both atrial sensing and pacing

and ventricular sensing and pacing, a variety of ECG patterns may be seen, depending on the patient's intrinsic electrical activity. A schematic of these pacemaker patterns appears in Figure 21-6.

Dual-chamber pacing is helpful in maintaining physiologic timing between atrial and ventricular systole. When ventricular pacing alone is used, this physiologic timing is lost. In some patients, the loss of timed atrial contractions causes a marked reduction in cardiac output. Dual-chamber pacing produces a significant improvement in the cardiac performance of these individuals. In selected patients, dual-chamber pacing may allow a physiologic increase in ventricular rate during exercise. For example, consider the patient with complete heart block and underlying sinus rhythm whose ventricular rate with a ventricular pacemaker is constant (e.g., 72 beats/min) regardless of the atrial (P wave) rate. With a dual-chamber pacemaker, the ventricular rate can increase in tandem with the sinus rate during exercise, further increasing cardiac output. Atrial sensing or pacing is obviously of no use in patients with chronic atrial fibrillation or atrial flutter.

### PROGRAMMABILITY

In the early days of cardiac pacing, the pacemaker rate was not adjustable once the unit had been inserted. A major advance was the introduction of programmable pacemakers, in which the pacemaker rate could be externally changed.

In addition to rate, many other parameters can be externally programmed in modern pacemakers. These parameters include the voltage

## Dual-Chamber (DDD) Pacemaker Functions

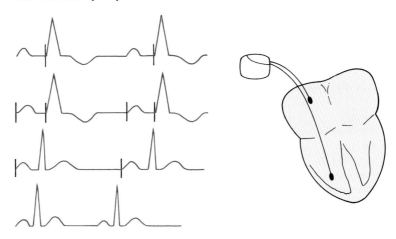

A. Atrial sensing
   Ventricular pacing

B. Atrial pacing
   Ventricular pacing

C. Atrial pacing
   Ventricular sensing

D. Atrial and ventricular
   sensing

**FIGURE 21-6**  Dual-chamber (DDD) pacemakers sense and pace in both atria and ventricles. The pacemaker emits a stimulus (spike) whenever a native P wave or QRS complex is not sensed within some programmed time interval.

of the pacemaker discharge, the sensitivity of the electrode to the intrinsic beats, the pacemaker refractory period, and the duration of the pacemaker spike.

## INDICATIONS FOR CARDIAC PACING

### Implanted (Permanent) Pacemakers

The major reason for implanting a pacemaker is the presence of a symptomatic bradyarrhythmia. In particular, electronic pacemakers may be indicated for numerous conditions, including syncope, light-headedness, weakness, or congestive failure associated with complete heart block, second-degree AV block, marked sinus bradycardia or sinus pauses (sick sinus syndrome), slow junctional rhythms, or atrial fibrillation or flutter with an excessively slow ventricular response.

Pacemaker functions have also been incorporated in new generations of implantable cardioverter-defibrillator (ICD) devices, as described in the section to follow.

### Temporary Pacemakers

Temporary pacemakers may be *transvenous* or *transcutaneous*. With transvenous pacemakers, the battery is connected to a pacing electrode that has been threaded through a vein into the right ventricle. With transcutaneous temporary pacing, specially designed electrodes are pasted on the chest wall. Although this technique is not successful in all patients and may cause some discomfort, it may be useful in certain critical circumstances when transvenous pacing is not available (see Chapter 19).

Temporary pacemakers are often employed during cardiac emergencies (e.g., myocardial infarction [MI]) when an extremely slow heart rate occurs. For example, they may be used immediately after open heart surgery or during cardiac arrest (see Chapter 19) when the ECG shows asystole or a slow escape rhythm that does not respond to drug therapy. Occasionally, temporary pacemakers are needed in patients with digitalis or other drug toxicity that is causing profound bradycardia.

As noted, temporary or permanent pacemakers are usually employed when the heart rate is too slow. Sometimes, a pacemaker is implanted to treat a tachyarrhythmia (e.g., ventricular tachycardia). The use of temporary pacing to treat atrial flutter is mentioned in Chapter 15. The use of overdrive pacemaking as part of ICD devices is discussed in this chapter.

## Pacemaker Malfunction: Failure to Sense

Monitor

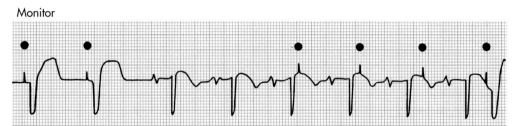

**FIGURE 21-7**  Notice that after the first two paced complexes, a series of sinus beats with a prolonged PR interval is seen. Failure of the pacemaker unit to sense these intrinsic QRS complexes leads to inappropriate pacemaker spikes (●), which sometimes fall on T waves. Three of these spikes do not capture the ventricle because they occur during the refractory period of the cardiac cycle.  (Adapted from Conover MB: Understanding Electrocardiography, 4th ed. St. Louis, Mosby, 1996.)

## Pacemaker Malfunction: Failure to Sense and Capture

Monitor

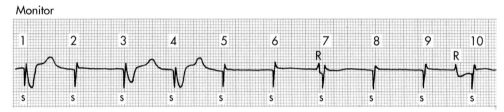

**FIGURE 21-8**  Notice that beats 1, 3, and 4 show pacemaker spikes (s) and normally paced wide QRS complexes and T waves. The remaining beats show only pacemaker spikes without capture. (R represents the patient's slow spontaneous QRS complexes, which the pacemaker also fails to sense.)

## PACEMAKER MALFUNCTION

Pacemaker malfunctions occur when either the sensing or pacing function is impaired. For example, when the pacemaker battery runs down, the pacing rate generally slows and *failure to sense or pace* may also occur. Failure to sense can be diagnosed by observing pacemaker spikes despite the patient's own adequate rate (Fig. 21-7). The two most common causes of failure to sense (without actual battery failure) are dislodgment of the pacemaker wire and excessive fibrosis around the tip of the pacing wire.

Pacemaker malfunction can also result from *failure to pace.* This problem is diagnosed by observing pacemaker spikes without subsequent QRS complexes (failure to "capture") (Fig. 21-8), or by finding no pacemaker spikes even though the patient has an excessively slow heart rate (Fig. 21-9). Failure to pace can also be caused by dislodgment of the pacemaker wire or by fibrosis around the tip of the pacing wire. In such cases, pacemaker spikes occur without associated QRS complexes. In other cases (particularly with a broken electrode wire, a short circuit in the pacing circuit, electrical interference from the muscles of the chest wall, or battery failure), failure to pace occurs without any pacemaker spike.

Pacemaker malfunction in patients with temporary pacemakers should always prompt an immediate search for loose connections

## Pacemaker Malfunction: Failure to Pace

Lead II

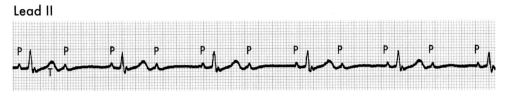

**FIGURE 21-9** The underlying rhythm is second-degree (2:1) AV block. Despite the very slow QRS, the pacemaker fails to function.

between the battery and the pacing wire, a faulty battery, or a dislodged wire.

### COMPLICATIONS OF PACEMAKER THERAPY

Pacemakers are not without potential harm. Therefore careful thought should be given before a temporary or particularly a permanent pacemaker is inserted. Infection may occur at the pacemaker site. The electrode may perforate the ventricular wall. The pacemaker itself may cause serious arrhythmias. For example, dual-chamber pacemakers may facilitate runs of supraventricular tachycardia ("endless loop" pacemaker-mediated arrhythmias). Occasionally, a pacemaker also paces the muscles of the chest wall or the diaphragm, resulting in patient discomfort.

Patients with ventricular demand-type pacemakers also lose the normal physiologic timing afforded by the sequential contraction of the atria and ventricles. In some cases, patients will develop symptoms (so-called *pacemaker syndrome*) due to this loss of physiologic timing. Complaints may include light-headedness, fainting, shortness of breath, and cough. Upgrading the pacemaker unit to a dual-chamber device with atrial and ventricular sensing and pacing will generally alleviate these symptoms. Right ventricular pacing may also reduce cardiac functions by causing asynchronous ventricular activation.

### DIAGNOSIS OF MYOCARDIAL INFARCTION WITH PACEMAKERS

The ECG diagnosis of MI may be difficult or impossible when all the QRS complexes are paced. With a right ventricular electrode, the ECG shows a left bundle branch block (LBBB) configuration. As described in Chapter 8, LBBB generally masks both the QRS and the ST-T changes of MI. Therefore, unless you see spontaneous QRS-T complexes, you may not be able to diagnose acute or prior MI based on the ECG alone.

Finally, pacemakers may also produce ECG changes simulating MI. After periods of ventricular pacing, the ECG may show deep T wave inversions in the nonpaced beats. These so-called *postpacemaker ("memory") T wave inversions* can be mistaken for primary ischemic ST-T changes.

### PACEMAKERS AND CARDIAC RESYNCHRONIZATION THERAPY IN CHRONIC HEART FAILURE

As noted, the major use of implanted pacemakers is to treat symptomatic bradycardias (Chapter 20). A more recent and innovative use of electronic pacemakers is to help improve ventricular function in selected patients with heart failure. This therapy was designed specifically to increase the low cardiac output by coordinating the contraction pattern of the two ventricles. Therefore this approach, which employs simultaneous pacing of the right and left ventricles, is referred to as *cardiac resynchronization therapy (CRT)* or *biventricular (BiV) pacing.*

As the name implies, BiV pacemaker technology is based on positioning one pacemaker lead (electrode wire) in the right ventricle and a second one in a position to stimulate simulta-

## Biventricular Pacemaker

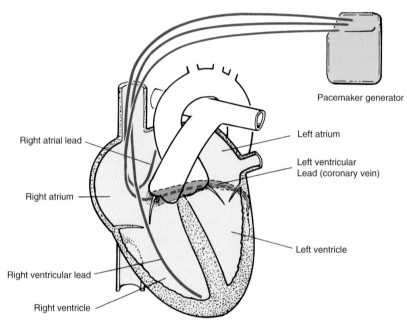

Pacemaker generator

Left atrium

Left ventricular
Lead (coronary vein)

Right atrial lead

Right atrium

Left ventricle

Right ventricular lead

Right ventricle

**FIGURE 21-10** Biventricular (BiV) pacemaker. Note the pacemaker lead in the coronary sinus vein that allows pacing of the left ventricle simultaneously with the right ventricle. BiV pacing is used in selected patients with congestive heart failure with left ventricular conduction delays to help "resynchronize" cardiac activation and thereby improve cardiac function.

neously the left ventricle. The pacing wire for the left ventricle is placed in a cardiac vein on the lateral surface of the heart. This site can be accessed via the coronary sinus, the heart's main venous blood vessel that delivers blood from the heart back to the right ventricle, as shown in Figure 21-10. Except in patients with atrial fibrillation or flutter, an atrial pacing electrode is also placed to allow for atrial sensing and, if needed, atrial pacing. In this way, the unit can be programmed such that the BiV stimulus is delivered at an optimal interval after the P wave.

Currently, the major indication for CRT is for patients with severe chronic heart failure who: (1) are still symptomatic on conventional medical therapy, and (2) have a wide QRS complex due to complete LBBB (or a similar) pattern. The LBBB results in an asynchronous pattern of ventricular contraction. Pacing the right and left ventricles at the same time with this kind of intraventricular conduction delay may help restore a more coordinated sequence of cardiac activation and contraction.

CRT has proven to be useful in improving symptoms (e.g., fatigue, shortness of breath) and objective measures of ventricular performance in appropriately selected groups of patients. Further, such therapy may also decrease the number of hospitalizations and even improve survival in some patients with heart failure.

## A. Right ventricular pacing      B. Biventricular pacing

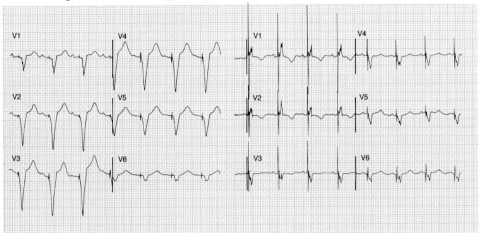

**FIGURE 21-11** Right ventricular and biventricular pacing. **A,** Patient with heart failure who had a standard dual chamber (right atrial and right ventricular) pacemaker. **B,** To improve cardiac function, the pacemaker was upgraded to a biventricular (BiV) device. Note that during right ventricular pacing **(A),** the ECG shows a left bundle branch block morphology. The preceding sinus P waves are sensed by the atrial lead. In contrast, during biventricular pacing **(B),** the QRS complexes show a right bundle branch block morphology. Also, the QRS duration is somewhat shorter during biventricular pacing, due to the cardiac resynchronization effects of pacing the ventricles in a nearly simultaneous fashion.

As described, the ECG during standard pacing of the right ventricle shows an LBBB type pattern. In contrast, with BiV during CRT, the ECG usually shows an RBBB type pattern (Fig. 21-11).

BiV pacing in patients with heart failure can be combined with implantable cardioverter-defibrillator (ICD) therapy, which is described in the next section.

## IMPLANTABLE CARDIOVERTER-DEFIBRILLATOR THERAPY

Sudden cardiac arrest, occurring unexpectedly, is most commonly due to the abrupt onset of ventricular fibrillation, often preceded by a run of ventricular tachycardia (Chapter 19). Less common causes are asystole and pulseless electrical activity. A major challenge in contemporary cardiology is how to prevent or interrupt episodes of ventricular arrhythmias that will otherwise lead to sudden cardiac death in high-risk patients.

The three major approaches to this problem used currently are: (1) antiarrhythmic drug therapy; (2) radiofrequency catheter ablation, designed to destroy arrhythmogenic areas of the ventricles; and (3) implantable cardioverter-defibrillators (ICDs). The rapid development of ICD therapy over the past few decades has been propelled by the findings that antiarrhythmic drug therapy is often ineffective or even dangerous and that catheter ablation has major limitations.

ICD therapy, as the name implies, involves the internal placement of a device, resembling a pacemaker, capable of delivering electrical shocks to the heart to terminate (cardiovert or defibrillate) a life-threatening run of ventricular tachycardia or ventricular fibrillation. This approach is modeled on conventional external cardioversion/defibrillation devices used in advanced cardiopulmonary resuscitation (CPR), which deliver an electrical shock via paddles placed on the chest wall to treat these types of tachycardias.

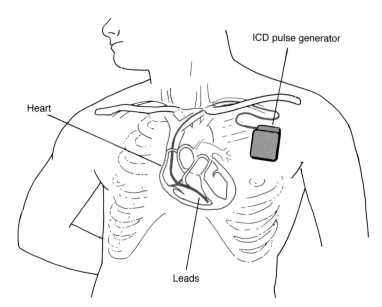

**FIGURE 21-12** An implanted cardioverter-defibrillator (ICD) device resembles a pacemaker with a pulse generator and a lead system. The device can sense potentially lethal ventricular arrhythmias and deliver appropriate electrical therapy, including defibrillatory shocks.

## ICD TECHNOLOGY

ICD devices resemble pacemakers and have two major components: a lead system and a pulse generator (Fig. 21-12). The lead system is used to sense cardiac electrical activity in the ventricles (and sometimes atria) and also to deliver shocks produced by the pulse generator. The ICD generator (about the size of a small pager) is usually inserted in the area of the pectoral muscle under the left collarbone, with the attached leads advanced through veins into the right side of the heart, like a pacemaker.

Contemporary ICD devices have many programmable features and have the capacity to deliver *tiered* (staged) therapy when they detect a tachyarrhythmia (Fig. 21-13). For example, the device may be programmed to perform antitachycardia (overdrive) pacing if it detects a presumed episode of ventricular tachycardia. This type of pacing may convert the arrhythmia without the need for an electrical cardioversion shock. If the arrhythmia persists or degenerates into ventricular fibrillation, actual shocks are delivered at increasing intensities. Newer ICD models also function as pacemakers in case of bradycardia. The ICD units have a storage

capability, allowing cardiac electrophysiologists to interrogate the device periodically and obtain a detailed record of any arrhythmias sensed and any antitachycardia pacing or shocks delivered.

## INDICATIONS FOR ICD THERAPY

The indications for ICD therapy have been expanding over recent years, based on miniaturization of the device, ease of implantation, and compelling clinical data showing a high degree of efficacy and safety compared with drug therapy.

A major and compelling indication is in *secondary prevention* of recurrent sudden death risk in patients who have already been resuscitated from an episode of cardiac arrest with ventricular fibrillation or ventricular tachycardia *not* due to a transient or reversible cause. Examples of transient or reversible causes of cardiac arrest include electrolyte abnormalities such as hypokalemia, acute myocardial infarction, and the use of drugs such as epinephrine or cocaine.

ICD therapy is also recommended in *primary prevention* of sudden death in very high–risk patients who have *spontaneous* episodes of sustained ventricular tachycardia with underlying structural heart disease (e.g., prior infarc-

## ICD: Tiered Therapy

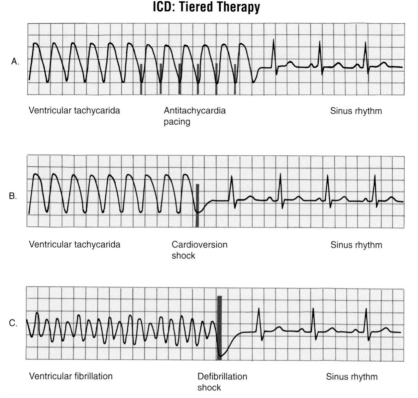

**FIGURE 21-13**  Tiered arrhythmia therapy and implanted cardioverter-defibrillators (ICDs). These devices are capable of automatically delivering staged therapy in treating ventricular tachycardia (VT) or ventricular fibrillation (VF), including antitachycardia pacing **(A)** and cardioversion shocks **(B)** for VT, and defibrillation shocks **(C)** for VF.

tion, cardiomyopathy) or in selected patients without evident structural heart disease. In addition, ICD therapy is used prophylactically in certain patients with syncope or chronic heart disease who have ventricular fibrillation or sustained ventricular tachycardia that is *induced* during an electrophysiologic study, as well as in selected patients with documented inherited or familial conditions with a high risk of a first episode of life-threatening ventricular tachyarrhythmia, especially long QT syndrome and hypertrophic cardiomyopathy.

Expanded indications for ICD placement for primary prevention of sudden cardiac death now also include selected patients with ischemic or nonischemic cardiomyopathy and other patients with coronary artery disease and a low left ventricular ejection fraction due to myocardial infarction, even in the absence of spontaneous or inducible ventricular tachyarrhythmia.

For detailed and updated guidelines to current and evolving indications for ICD therapy, and also pacemaker therapy, readers are referred to the websites of the American Heart Association, the American College of Cardiology, and the Heart Rhythm Society.

## COMPLICATIONS OF ICD THERAPY

ICD devices, despite their utility, are not without risk. The implantation procedure carries a small risk of death and serious morbidity related to vascular or myocardial perforation, infection, and thrombosis. After implantation, patients may suffer from inap-

| TABLE 21-1 | **Three-Position (Simplified) Pacemaker Code** | |
| --- | --- | --- |
| Position | Category | Letters used |
| I | Chamber(s) paced | |
| | Ventricle | V |
| | Atrium | A |
| | Dual (atrium and ventricle) | D |
| | None | O |
| II | Chamber(s) sensed | |
| | Ventricle | V |
| | Atrium | A |
| | Dual (atrium and ventricle) | D |
| | None | O |
| III | Mode of response(s) to sensing | |
| | Triggered | T |
| | Inhibited | I |
| | Dual (triggered and inhibited)* | D |
| | None | O |

*Dual* mode of response refers to dual-chamber pacemakers in which atrial pacing may be inhibited by the patient's own P waves and a ventricular spike may be inhibited by the patient's P wave if atrioventricular block is present. A single-chamber (VVI) pacemaker and a dual-chamber (DDD) pacemaker are depicted schematically below.

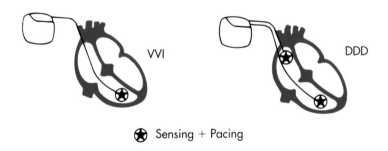

VVI          DDD

★ Sensing + Pacing

propriate and painful shocks delivered in response to electrical artifacts or non–life-threatening rhythms.

## APPENDIX: THE THREE- AND FIVE-LETTER PACEMAKER CODE

A simple three-position pacemaker code is often used to describe a particular pacemaker's functions and mode of response. As shown in Table 21-1, the letter in the first position indicates the chamber(s) being paced—the *atrium (A), ventricle (V),* or *both (D).* The letter in the second posi-

tion indicates the chamber(s) where sensing occurs—again the atrium (A), ventricle (V), or both (D). Finally, the letter in the third position refers to the mode of response of the pacemaker—*triggered (T), inhibited (I),* or *dual (D).*

Thus a VVI unit is identified as a single-chamber pacemaker that both paces (V) and senses (V) exclusively in the *ventricle* and is *inhibited* (I) by the patient's own QRS complexes.

The most versatile pacemakers are the DDD units. These are dual-chamber pacemakers that can pace the atrium or ventricle (D) and sense in the atrium or ventricle (D). In addition, the mode of response is dual (D). Consequently, atrial pacing can be inhibited by the patient's P waves, and a ventricular pacer spike is triggered by the patient's P waves if a native QRS complex does not appear within a preset time because of AV block.

The basic three-letter pacemaker code has been expanded to five letters, reflecting ongoing advances in pacemaker electronics. The fourth letter indicates the *programming* features of the pacemaker, including rate responsiveness (R).

Contemporary *rate-responsive pacemakers* are designed with special sensors to detect muscle activity, breathing, or other variables that correlate with increased activity. The pacing rate automatically increases with exercise to accommodate the need for increased cardiac output.

Thus a pacemaker that paces and senses only in the right ventricle and has rate-responsive capabilities is designated VVI-R. The fifth letter (less frequently used) indicates whether there is multisite pacing in the atria or ventricles (e.g., biventricular pacing).

# REVIEW

Electronic pacemakers are battery-powered devices used to stimulate the heart electrically, particularly when a patient's own heart rate is excessively slow. When the pacemaker wire is attached to the right ventricular endocardium, the ECG shows a left bundle branch block pattern because of delayed left ventricular stimulation. Each QRS complex is preceded by a pacemaker spike. Cardiac pacing can be done in a *fixed-rate* or *demand* mode. Demand pacemakers are inhibited when the heart rate is faster than the escape rate of the pacemaker.

A temporary pacemaker is a unit with an external battery. Temporary pacing wires can be inserted during cardiac emergencies (e.g., cardiac arrest caused by asystole or myocardial infarction [MI] complicated by high-degree heart block or sinus arrest). An implanted permanent pacemaker, in which the battery is inserted subcutaneously (usually in the chest wall) is indicated for patients with symptomatic second- or third-degree AV block or other major bradyarrhythmias (e.g., sinus arrest or slow junctional escape rhythm) leading to inadequate cardiac output.

*Dual-chamber* (atrial and ventricular) pacemakers were developed to maintain physio-

logic timing between atrial and ventricular contractions, thereby increasing cardiac output.

When the pacemaker battery starts to run down, the pacemaker rate slows. Dislodgment of the pacemaker wire or excessive fibrosis around the tip of the wire can cause failure to sense or failure to pace. Pacing failure in permanent units can also be caused by electrode fracture, short circuits, or electrical interference from skeletal muscles.

Pacemakers may obscure the ECG diagnosis of MI. Conversely, after electronic pacing of the ventricles, deep noninfarctional T wave inversions may appear in spontaneous QRS complexes (*postpacemaker T wave pattern*).

*Biventricular pacing*, designed to coordinate (resynchronize) the contraction of the left and right ventricles, is used primarily in selected patients with chronic heart failure.

*Implantable cardioverter-defibrillator* (ICD) therapy involves the internal placement of a device capable of delivering electrical shocks to the heart to interrupt a life-threatening run of ventricular tachycardia or ventricular fibrillation and thereby prevent syncope or sudden death. This therapy is used as secondary prevention in patients who have already been resuscitated from an episode of cardiac arrest due to ventricular fibrillation or ventricular tachycardia *not* due to a transient or reversible cause or in carefully selected patients at high risk for experiencing a sustained ventricular tachyarrhythmia (primary prevention).

# QUESTIONS

1. Which of the following is the major indication for a *permanent* pacemaker?
   a. History of multiple prior myocardial infarctions
   b. Symptomatic bradyarrhythmia
   c. Digitalis toxicity
   d. Ventricular bigeminy
   e. Paroxysmal supraventricular tachycardia

2. What does the following rhythm strip show?

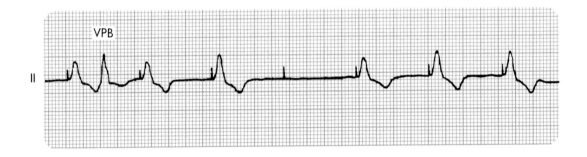

   a. Failure to sense
   b. Failure to pace
   c. Normal pacemaker function with a ventricular premature beat
   d. Failure to sense and pace

3. What is shown in the following rhythm strip?

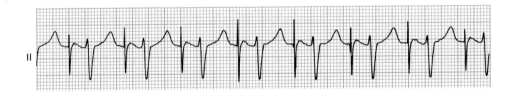

4. Biventricular (BiV) pacing is used primarily in which of the following conditions?
   a. Recurrent ventricular tachycardia
   b. Chronic heart failure with left bundle branch block
   c. Long QT syndromes
   d. Acute myocardial infarction with cardiogenic shock

5. *True or false:* Implantable cardioverter-defibrillators (ICDs) are most often employed with acute MI.

# Overview and Review

## CHAPTER 22

# How to Interpret an ECG

P art One of this book discussed the fundamentals of the normal ECG, and Part Two described the major abnormal patterns and arrhythmias. Drawing on those concepts and information, this chapter provides a systematic approach to ECG interpretation.

## ECG INTERPRETATION

Accurate interpretation of ECGs requires thoroughness and care. Therefore you must develop a systematic method of reading ECGs that is applied in every case. Many of the most common mistakes are errors of omission, specifically the failure to note certain subtle but critical findings. For example, overlooking a short PR interval may cause you to miss the important Wolff-Parkinson-White pattern. Marked prolongation of the QT interval, a potential precursor of torsades de pointes (see Chapter 16) and sudden cardiac death (see Chapter 19), sometimes goes unnoticed. These and other common pitfalls in ECG diagnosis are reviewed in Chapter 23.

## ECG FEATURES TO ANALYZE

On every ECG, 14 features should be analyzed. These features are listed in Box 22-1 and discussed in the following sections.

### Standardization and Technical Features

Make sure that the electrocardiograph has been properly calibrated so that the standardization mark is 10 mm tall (1 mV = 10 mm) (see Chapter 2).* Also check for limb lead reversal (see Chapter 23) and ECG artifacts (discussed later in this chapter).

### Heart Rate

Calculate the heart rate (see Chapter 2). If the rate is faster than 100 beats/min, a tachycardia is present. A rate slower than 60 beats/min means that a bradycardia is present.

### Rhythm

The cardiac rhythm can almost always be described in one of the following four categories: (1) sinus rhythm (or a sinus variant such as sinus bradycardia or sinus tachycardia); (2) sinus rhythm with extra (ectopic) beats such as atrial premature beats (APBs) or ventricular premature beats (VPBs); (3) an entirely ectopic (nonsinus) mechanism such as atrial fibrillation or flutter, ventricular tachycardia, or an atrioventricular (AV) junctional escape rhythm; or

---

*In special cases, the ECG may be intentionally recorded at one-half standardization (1 mV = 5 mm) or two-times normal standardization (1 mV = 20 mm).

---

| BOX 22-1 | **14 Features to Analyze on Every ECG** |

Standardization (calibration) and technical
quality
Heart rate
Rhythm
PR interval
P wave size
QRS width (interval)
QT interval
QRS voltage
Mean QRS electrical axis
R wave progression in chest leads
Abnormal Q waves
ST segments
T waves
U waves

---

(4) sinus rhythm or some ectopic rhythm (e.g., atrial fibrillation) with second- or third-degree heart block or other AV dissociation mechanism.

Sometimes, the ECG will show an abrupt change between two of these mechanisms, for example, paroxysmal atrial fibrillation spontaneously converting to sinus rhythm.

Be particularly careful not to overlook hidden P waves. These waves may be present, for example, in some cases of second- or third-degree AV block, atrial tachycardia (AT) with block, or blocked atrial premature beats (APBs). Also, whenever the ventricular rate is about 150 per minute, always consider the possibility of atrial flutter because the flutter waves may mimic the P waves of AT or sinus tachycardia.

## PR Interval

The normal PR interval (measured from the beginning of the P wave to the beginning of the QRS complex) is 0.12 to 0.2 second. A uniformly prolonged PR interval is often referred to as *first-degree AV block* (see Chapter 17). A short PR interval with sinus rhythm and with a wide QRS complex and a delta wave is seen in the Wolff-Parkinson-White pattern. By contrast, a short PR interval with retrograde P waves (negative in lead II) generally indicates an ectopic (atrial or AV junctional) pacemaker.

## P Wave Size

Normally, the P wave does not exceed 2.5 mm in amplitude and is less than 3 mm wide in all leads. Tall peaked P waves may be a sign of right atrial overload (P pulmonale). Wide P waves are seen with left atrial abnormality.

## QRS Width (Interval)

Normally, the QRS width is 0.1 second (100 msec) or less in all leads. The differential diagnosis of a wide QRS complex is described in Chapter 24.

## QT Interval

A prolonged QT interval may be a clue to electrolyte disturbances (hypocalcemia or hypokalemia), drug effects (quinidine, procainamide, amiodarone, or sotalol), or myocardial ischemia (usually with prominent T wave inversions). Shortened QT intervals are seen with hypercalcemia and digitalis effect.

## QRS Voltage

Look for signs of right or left ventricular hypertrophy (see Chapter 6). Remember that thin-chested people, athletes, and young adults frequently show tall voltage without left ventricular hypertrophy (LVH). Do not forget about low voltage, which may result from pericardial effusion or pleural effusion, hypothyroidism, emphysema, obesity, myocardial disease, or other factors (see Chapter 24).

## Mean QRS Electrical Axis

Estimate the mean QRS axis in the frontal plane. Decide by inspection whether the axis is normal (between −30° and +100°) or whether left or right axis deviation is present (see Fig. 5-13).

## R Wave Progression in Chest Leads

Inspect leads $V_1$ to $V_6$ to see if the normal increase in the R/S ratio occurs as you move across the chest (see Chapter 4). The terms "poor" or preferably "slow" R wave progression (small or absent R waves in leads $V_1$ to $V_3$)* refer to a finding that may be a sign of anterior myocardial infarction (MI), but may also be seen in many other settings, including: altered lead placement, LVH, chronic lung disease, left bundle branch block, and many other conditions in the absence of infarction.

### Abnormal Q Waves

Prominent Q waves in leads II, III, and $aV_F$ may indicate inferior wall infarction. Prominent Q waves in the anterior leads (I, $aV_L$, and $V_1$ to $V_6$) may indicate anterior wall infarction (see Chapter 8).

### ST Segments

Look for abnormal ST segment elevations or depressions.

### T Waves

Inspect the T waves. Normally, they are positive in leads with a positive QRS complex. They are also normally positive in leads $V_3$ to $V_6$ in adults, negative in lead $aV_R$, and positive in lead II. The polarity of the T waves in the other extremity leads depends on the QRS electrical axis. (T waves may be normally negative in lead III even in the presence of a vertical QRS axis.)

### U Waves

Look for prominent U waves. These waves may be a sign of hypokalemia or drug effect or toxicity (e.g., amiodarone, dofetilide, quinidine, sotalol).

**Memory aid:** Students looking for a mnemonic to help recall key features of the ECG can try using "IR-WAX." *I* is for the four basic intervals (Heart rate, PR, QRS, QT); *R* is for rhythm (sinus or other), *W* is for the five alphabetic waves (P, QRS, ST, T and U), and *AX* is for electrical axis.

---

*The term *reversed R wave progression* is used to describe abnormally tall R waves in lead $V_1$ that progressively decrease in amplitude. This pattern may occur with a number of conditions, including right ventricular hypertrophy, posterior (or posterolateral) infarction, and dextrocardia.

## FORMULATING AN INTERPRETATION

After you have analyzed the 14 ECG features, you should formulate an overall interpretation. The final ECG reading actually consists of three sections:

1. A list of notable findings

2. An interpretive summary that attempts to integrate or explain these findings

3. A comparison with prior ECGs, if available.

For example, the ECG might show a prolonged QT interval and prominent U waves. The interpretation could be "Repolarization abnormalities consistent with drug effect or toxicity or hypokalemia. Clinical correlation suggested." Another ECG might show wide P waves, right axis deviation, and a tall R wave in lead $V_1$ (see Fig. 23-1). The interpretation could be "Findings consistent with left atrial abnormality (enlargement) and right ventricular hypertrophy. This combination is highly suggestive of mitral stenosis." In yet a third case, the interpretation might simply be "Within normal limits."

You should also formulate a statement comparing the present ECG with previous ECGs (when available). The absence of a comparison ECG should be noted.

Thus the ECG report is analogous to a newspaper account that consists of the hard facts and then the editorial comment. Like the editorialist, the ECG interpreter may sometimes offer suggestions such as "Serial tracings advisable to evaluate possible evolving ischemic T wave changes." Figure 22-1 illustrates this systematic approach to ECG interpretation.

Every ECG abnormality you identify should summon up a list of differential diagnostic possibilities (see Chapter 24). *You should search for an explanation of every abnormality found.* For example, if the ECG shows sinus tachycardia, you need to find the cause of the arrhythmia. Is it a result of anxiety, hyperthyroidism, congestive heart failure, hypovolemia, sympathomimetic drugs, alcohol withdrawal, or other causes? If you find ventricular tachycar-

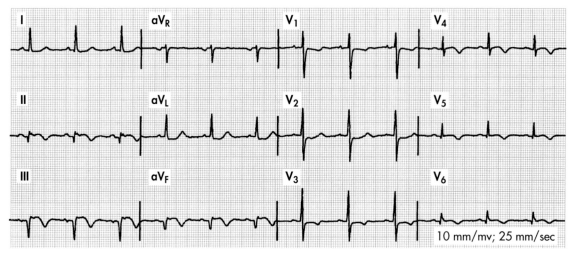

**FIGURE 22-1** ECG for interpretation: (1) standardization—10 mm/mV; 25 mm/sec (electronic calibration); (2) heart rate—75 beats/min; (3) rhythm—normal sinus; (4) PR interval—0.16 sec; (5) P waves—normal size; (6) QRS width—0.08 sec (normal); (7) QT interval—0.4 sec (slightly prolonged for rate); (8) QRS voltage—normal; (9) mean QRS axis—about –30° (biphasic QRS complex in lead II with positive QRS complex in lead I); (10) R wave progression in chest leads—early precordial transition with relatively tall R wave in lead $V_2$; (11) abnormal Q waves—leads II, III, and $aV_F$; (12) ST segments—slightly elevated in leads II, III, $aV_F$, $V_4$, $V_5$, and $V_6$; slightly depressed in leads $V_1$ and $V_2$; (13) T waves—inverted in leads II, III, $aV_F$, and $V_3$ through $V_6$; and (14) U waves—not prominent. *Impression: This ECG is consistent with an inferolateral (or inferoposterolateral) wall myocardial infarction of indeterminate age, possibly recent or evolving.* Comment: The relatively tall R wave in lead $V_2$ could reflect loss of lateral potentials or actual posterior wall involvement.

dia, what are the diagnostic possibilities? Is it due to MI or some promptly reversible cause such as hypoxemia, digitalis toxicity, toxic effects of another drug, hypokalemia, or hypomagnesemia? If you see signs of LVH, is the likely cause valvular heart disease, hypertensive heart disease, or cardiomyopathy? In this way, the interpretation of an ECG becomes an integral part of clinical diagnosis and patient care.

## COMPUTERIZED ECG INTERPRETATIONS

Computerized ECG systems are now widely used. These systems provide interpretation and storage of ECG records. The computer programs (software) for ECG analysis have become more sophisticated and accurate.

Despite these advances, computer ECG analyses have important limitations and not infrequently are subject to error. Diagnostic

errors are most likely with arrhythmias or more complex abnormalities. Therefore computerized interpretations (including measurements of basic ECG intervals and electrical axes) must never be accepted without careful review.

## ECG ARTIFACTS

The ECG, like any other electronic recording, is subject to numerous artifacts that may interfere with accurate interpretation. Some of the most common of these are described here.

### 60-HERTZ (CYCLE) INTERFERENCE

Interference from alternating-current generators produces the characteristic pattern shown in Figure 22-2. Notice the fine-tooth comb 60-hertz (Hz) artifacts. You can usually eliminate 60-Hz interference by switching the electrocardiograph plug to a different outlet or turning off other electrical appliances in the room.

Monitor lead

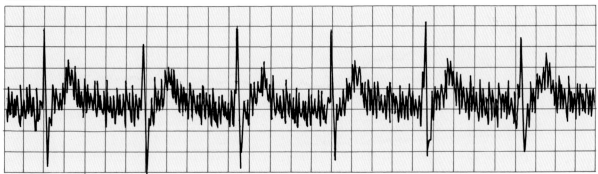

**FIGURE 22-2**   Common ECG artifact produced by 60-Hz electrical interference.

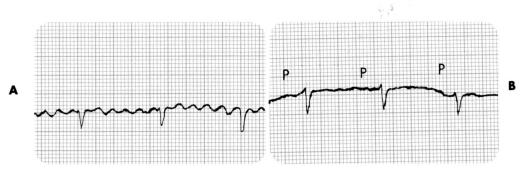

**FIGURE 22-3**   Common ECG artifact produced by muscle tremor. *A,* Wavy baseline simulating atrial flutter. *B,* Same recording without the artifact, showing normal P waves.

## MUSCLE TREMOR

Involuntary muscle tremor (e.g., parkinsonism) can produce undulations in the baseline that may be mistaken for atrial flutter or fibrillation (Fig. 22-3).

## WANDERING BASELINE

Upward or downward movement of the baseline may produce spurious ST segment elevations or depressions (Fig. 22-4).

## POOR ELECTRODE CONTACT OR PATIENT MOVEMENT

Poor electrode contact or patient movement (Fig. 22-5) can produce artifactual deflections in the baseline that may obscure the underlying pattern or be mistaken for abnormal beats.

## IMPROPER STANDARDIZATION

The electrocardiograph, as mentioned, should be standardized before each tracing so that a 1-mV pulse produces a square wave 10 mm high (see Fig. 2-5). Failure to standardize properly results in complexes that are either spuriously low or spuriously high. Furthermore, most electrocardiographs are equipped with half-standardization and double-standardization settings. Unintentional recording of an ECG on either of these settings also results in misleading low or high voltage.

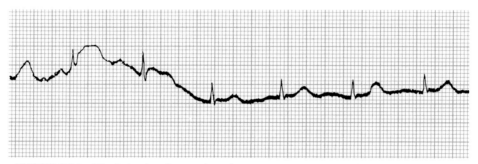

**FIGURE 22-4** Wandering baseline resulting from patient movement or loose electrode contact.

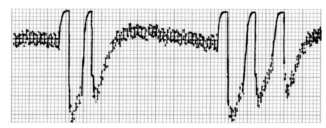

**FIGURE 22-5** Deflections simulating ventricular premature beats, produced by patient movement. An artifact produced by 60-Hz interference is also present.

# REVIEW

The following 14 points should be evaluated on every ECG: standardization, heart rate, rhythm, PR interval, P wave size, QRS width (interval), QT interval, QRS voltage, mean QRS axis, R wave progression in chest leads, abnormal Q waves, ST segments, T waves, and U waves. Any ECG abnormality should be related to the clinical status of the patient.

Computer interpretations of ECGs are subject to error and must be carefully reviewed. The ECG can also be affected by numerous artifacts, including 60-Hz interference, patient movement, poor electrode contact, and muscle tremor.

## CHAPTER 23

# Limitations and Uses of the ECG

Throughout this book, the clinical uses of the ECG have been stressed. This review chapter underscores some important *limitations* of the ECG, reemphasizes its *utility*, and reviews some common *pitfalls* in its interpretation.

## IMPORTANT LIMITATIONS OF THE ECG

Like most clinical tests, the ECG yields both *false-positive* and *false-negative* results. A false-positive result is an apparently abnormal ECG in a normal subject. For example, prominent precordial voltage may occur in the absence of left ventricular hypertrophy (see Chapter 6). Furthermore, Q waves may occur as a normal variant and therefore do not always indicate heart disease (see Chapters 8 and 9). False-negative results, on the other hand, occur when the ECG fails to show evidence of some cardiac abnormality. For example, some patients with acute myocardial infarction (MI) may not show diagnostic ST-T changes, and patients with severe coronary artery disease may not show diagnostic ST depressions during stress testing (Chapter 9).

The diagnostic accuracy of any test is determined by the percentages of false-positive and false-negative results. The *sensitivity* of a test is a measure of the percentage of patients with a particular abnormality that can be identified by an abnormal test result. For example, a test with 100% sensitivity has no false-negative results. The more false-negative results, the less sensitive is the test. The *specificity* of a test is a measure of the percentage of false-positive results. The more false-positive test results, the less specific is the test.

As just noted, both the sensitivity and specificity of the ECG in diagnosing a variety of conditions, including MI, are limited. Clinicians need to be aware of these diagnostic limitations. The following are some important problems that *cannot* be excluded simply because the ECG is normal or shows only nondiagnostic abnormalities:

- Prior MI

- Acute MI*

- Severe coronary artery disease

- Significant left ventricular hypertrophy (LVH)

---

*The pattern of acute MI may also be masked in patients with left bundle branch block, Wolff-Parkinson-White preexcitation patterns, or electronic ventricular pacemakers.

- Significant right ventricular hypertrophy (RVH)

- Intermittent arrhythmias such as paroxysmal atrial fibrillation (AF), paroxysmal supraventricular tachycardia (PSVT), ventricular tachycardia (VT), and bradycardias

- Acute pulmonary embolism

- Pericarditis, acute or chronic

## UTILITY OF THE ECG IN SPECIAL SETTINGS

Although the ECG has definite limitations, it often helps in the diagnosis of specific cardiac conditions and sometimes aids in the evaluation and management of general medical problems such as life-threatening electrolyte disorders (Box 23-1). Some particular areas in which the ECG may be helpful are as follows:

- *Myocardial infarction*

   Most patients with acute MI show diagnostic ECG changes (i.e., new Q waves and/or ST elevations, hyperacute T waves, ST depressions, or T wave inversions). In the weeks and months after an acute MI, however, these changes may become less apparent and, in some cases, may disappear.

   ST segment elevation in a right chest lead (e.g., $V_4R$) in a patient with acute inferior infarction suggests associated right ventricular ischemia or infarction (see Chapter 8).

   Persistent ST elevations several weeks after an MI should suggest a ventricular aneurysm.

- *Pulmonary embolism*

   A new $S_IQ_{III}$ or right bundle branch block pattern, particularly in association with sinus tachycardia, should suggest the possibility of acute cor pulmonale resulting from, for example, pulmonary embolism (see Chapter 11).

- *Pericardial tamponade*

   Low QRS voltage in a patient with elevated central venous pressure (distended neck veins) and sinus tachycardia suggests possible pericardial tamponade. Sinus tachycardia with electrical alternans is virtually diagnostic of pericardial effusion with tamponade (see Chapter 11).

- *Aortic valve disease*

   LVH is seen in most patients with critical aortic stenosis or severe aortic regurgitation.

- *Mitral valve disease*

   ECG signs of left atrial enlargement (abnormality) and RVH strongly suggest mitral stenosis (Fig. 23-1).

   Frequent ventricular premature beats (VPBs) and nonspecific ST-T changes, particularly in a younger patient, should prompt a search for mitral valve prolapse.

- *Atrial septal defect*

   Most patients with a moderate to large atrial septal defect have a right bundle branch block pattern.

| BOX 23-1 | ECG as a Clue to Acute Life-Threatening Conditions without Primary Heart or Lung Disease |
|---|---|

Cerebrovascular accident (especially intracranial bleed)
Drug toxicity
   Tricyclic antidepressant overdose
Electrolyte disorders
   Hypokalemia
   Hyperkalemia
   Hypocalcemia
   Hypercalcemia
Endocrine disorders
   Hypothyroidism
   Hyperthyroidism
Hypothermia

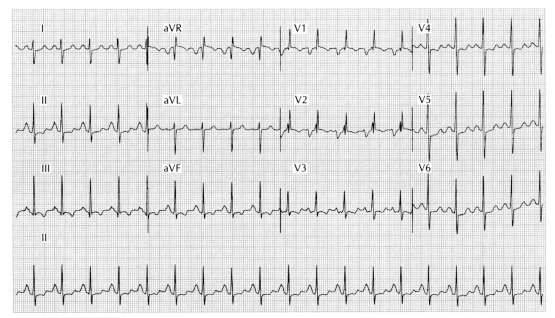

**FIGURE 23-1** This ECG from a 45-year-old woman with severe mitral stenosis shows multiple abnormalities. The rhythm is sinus tachycardia. Right axis deviation and a tall R wave in lead $V_1$ indicate right ventricular hypertrophy. The prominent biphasic P wave in lead $V_1$ indicates left atrial abnormality (enlargement). The tall P wave in lead II may indicate concomitant right atrial enlargement (biatrial abnormality). Nonspecific ST-T changes and incomplete right bundle branch block are also present. The combination of right ventricular hypertrophy and left atrial abnormality (enlargement) is highly suggestive of mitral stenosis.

- *Hyperkalemia*

Severe hyperkalemia, a life-threatening electrolyte abnormality, virtually always produces ECG changes, beginning with T wave peaking, loss of P waves, QRS widening, and finally asystole (see Chapter 10).

- *Renal failure*

The triad of LVH (caused by hypertension), peaked T waves (caused by hyperkalemia), and prolonged QT interval (caused by hypocalcemia) should suggest chronic renal failure.

- *Thyroid disease*

The combination of low voltage and sinus bradycardia should suggest possible *hypothyroidism*. ("Low and slow—think hypo.")

Unexplained AF (or sinus tachycardia at rest) should prompt a search for *hyperthyroidism*.

- *Chronic lung disease*

The combination of low voltage and slow precordial R wave progression is commonly seen with chronic obstructive lung disease.

- *Cardiomyopathy*

The ECG-CHF (congestive heart failure) triad of relatively low limb lead voltage, prominent precordial voltage, and slow R wave progression suggests an underlying dilated cardiomyopathy (see Chapter 11).

## COMMON APPLICATIONS OF THE ECG

The ECG may also provide important and immediately available clues in the evaluation of such major medical problems as *syncope*, *coma*, *shock*, and *weakness*.

## SYNCOPE

Fainting (transient loss of consciousness) can result from primary cardiac factors and various noncardiac causes. The primary cardiac causes can be divided into mechanical obstructions (aortic stenosis, primary pulmonary hypertension, or atrial myxoma) and electrical problems (bradyarrhythmias or tachyarrhythmias). The noncardiac causes of syncope include neurogenic mechanisms (e.g., vasovagal attacks), orthostatic (postural) hypotension, and brain dysfunction from vascular insufficiency or metabolic derangements (e.g., from alcohol or hypoglycemia).

Patients with syncope resulting from aortic stenosis generally show LVH on their resting ECG. Primary pulmonary hypertension is most common in young and middle-aged adult women. The ECG generally shows RVH. The presence of frequent VPBs may be a clue to intermittent sustained VT. Evidence of previous Q wave MI with syncope should suggest the possibility of sustained monomorphic VT. Syncope with QT(U) prolongation should suggest torsades de pointes, a potentially lethal ventricular arrhythmia (see Chapter 16). A severe bradycardia (usually from heart block or sick sinus syndrome) in a patient with syncope constitutes the Stokes-Adams syndrome (see Chapter 17). In some cases, serious arrhythmias can be detected only when long-term monitoring is performed. Syncope in a patient with ECG evidence of bifascicular block (e.g., RBBB with left anterior fascicular block) should prompt a search for intermittent second- or third-degree heart block or other arrhythmias. Syncope in patients taking dofetilide, quinidine, sotalol, and related drugs may be associated with torsades de pointes or other arrhythmias.

Selected patients with *unexplained syncope* may benefit from invasive electrophysiologic testing. During these studies, the placement of intracardiac electrodes permits more direct and controlled assessment of sinoatrial (SA) node function, atrioventricular (AV) conduction, and the susceptibility to sustained ventricular or supraventricular tachycardias.

## COMA

An ECG should be obtained in all comatose patients. If coma is from MI with subsequent cardiac arrest (anoxic encephalopathy), diagnostic ECG changes related to the infarct are usually seen. Subarachnoid hemorrhage or certain other types of central nervous system pathology may cause very deep T wave inversions (see Fig. 9-11), simulating the changes of MI. When coma is associated with hypercalcemia, the QT interval is often short. Myxedema coma generally presents with ECG evidence of sinus bradycardia and low voltage. Widening of the QRS complex in a comatose patient should also always raise the possibility of drug overdose (tricyclic antidepressant or phenothiazine) or hyperkalemia. The triad of a wide QRS, a prolonged QT interval, and sinus tachycardia is particularly suggestive of tricyclic antidepressant overdose (see Fig. 10-5A).

## SHOCK

An ECG should be obtained promptly in patients with severe hypotension because MI is a major cause of shock (cardiogenic shock). In other cases, hypotension may be caused or worsened by a bradyarrhythmia or tachyarrhythmia. Finally, some patients with shock from noncardiac causes (e.g., hypovolemia or diabetic ketoacidosis) may have myocardial ischemia and sometimes MI as a *consequence* of their initial problem.

## WEAKNESS

An ECG may be helpful in evaluating patients with unexplained weakness. Elderly or diabetic patients, in particular, may have relatively "silent" MIs with minimal or atypical symptoms, such as the onset of fatigue or general weakness. Distinctive ECG changes may also occur with certain pharmacologic and metabolic factors (e.g., hypokalemia or hypocalcemia) that cause weakness (Chapter 10).

## COMMON PITFALLS IN ECG INTERPRETATION

You can minimize errors in interpreting ECGs by taking care to analyze *all* the points listed in the first section of Chapter 22. Many mistakes result from the failure to be systematic. Other mistakes result from confusing ECG patterns that are "look-alikes." Important reminders are provided in Box 23-2. Some common pitfalls in ECG interpretation are discussed in the following sections.

| BOX 23-2 | **Some Important Reminders** |
|---|---|

Check standardization.

Exclude limb lead reversal. (For example, a negative P wave with a negative QRS complex in lead I suggests a left/right arm electrode switch.)

Look for hidden P waves, which may indicate atrioventricular (AV) block, blocked atrial premature beats, or atrial tachycardia with block.

With a regular narrow-complex tachycardia at about 150 beats/min at rest, consider atrial flutter with 2:1 block versus paroxysmal supraventricular tachycardia or (less likely) sinus tachycardia.

With group beating (clusters of QRS complexes), consider Mobitz type I (Wenckebach) block or blocked atrial premature beats.

With wide QRS complexes and with short PR intervals, consider the Wolff-Parkinson-White preexcitation pattern.

With wide QRS complexes without P waves or with AV block, think of hyperkalemia.

Unless recognized and corrected, inadvertent reversal of limb lead electrodes can cause diagnostic confusion. For example, reversal of the left and right arm electrodes can cause an apparent rightward QRS axis shift as well as an abnormal P wave axis that simulates an ectopic atrial or junctional rhythm (Fig. 23-2). As a general rule, *when lead I shows a negative P wave and a negative QRS, reversal of the left and right arm electrodes should be suspected.*

Voltage can appear abnormal if standardization is not checked. Many ECGs are mistakenly thought to show "high" or "low" voltage when the voltage is actually normal but the standardization marker is set at half standardization or two-times normal sensitivity.

Atrial flutter with 2:1 block is one of the most commonly missed diagnoses. The rhythm is often misdiagnosed as sinus tachycardia (mistaking part of a flutter wave for a true P wave) or PSVT. *When you see a narrow-complex tachycardia with a ventricular rate of about 150 beats/min, you should always consider atrial flutter* (see Fig. 15-3).

Coarse atrial fibrillation and atrial flutter are sometimes confused. When the fibrillatory (f) waves are prominent (coarse), the rhythm is commonly mistaken for atrial flutter. With AF, however, the ventricular rate is erratic, and the atrial waves are not exactly consistent from one segment to the next. With pure atrial flutter, the atrial waves are identical from one moment to the next, even when the ventricular response is variable (Fig 23-3).

The Wolff-Parkinson-White (WPW) pattern is frequently mistaken for bundle branch block, hypertrophy, or infarction because the preexcitation results in a wide QRS complex and may cause increased QRS voltage, T wave inversions, and pseudoinfarction Q waves (see Fig. 12-3).

Isorhythmic AV dissociation and complete heart block can be confused. With isorhythmic AV dissociation, the SA and AV node pacemakers become "desynchronized," and the QRS rate

## Lead Reversal

ARM ELECTRODES
REVERSED                                          CORRECTED ECG

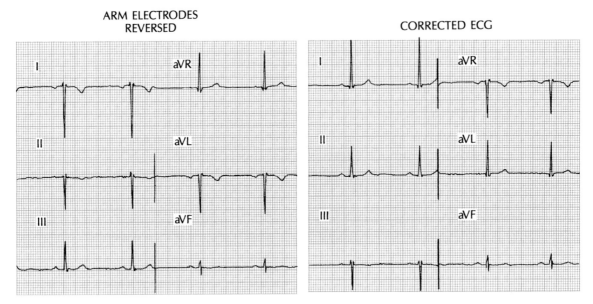

**FIGURE 23-2**   Whenever the QRS axis is unusual, limb lead reversal may be the problem. Most commonly, the left and right arm electrodes become switched so that lead I shows a negative P wave and a negative QRS complex.

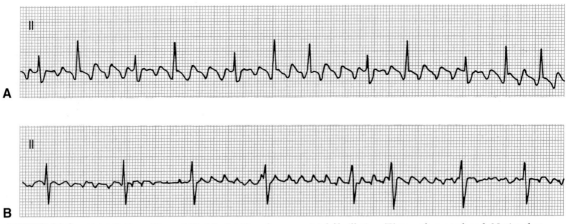

**FIGURE 23-3**   Atrial flutter with variable block **(A)** and coarse atrial fibrillation **(B)** are often confused. Notice that with atrial fibrillation the ventricular rate is completely erratic and the atrial waves are not identical from segment to segment, as they are with atrial flutter.

is the same as or slightly faster than the P wave rate (see Chapter 17). With complete heart block, the atria and ventricles also beat independently, but the ventricular rate is much slower than the atrial (sinus) rate. Isorhythmic AV dissociation is usually a minor arrhythmia, although it may reflect conduction disease or drug toxicity (e.g., digitalis, diltiazem, verapamil, and beta blockers). Complete heart block is always a major arrhythmia and generally requires pacemaker therapy.

Normal-variant and pathologic Q waves require special attention. Remember that Q waves may be a normal variant as part of QS waves in leads $aV_R$, $aV_L$, $aV_F$, III, $V_1$, and occasionally $V_2$ (see Chapter 8). Small q waves (as part of qR waves) may occur in leads I, II, III, $aV_L$, and $aV_F$ as well as in the left chest leads ($V_4$ to $V_6$). These "septal" Q waves are less than 0.04 second in duration. On the other hand, small pathologic Q waves may be overlooked because they are not always very deep. In some cases, it may not be possible to state definitively whether or not a Q wave is pathologic.

Mobitz type I (Wenckebach) AV block is a commonly missed diagnosis. "Group beating" is an important clue to the diagnosis of this finding (see Chapter 17). The QRS complexes become grouped in clusters because of the intermittent failure of AV nodal conduction.

Hidden P waves may lead to mistakes in the diagnosis of a number of arrhythmias, including blocked APBs, atrial tachycardia with block, and second- or third-degree (complete) AV block. Therefore you must search the ST segment and T wave for buried P waves (see Fig. 18-3).

Multifocal atrial tachycardia (MAT) and AF are often confused because the ventricular response in both is usually rapid and irregular. With MAT, you need to look for multiple different P waves. With AF, you must be careful not to mistake the sometimes "coarse" f waves for actual P waves.

LBBB may be mistaken for infarction because it is associated with poor R wave progression and, often, ST segment elevation in the right chest leads.

U waves are sometimes overlooked. Small U waves are a physiologic finding, but large U waves (which may only be apparent in the chest leads) are sometimes an important marker of hypokalemia or drug toxicity (e.g., sotalol). Large U waves may be associated with increased risk of torsades de pointes (see Fig. 16-17).

Severe hyperkalemia must be considered immediately in any patient with an unexplained wide QRS complex, particularly if P waves are not apparent. Delay in making this diagnosis can be fatal because severe hyperkalemia may lead to asystole and cardiac arrest while the clinician is waiting for the laboratory report (see Figs. 10-5 and 10-6).

## SPECIAL TOPIC: PEDIATRIC ELECTROCARDIOGRAPHY

The normal ECG patterns seen in children differ considerably from those in adults. The topic of pediatric electrocardiography falls outside the scope of this book (see Bibliography), but a few critical points of difference between pediatric and adult ECGs are mentioned briefly. The normal ECG of a neonate resembles the pattern seen in RVH, with tall R waves in the right chest leads and right axis deviation. The QRS complex, however, is very narrow at about 0.04 sec (Fig. 23-4).

During the first decade of life, the T waves in the right to middle chest leads are normally inverted. This pattern, which sometimes persists into adolescence and adulthood, is called the *juvenile T wave variant*. Children and young adults may also have high voltage in the chest leads as a normal variant (see Chapter 6).

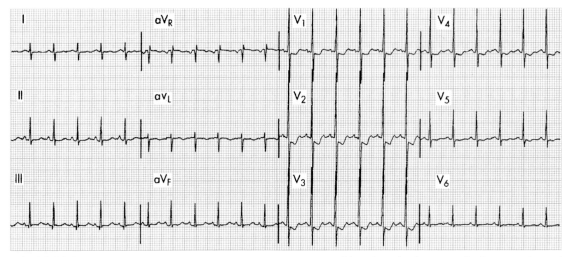

**FIGURE 23-4** The ECG of this healthy neonate shows a pattern resembling that of right ventricular hypertrophy, with tall right precordial R waves and right axis deviation. This pattern reflects the physiologic predominance of the right ventricle during fetal development. Notice also the sinus tachycardia and relatively narrow QRS complexes.

## REVIEW

Like most clinical tests, the ECG yields both *false-positive* and *false-negative* diagnoses. For example, not all Q waves indicate myocardial infarction (MI) and not all patients with actual MI show diagnostic ECG changes. A normal or nondiagnostic ECG also does not exclude left ventricular hypertrophy, right ventricular hypertrophy, intermittent life-threatening bradyarrhythmias or tachyarrhythmias, pulmonary embolism, or pericarditis.

Despite limitations in sensitivity and specificity, the ECG can provide valuable information in a wide range of clinical situations, including the evaluation of general major medical problems such as syncope, coma, weakness, and shock.

## QUESTIONS

1. Which arrhythmias can lead to syncope (fainting)?

   *True or false* (Questions 2 and 3):

2. A normal exercise tolerance test excludes significant coronary disease.

3. The more false-positive results associated with a particular test, the less sensitive the test is.

# CHAPTER 24

# ECG Differential Diagnoses

Instant reviews

This chapter presents 15 boxes that review selected aspects of ECG differential diagnosis for easy reference. For the most part, the boxes recap topics covered in this book. Some advanced topics are briefly mentioned, with additional discussion available in references cited in the Bibliography.

---

**Wide QRS Complex**

I. Intrinsic intraventricular delay (IVCD)*
  A. Left bundle branch block and variants
  B. Right bundle branch block and variants
  C. Other (nonspecific) patterns of IVCD
II. Extrinsic ("toxic") intraventricular delay
  A. Hyperkalemia
  B. Drugs: class I antiarrhythmic drugs and other sodium-channel blocking agents (e.g., tricyclic antidepressants and phenothiazines)
III. Ventricular beats: premature, escape, or paced
IV. Ventricular preexcitation: Wolff-Parkinson-White pattern and variants

---

*Bundle branch block patterns may occur transiently. Note also that a spuriously wide-appearing QRS complex occurs if the ECG is unintentionally recorded at fast paper speeds (e.g., 50 mm/sec).

---

**Low-Voltage QRS Complexes**

1. Artifactual or spurious (especially unrecognized standardization of the ECG at half the usual gain, i.e., 5 mm/mV). Always check this first!
2. Adrenal insufficiency (Addison's disease)
3. Anasarca (generalized edema)
4. Cardiac infiltration or replacement (e.g., amyloid, tumor)
5. Cardiac transplantation, especially with acute or chronic rejection
6. Cardiomyopathies*
7. Chronic obstructive pulmonary disease
8. Constrictive pericarditis
9. Hypothyroidism/myxedema (usually with sinus bradycardia)
10. Left pneumothorax (mid-left chest leads)
11. Myocardial infarction, usually extensive
12. Myocarditis, acute or chronic
13. Normal variant
14. Obesity
15. Pericardial effusion/tamponade (latter usually with sinus tachycardia)
16. Pleural effusions

---

*Dilated cardiomyopathies may be associated with a combination of relatively low limb-lead voltage and prominent precordial voltage.

## Right Axis Deviation

I. Spurious: left-right arm electrode reversal (look for negative P wave and negative QRS complex in lead I)
II. Normal variant
III. Dextrocardia
IV. Right ventricular overload
   A. Acute (e.g., pulmonary embolus or severe asthmatic attack)
   B. Chronic
      1. Chronic obstructive pulmonary disease
      2. Any cause of right ventricular hypertrophy (e.g., pulmonic stenosis or primary pulmonary hypertension)
V. Lateral wall myocardial infarction
VI. Left posterior fascicular block (exclude all other causes of right axis deviation)

## QT Prolongation (Long QT Syndromes)

I. Acquired long QT syndromes
   A. Electrolyte abnormalities
      1. Hypocalcemia
      2. Hypokalemia
      3. Hypomagnesemia
   B. Drugs
      1. Class IA or III antiarrhythmic agents (e.g., amiodarone, disopyramide, dofetilide, ibutilide, procainamide, quinidine, and sotalol)
      2. Psychotropic agents (e.g., phenothiazines, tricyclic antidepressants, tetracyclic agents, and haloperidol)
      3. Others: astemizole, terfenadine, bepridil, certain antibiotics (e.g., erythromycin and pentamidine), probucol, cisapride, etc.
   C. Myocardial ischemia or infarction (with deep T wave inversions)
   D. Cerebrovascular injury
   E. Bradyarrhythmias (especially high-grade AV heart block)
   F. Systemic hypothermia
   G. Miscellaneous conditions
      1. Liquid protein diets
      2. Starvation
      3. Myocarditis
      4. Arsenic poisoning
II. Congenital (hereditary) long QT syndromes
   A. Romano-Ward syndrome (autosomal dominant)
   B. Jervell and Lange-Nielsen syndrome (autosomal recessive with congenital deafness)

## Q Waves

I.  Physiologic or positional factors
   A.  Normal-variant septal Q waves
   B.  Normal-variant Q waves in leads V1, V2, aV$_L$, III, and aV$_F$
   C.  Left pneumothorax (acute loss of lateral R wave progression)
   D.  Dextrocardia (chronic loss of lateral R wave progression)
II.  Myocardial injury or infiltration
   A.  Acute processes
      1.  Myocardial ischemia or infarction
      2.  Myocarditis
      3.  Hyperkalemia
   B.  Chronic processes
      1.  Myocardial infarction
      2.  Idiopathic cardiomyopathy
      3.  Myocarditis
      4.  Amyloid
      5.  Tumor
      6.  Sarcoid
III.  Ventricular hypertrophy or enlargement
   A.  Left ventricular hypertrophy (slow R wave progression*)
   B.  Right ventricular hypertrophy (reversed R wave progression†) or slow R wave progression (particularly with chronic obstructive lung disease)
   C.  Hypertrophic cardiomyopathy (may simulate anterior, inferior, posterior, or lateral infarcts)
IV.  Conduction abnormalities
   A.  Left bundle branch block (slow R wave progression*)
   B.  Wolff-Parkinson-White patterns

*Small or absent R waves are seen in the right to mid-precordial leads.
†The R wave amplitude decreases progressively from lead V1 to the mid-lateral precordial leads.

## Tall R Wave in Lead V$_1$

I.  Physiologic and positional factors
   A.  Misplacement of chest leads
   B.  Normal variants
   C.  Displacement of heart toward right chest
II.  Myocardial injury
   A.  Posterior and/or lateral myocardial infarction
   B.  Duchenne's muscular dystrophy
III.  Ventricular enlargement
   A.  Right ventricular hypertrophy (usually with right axis deviation)
   B.  Hypertrophic cardiomyopathy
IV.  Altered ventricular depolarization
   A.  Right ventricular conduction abnormalities
   B.  Wolff-Parkinson-White patterns (caused by posterior or lateral wall preexcitation)

## ST Segment Elevations

I.  Myocardial ischemia/infarction
   A.  Noninfarction, transmural ischemia (Prinzmetal's angina pattern)
   B.  Acute myocardial infarction
   C.  Post–myocardial infarction (ventricular aneurysm pattern)
II.  Acute pericarditis
III.  Normal variant ("early repolarization" pattern)
IV.  Left ventricular hypertrophy (LVH)/left bundle branch block (LBBB) (V$_1$–V$_2$ or V$_3$ and other leads with QS or rS waves, only)
V.  Brugada pattern (right bundle branch block (RBBB)–like pattern with ST elevations in right precordial leads)
VI.  Other (rarer)
   A.  Myocardial injury (non-infarction)
      1.  Myocarditis (ECG may resemble myocardial infarction or pericarditis patterns)
      2.  Tumor invading the left ventricle
      3.  Trauma to the ventricles
   B.  Hypothermia (J waves/Osborn waves)
   C.  Hyperkalemia (usually localized to V$_1$ and V$_2$)

## ST Segment Depressions

I.   Myocardial ischemia or infarction
   A. Acute subendocardial ischemia or non–Q wave myocardial infarction
   B. Reciprocal change with acute transmural ischemia
II.  Abnormal noncoronary patterns
   A. Left or right ventricular hypertrophy (formerly called "strain" pattern)
   B. Secondary ST-T changes
     1. Left bundle branch block
     2. Right bundle branch block
     3. Wolff-Parkinson-White preexcitation pattern
   C. Drugs (e.g., digitalis)
   D. Metabolic conditions (e.g., hypokalemia)
   E. Miscellaneous conditions (e.g., cardiomyopathy)
III. Physiologic and normal variants*

*With physiologic and normal variants, the often-transient ST segment/J point depressions are usually less than 1 mm and are seen especially with exertion or hyperventilation.

## Prominent T Wave Inversions

I.    Normal variants
   A. "Juvenile" T wave pattern
   B. Early repolarization variants
II.   Myocardial ischemia/infarction
III.  Cerebrovascular accident (especially intracranial bleeds) and related neurogenic patterns
IV.   Left or right ventricular overload/dysfunction
   A. Typical patterns (formerly referred to as "strain" patterns)
   B. Apical hypertrophic cardiomyopathy (Yamaguchi syndrome)
   C. Other cardiomyopathies
V.    Idiopathic global T wave inversion syndrome
VI.   Secondary T wave alterations: bundle branch blocks, Wolff-Parkinson-White patterns
VII.  Intermittent left bundle branch block, preexcitation, or ventricular pacing ("memory T waves")

## Tall Positive T Waves

I.   Nonischemic causes
   A. Normal variants (early repolarization patterns)
   B. Hyperkalemia
   C. Cerebrovascular hemorrhage (more commonly, T wave inversions)
   D. Left ventricular hypertrophy
   E. Right precordial leads, usually in conjunction with left precordial ST depressions and T wave inversions
   F. Left precordial leads, particularly in association with "diastolic overload" conditions (e.g., aortic or mitral regurgitation)
   G. Left bundle branch block (right precordial leads)
   H. Acute pericarditis (occasionally)
II.  Ischemic causes
   A. Hyperacute phase of myocardial infarction
   B. Acute transient transmural ischemia (Prinzmetal's angina)
   C. Chronic (evolving) phase of myocardial infarction (tall positive T waves reciprocal to primary deep T wave inversions)

## Major Bradycardias

I.   Sinus bradycardia and its variants, including sinoatrial block
II.  Atrioventricular (AV) heart block* or dissociation
   A. Second- or third-degree AV block
   B. Isorhythmic AV dissociation and related variants
III. Junctional (AV nodal) escape rhythms
IV.  Atrial fibrillation or flutter with a slow ventricular response
V.   Ventricular escape rhythms (idioventricular rhythms)

*AV heart block may occur with sinus rhythm or other rhythms (e.g., atrial fibrillation or flutter).

## Major Tachycardias

I. Narrow QRS complex
 A. Sinus tachycardia
 B. Paroxysmal supraventricular tachycardias (PSVTs),* a class of arrhythmias with three major mechanisms:
  1. Atrial tachycardias, including single-focus or multifocal (MAT) variants
  2. AV nodal reentrant tachycardia (AVNRT)
  3. AV reentrant tachycardia (AVRT) involving a bypass tract
 C. Atrial flutter
 D. Atrial fibrillation
II. Wide QRS complex
 A. Ventricular tachycardia (three or more consecutive premature ventricular beats at a rate ≥ 100 beats/min)
 B. Supraventricular tachycardia or atrial fibrillation or flutter, with aberrant ventricular conduction usually caused by either of the following:
  1. Bundle branch block patterns
  2. Atrioventricular bypass tract (Wolff-Parkinson-White preexcitation patterns)

*Nonparoxysmal supraventricular tachycardias may also occur, including certain types of junctional tachycardia, as well as incessant tachycardias caused by increased atrial automaticity or a slowly conducting bypass tract.

## Atrial Fibrillation: Causes and Contributors

1. Alcohol abuse ("holiday heart")
2. Autonomic factors
 a. Sympathetic (occurring during exercise or stress)
 b. Vagotonic (occurring during sleep)
3. Cardiothoracic surgery
4. Cardiomyopathies or myocarditis
5. Congenital heart disease
6. Coronary artery disease
7. Hypertensive heart disease
8. Idiopathic ("lone" atrial fibrillation)
9. Obstructive sleep apnea
10. Paroxysmal supraventricular tachycardias or the Wolff-Parkinson-White preexcitation syndrome
11. Pericardial disease (usually chronic)
12. Pulmonary disease (e.g., chronic obstructive pulmonary disease)
13. Pulmonary emboli
14. Sick sinus syndrome (brady-tachy variants)
15. Thyrotoxicosis (hyperthyroidism)
16. Valvular heart disease (particularly mitral valve disease)

## Digitalis Toxicity: Major Arrhythmias

I. Bradycardias
  A. Sinus bradycardia, including sinoatrial block
  B. Junctional (nodal) escape rhythms*
  C. Atrioventricular (AV) heart block,* including the following:
    1. Mobitz type I (Wenckebach) AV block
    2. Complete heart block*
II. Tachycardias
  A. Accelerated junctional rhythms and nonparoxysmal junctional tachycardia
  B. Atrial tachycardia with block
  C. Ventricular ectopy
    1. Ventricular premature beats
    2. Monomorphic ventricular tachycardia
    3. Bidirectional ventricular tachycardia
    4. Ventricular fibrillation

*Junctional rhythms may occur with underlying atrial fibrillation leading to slow or regularized ventricular response. AV dissociation without complete heart block may also occur.

## Cardiac Arrest: Three Basic ECG Patterns

1. Ventricular tachyarrhythmia
  a. Ventricular fibrillation (or ventricular flutter)
  b. Sustained ventricular tachycardia (monomorphic or polymorphic)
2. Ventricular asystole (standstill)
3. Pulseless electrical activity (electromechanical dissociation)

# Self-Assessment Problems

# FOUR

The final section of this textbook is a collection of 50 ECGs for review and self-assessment. These unknowns have been selected to challenge students and others who have completed the text or to serve as a stand-alone examination for clinicians who wish to take a board review–type "pretest."

Each question comes with a short case description. (Helpful clues are sometimes provided.) Students are encouraged to write down their findings and compare their interpretations with the "official" answers given at the end of the section. Each question is worth 2 points. A perfect score is 100!

This section also gives answers to questions posed at the end of most chapters. Additional ECG questions and answers are freely available at a number of Internet sites including the *ECG Wave-Maven: Self-Assessment Program for Students and Clinicians* (http://ecg.bidmc.harvard.edu). This site includes more than 250 practice ECGs.

# Questions

## LIFE SAVERS: STAT ECG DIAGNOSES

The following five patients all have different life-threatening problems that you can diagnose from their ECGs without any further history.

*Case 1* 60-year-old man

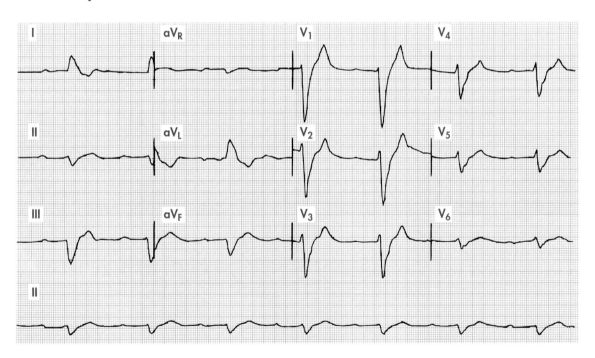

## Case 2 50-year-old man

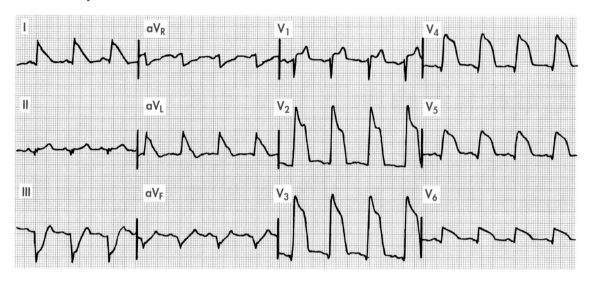

## Case 3 68-year-old man

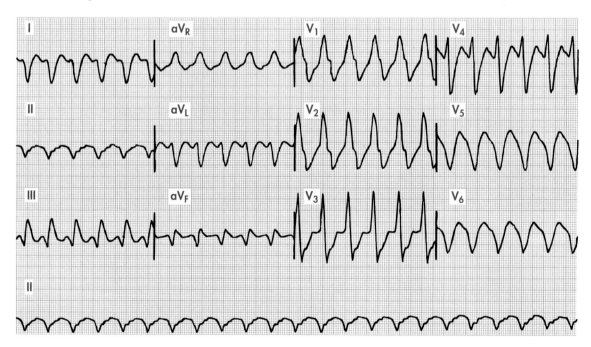

*Case 4* 75-year-old woman

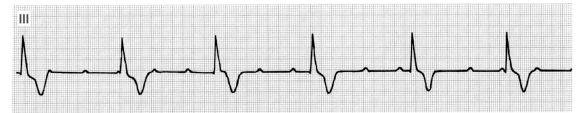

*Case 5* 52-year-old man

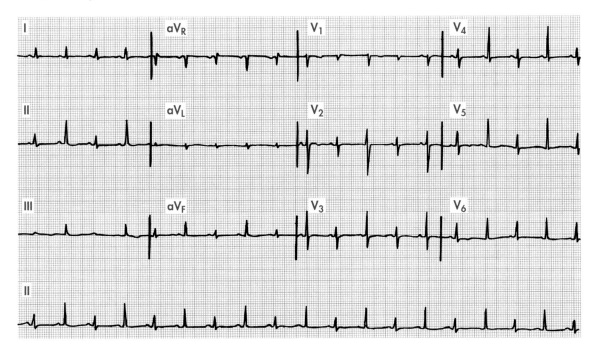

## TRIAGE TRYOUT

These patients arrive in your office at the same time. Both complain of severe chest pain. One ambulance and one taxicab are available for transporting them to the nearest hospital, which is five miles away. What do you do?

*Case 6* 50-year-old man with chest pain

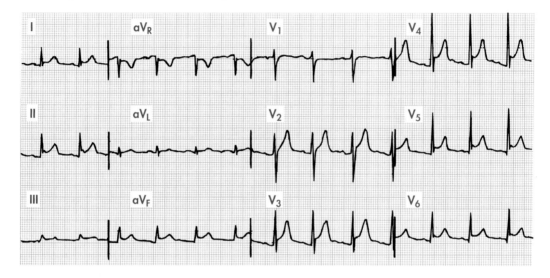

*Case 7* 50-year-old man with chest pain

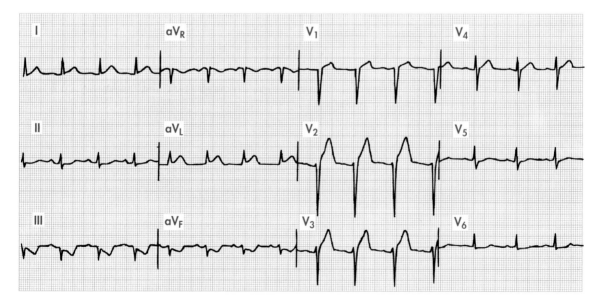

## FOUR CASES OF MISTAKEN IDENTITY

The following ECGs are commonly incorrectly identified as shown. For each ECG, what is your correct diagnosis?

*Case 8* "Left bundle branch block or left ventricular hypertrophy with inferior myocardial infarction"

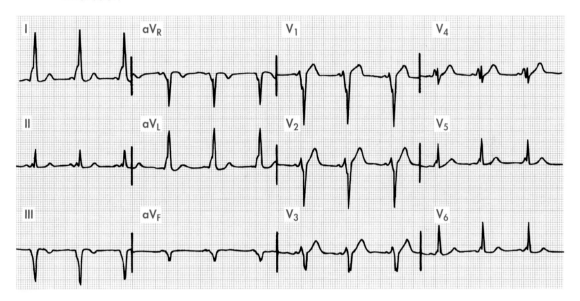

*Case 9* "Complete heart block"

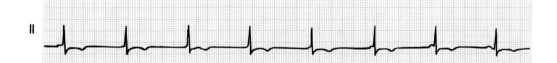

*Case 10* "Sinus (or ectopic atrial) tachycardia"

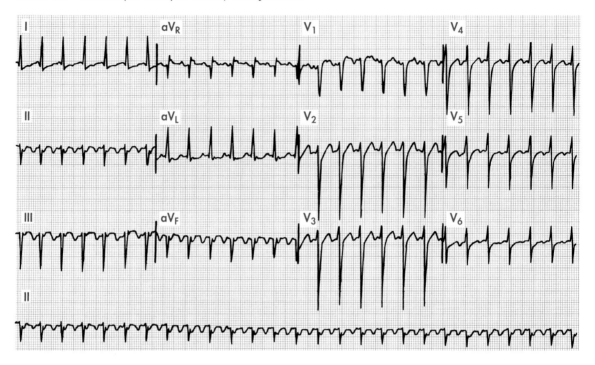

*Case 11* "Right axis deviation resulting from lateral wall infarction"

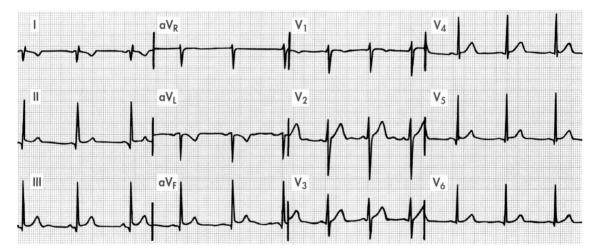

## SYNCOPATED RHYTHMS

Both of these patients are complaining of an irregular heartbeat. What are the diagnoses?

*Case 12*

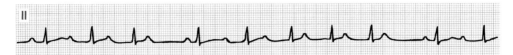

*Case 13*

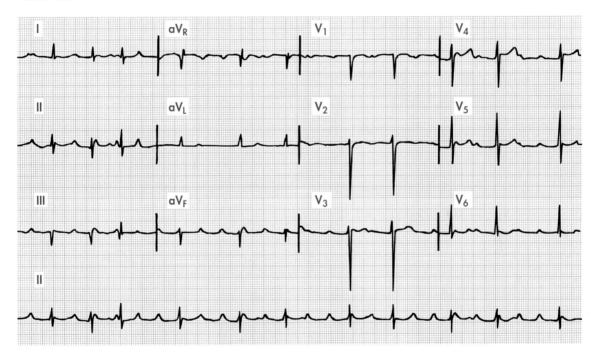

## INCOMPLETE DIAGNOSES OF COMPLETE RIGHT BUNDLE BRANCH BLOCK

Right bundle branch block was correctly diagnosed in these two patients with chest pain. That is only part of the story, however. What else is going on?

*Case 14*

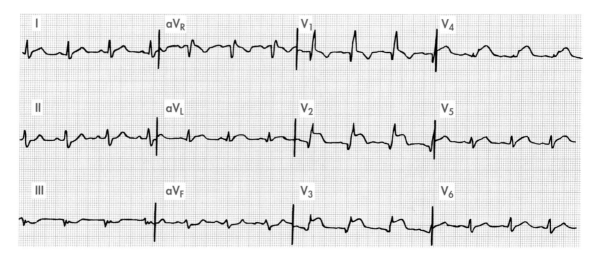

*Case 15*

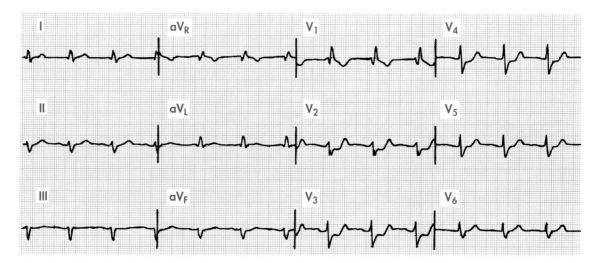

## MORPHING P WAVES

What subtle arrhythmia is present in this ECG?

*Case 16*

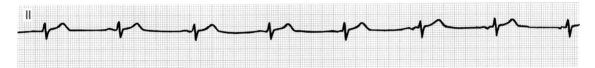

## TEARFUL PATIENT

Why is this very healthy female crying? (Clue: Consider QRS duration.)

*Case 17*

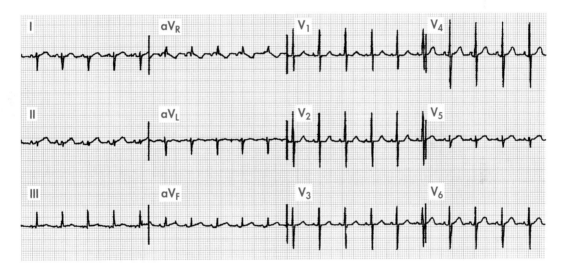

## TRICKY BUSINESS

An ECG is obtained in this 45-year-old businessman before he undergoes appendectomy. He complains of lower left quadrant pain. The ECG is unchanged from a previous one, at which time the workup revealed normal cardiac function. What is the diagnosis?

*Case 18*

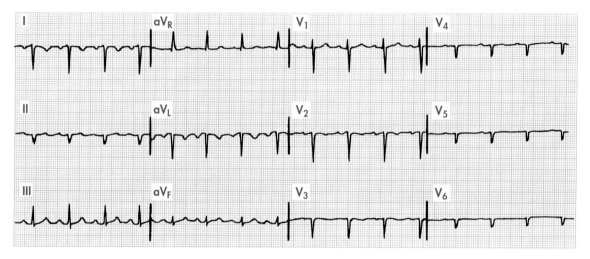

## HEART FAILURE AFTER MYOCARDIAL INFARCTION

Two months after having a myocardial infarction, this 75-year-old man presents with rales on chest auscultation and an S3 gallop. His ECG is unchanged from a month ago and cardiac enzymes are negative. What does the ECG show?

*Case 19*

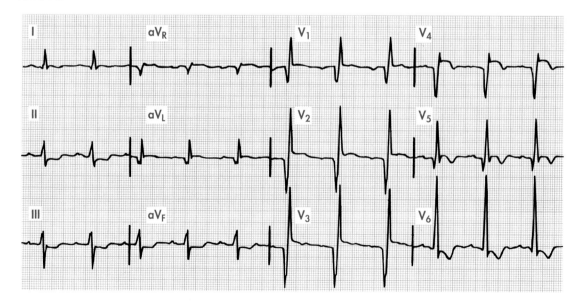

# COMMON THEME

These elderly women have heart failure, and both complain of nausea. What are the two arrhythmias? What is the probable common underlying problem?

*Case 20* (Clue: Previous ECGs showed atrial fibrillation with a rapid rate.)

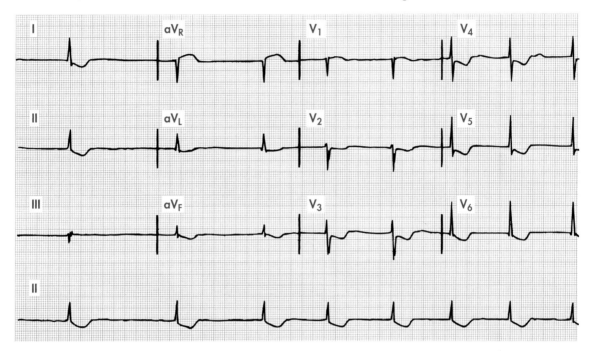

*Case 21* (Clue: Double-check leads II and $V_1$.)

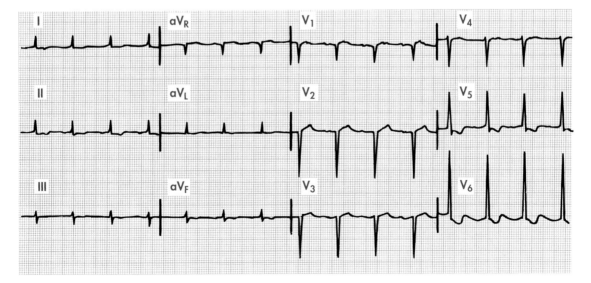

## DRUG DILEMMA

This ECG (from a patient with normal electrolytes) is most consistent with therapy using which one of the following drugs?

a. Digoxin

b. Captopril

c. Amiodarone

d. Metoprolol

e. Verapamil

f. None of the above

*Case 22*

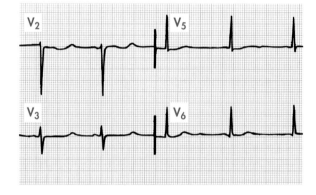

## NARROWED-DOWN DIFFERENTIAL DIAGNOSES

The following patients both have narrowed heart valves. One has mitral stenosis, and the other has pulmonic stenosis. Can you tell which is which?

*Case 23*

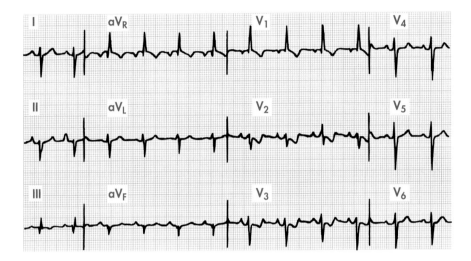

*Case 24*

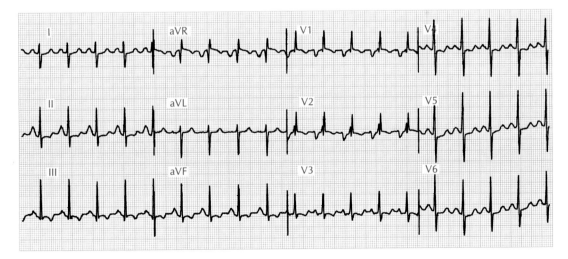

## PAUSE FOR THOUGHT

A 72-year-old woman has intermittent light-headedness. What does the ECG lead show?

*Case 25*

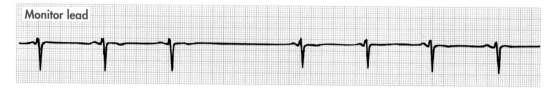

## LOOK-ALIKE TACHYCARDIAS

The following patients both complain of a fast heartbeat. One has atrial flutter with 2:1 block. The other has paroxysmal supraventricular tachycardia (PSVT) due to atrioventricular nodal reentrant tachycardia (AVNRT). Can you tell which is which?

*Case 26*

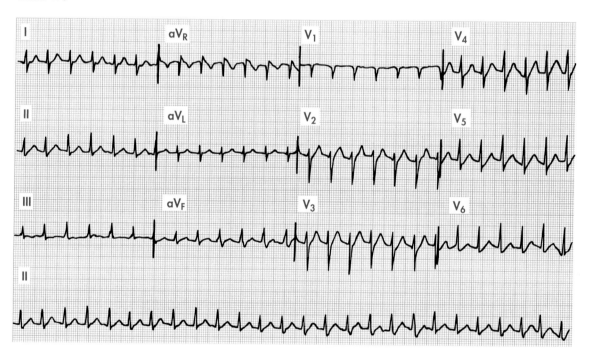

## Case 27

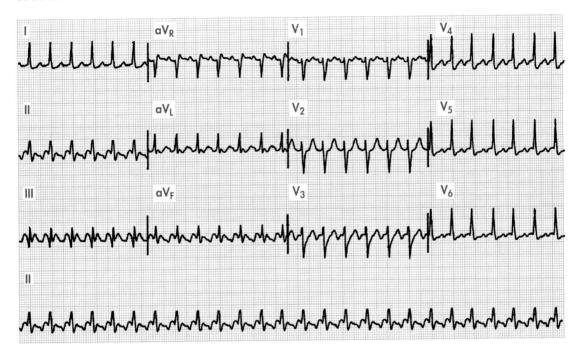

## SILENT HISTORY

A 75-year-old man has an ECG before undergoing cataract surgery. He denies previous cardiac problems. What does his ECG show?

## Case 28

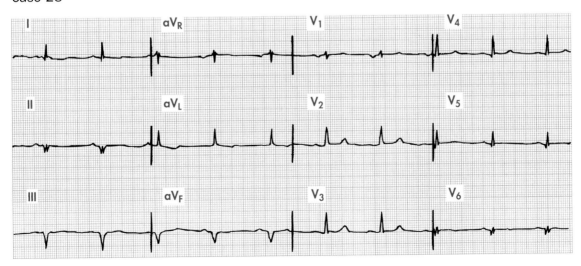

## THREE PATIENTS WITH RECURRENT SYNCOPE

The following three patients (Cases 29–31) had recurrent episodes of fainting. Can you diagnose the cause in each case?

*Case 29* 21-year-old woman on no medications with normal serum electrolyte values

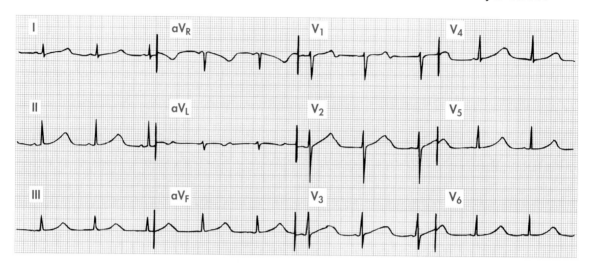

*Case 30* 37-year-old man

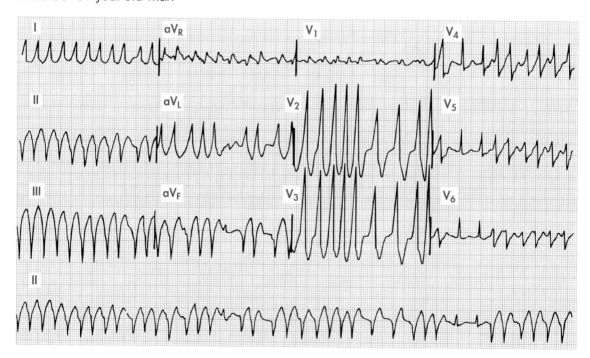

*Case 31* 75-year-old woman

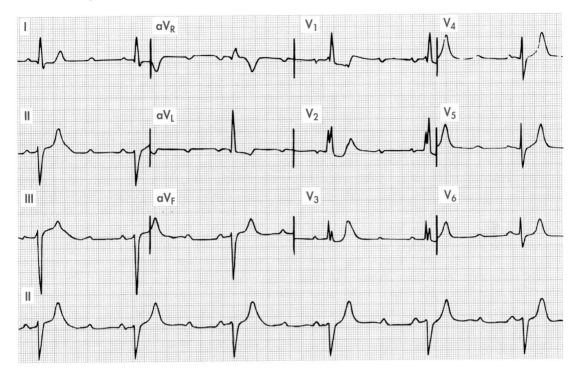

## HEARTBURN

This 52-year-old man has indigestion, nausea, and an irregular pulse. What is the rhythm? What is the underlying problem?

*Case 32*

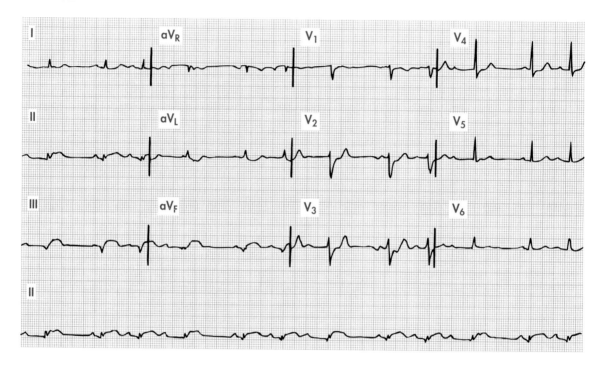

## HIDDEN P WAVE "ST-ORIES"

Can you diagnose these two arrhythmias?

*Case 33*

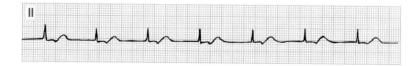

*Case 34*

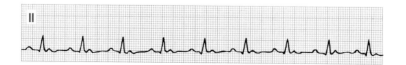

## MYOCARDIAL INFARCTION SIMULATOR

This 46-year-old man has chest pain and dyspnea. Initially, he was thought to have had a myocardial infarction. What alternative life-threatening diagnosis would account for all these findings?

*Case 35*

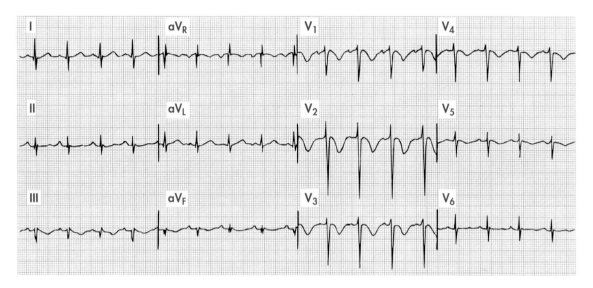

## IRREGULAR BEHAVIOR

The following highly irregular rhythms are often confused. What is the arrhythmia in each case?

*Case 36*

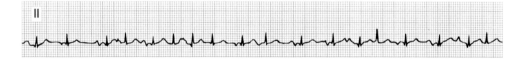

*Case 37*

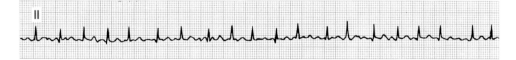

## QUICK CHANGES

These two rhythm strips show underlying sinus rhythm with abrupt changes in cardiac electrical activity and intermittent wide QRS complexes. What are the diagnoses?

*Case 38*

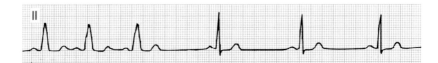

*Case 39*

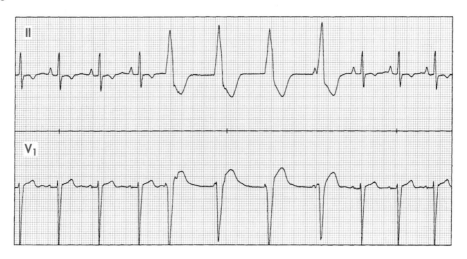

## MISSING BIFOCALS

A middle-aged cardiologist left his bifocals at home and missed the following diagnosis. (Clue: see arrow.)

*Case 40*

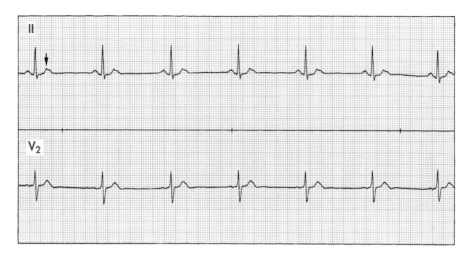

## LONG AND SHORT OF IT

Both of these patients have mental status changes. Can you diagnose the cause from the ECG alone? (Clue: The key to their treatable diagnoses relates to the beginning of the ST segment.)

*Case 41* 30-year-old woman

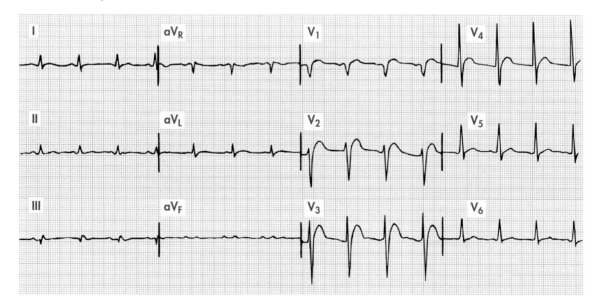

## Case 42 65-year-old man

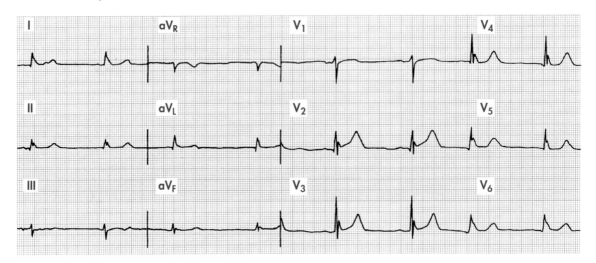

## PACEMAKER PLUS

This 78-year-old man has a VVI pacemaker for complete heart block. He comes into your office with shortness of breath and evidence of pulmonary edema. In addition to the expected pacemaker pattern, what does his ECG show?

## Case 43

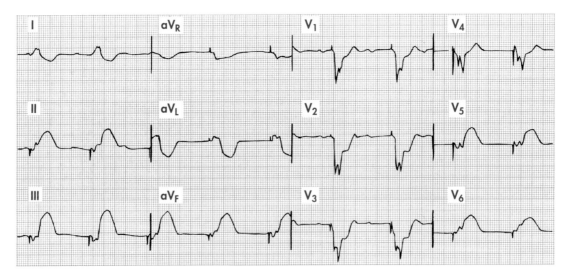

## ECG/CORONARY ARTERIOGRAM MATCHUP

Which ECG (A to D) goes best with which story for these four middle-aged men?

*Case 44* This man had chest pain 3 days ago. His creatine kinase level is now normal. He has an occluded large left circumflex coronary artery and a severe inferoposterolateral wall motion abnormality.

*Case 45* This man has had chest pain for the past 4 hours. His creatine kinase level is 800 U/L (normal: less than 200 U/L). He has three-vessel coronary disease with 80% to 90% proximal stenoses and anterior wall hypokinesis.

*Case 46* This man had chest pain 1 month ago, but his creatine kinase level is now normal. Currently, he is complaining of dyspnea. He has an occluded proximal left anterior descending coronary artery with an anterior wall aneurysm.

*Case 47* This man has had chest pain for 12 hours with a normal creatine kinase level. His coronary arteries and ventricular wall motion are normal.

**A**

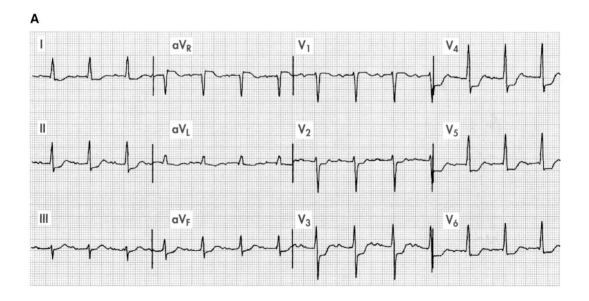

**B**

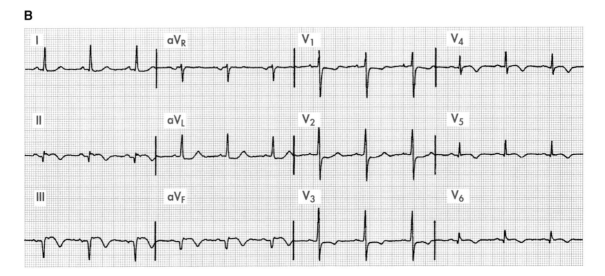

**C**

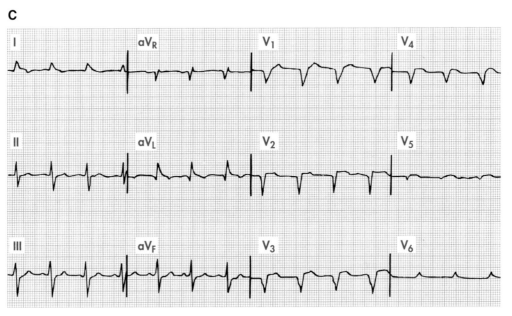

**D**

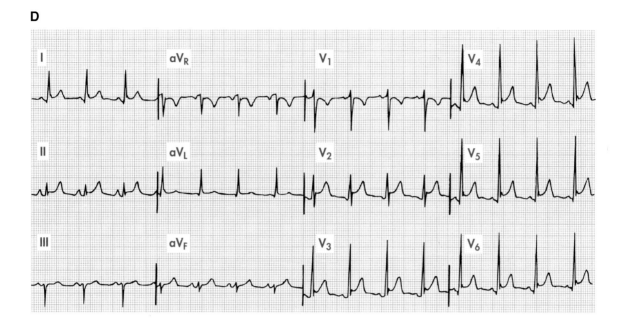

## CALCULATION LEADS TO DIAGNOSIS

A 40-year-old woman complains about feeling weak. She is not taking any medication. Based on the ECG, what laboratory values do you want checked?

*Case 48*

Lead II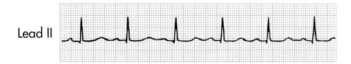

## INTEREST-PIQUING T WAVES

What underlying condition explains all findings? Additive clues: QRS voltage, P waves, and QT$_c$.

*Case 49*

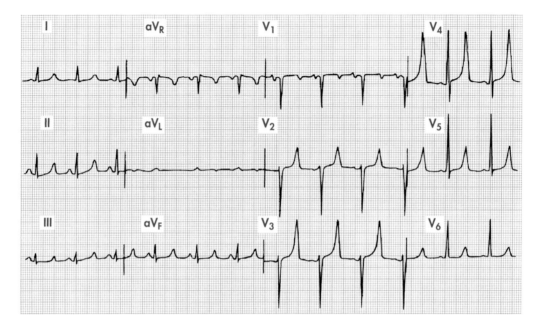

## FITTING FINALE

*Case 50*

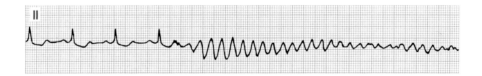

# Answers to Self-Assessment Problems

## Case 1

Severe hyperkalemia. Note the markedly prolonged PR interval peaked T waves and widened QRS complex.

## Case 2

Hyperacute phase of anterior wall ST elevation myocardial infarction. Note the marked ST elevations in leads $V_1$ through $V_6$, I, and $aV_L$, with reciprocal ST depressions in leads III and $aV_F$. Q waves are present in leads $V_3$ through $V_6$. Also note left axis deviation with possible prior inferior wall infarction.

## Case 3

Sustained monomorphic ventricular tachycardia. Note the wide-complex tachycardia (QRS duration up to 0.20 sec) with a wide R wave in lead $V_1$, a QS wave in lead $V_6$, and extreme axis deviation.

## Case 4

Sinus rhythm with complete (third-degree) heart block. Note the idioventricular (or very slow junctional) rhythm at about 33 beats/min.

## Case 5

Sinus tachycardia with *electrical alternans.* This combination is highly specific for pericardial effusion with tamponade. (See Chapter 11.)

## Case 6

Acute pericarditis. Note the *diffuse* ST elevations (leads I, II, III, $aV_F$, and $V_3$ through $V_6$) with PR segment deviations (up in lead $aV_R$, down in leads $V_4$, $V_5$, and $V_6$). This patient gets the taxi.

## Case 7

Acute ST elevation anterior myocardial infarction. ST elevations are *localized* to leads $V_1$, $V_2$, $V_3$, I, and $aV_L$, with poor R wave progression in leads $V_1$, $V_2$, and $V_3$. In addition, note the *reciprocal* ST depressions in leads II, III, and $aV_F$. This patient needs an ambulance *immediately.*

## Case 8

Wolff-Parkinson-White (WPW) pattern. Note the triad of short PR intervals, wide QRS complexes, and delta waves (i.e., slurring of the early part of the QRS complexes in leads I, $aV_L$, $V_1$, $V_2$, and so forth).

## Case 9

Sinus rhythm with isorhythmic AV dissociation.

## Case 10

Atrial flutter with 2:1 AV block.

## Case 11

Left-right arm lead reversal, which accounts for the negative P waves and negative QRS complexes in lead I.

## Case 12
Sinus rhythm with Wenckebach-type AV block.

## Case 13
Atrial tachycardia at 150 beats/min with variable AV block.

## Case 14
Right bundle branch block with acute anterior Q wave myocardial infarction. Note the Q waves in leads $V_1$, $V_2$, and $V_3$, with ST elevations in leads $V_1$ through $V_5$ and $aV_L$.

## Case 15
Right bundle branch block with anterior subendocardial ischemia. Note the ST depressions in leads $V_2$, $V_3$, and $V_4$.

## Case 16
Wandering atrial pacemaker.

## Case 17
Normal (and hungry) neonate. Note the very narrow QRS complex (about 0.06 sec) with a rightward axis, tall R wave in lead $V_1$, and fast sinus rate (125 beats/min). All of these findings are appropriate for the patient's age (see Chapter 23).

## Case 18
Dextrocardia with situs inversus. Note the apparently reversed limb and chest leads. This patient has a normal heart (right side of chest) and an inflamed appendix (left side of lower abdomen!).

## Case 19
Sinus rhythm with prolonged PR interval. The ECG shows left atrial abnormality, left ventricular hypertrophy, and right bundle branch block. Q waves and ST elevations are seen in leads $V_1$ through $V_5$, I, and $aV_L$. The findings are consistent with left ventricular aneurysm, which was confirmed with echocardiography.

## Case 20
Atrial fibrillation with a *slow* and at times *regularized* ventricular response should make you suspect digitalis toxicity. ST-T changes are consistent with digitalis toxicity or ischemia, in particular.

## Case 21
Atrial tachycardia with 2:1 AV block. (A very subtle "extra" P wave in the ST segment is best seen in leads $V_1$ and $V_2$.) An important cause of this arrhythmia is digitalis toxicity. The ECG shows low voltage in the extremity (limb) leads. Because of the poor R wave progression, this patient may have had a previous anterior myocardial infarction. Based on precordial voltage, left ventricular hypertrophy is present. ST-T changes are consistent with digitalis toxicity, ischemia, left ventricular hypertrophy, and so on.

The theme common to Cases 20 and 21, therefore, is *digitalis toxicity.*

## Case 22
c. Amiodarone. Note the markedly prolonged QT(U) interval.

## Case 23
Mitral stenosis. The ECG shows signs of right ventricular hypertrophy (i.e., relatively tall R waves in lead $V_1$ with right axis deviation) and left atrial abnormality.

## Case 24
Pulmonic stenosis. The ECG shows signs of right ventricular hypertrophy (relatively tall R waves in lead $V_1$ with right axis deviation) and right atrial abnormality.

## Case 25
2:1 sinoatrial (SA) block causes an entire P-QRS-T cycle to be "dropped." This patient has symptomatic *sick sinus syndrome* and requires a permanent pacemaker.

## Case 26
Atrioventricular nodal reentrant tachycardia (AVNRT). In some of the beats, small retrograde P waves (negative in lead II, positive in lead $aV_R$) are visible immediately after the QRS complex, at the very beginning of the ST segment.

## Case 27
Atrial flutter with 2:1 AV conduction. Note the flutter waves at a rate of 300 beats/min (e.g., leads $aV_R$ and $aV_L$).

## Case 28
Inferoposterolateral myocardial infarction. Note the Q waves in leads II, III, $aV_F$, $V_5$, and $V_6$, and the tall R waves in leads $V_1$ and $V_2$.

## Case 29

Sinus rhythm with a markedly prolonged QT(U) interval (about 0.6 sec). This patient has a hereditary type of long QT syndrome. Syncope was caused by recurrent episodes of a *torsades de pointes*–type of ventricular tachycardia.

## Case 30

Atrial fibrillation with Wolff-Parkinson-White (WPW) syndrome. The clue to the diagnosis is the *extremely rapid wide-complex tachycardia* (about 300 beats/min at times) with a very *irregular* rate.

## Case 31

Sinus rhythm at 100 beats/min with advanced second-degree atrioventricular block (3:1 conduction pattern). The QRS complexes show a bifascicular block pattern (right bundle branch block and left anterior fascicular block). Evidence of left atrial abnormality and left ventricular hypertrophy is also present. Note that one of the P waves is partly hidden in the T waves (see $V_1$). The patient required a permanent pacemaker.

## Case 32

Sinus rhythm at 95 beats/min with a 4:3 Wenckebach AV block. Note the group beating pattern. This arrhythmia was due to an acute/evolving Q wave inferior myocardial infarction.

## Case 33

Junctional rhythm at 60 beats/min. Note the negative P waves "hidden" at the end of the ST segments.

## Case 34

Atrial tachycardia with 2:1 AV block. Note the "hidden" P wave in the ST segments. The atrial rate is 160 beats/min with a ventricular rate of 80 beats/min.

## Case 35

Acute cor pulmonale, in this case due to massive pulmonary embolism. Note the sinus tachycardia, $S_1Q_{III}$ pattern, poor R wave progression, and prominent anterior T wave inversions, caused here by right ventricular overload (formerly called "strain").

## Case 36

Multifocal atrial tachycardia (MAT).

## Case 37

Atrial fibrillation (AF).

## Case 38

Sinus rhythm with intermittent left bundle branch block. First, three sinus beats are conducted with a left bundle branch block pattern; the next three beats occur with a normal QRS complex. Note the rate slowing, which is associated with normalization of the QRS complex. Therefore the left bundle branch block here is related to increase in the rate (acceleration- or tachycardia-dependent bundle branch block).

## Case 39

Sinus rhythm with transient accelerated idioventricular rhythm.

## Case 40

Sinus rhythm with *atrial bigeminy* and blocked atrial premature beats. The arrow points to a subtle P wave from an atrial premature beat. This beat came so early that it cannot conduct through the AV node, which is still refractory after the previous sinus beat.

## Case 41

Hypercalcemia. Note the short QT interval with very abbreviated ST segment; thus the T wave appears to take off right from the end of the QRS complex.

## Case 42

Hypothermia. Note the characteristic J (Osborn) waves, best seen in leads $V_3$, $V_4$, and $V_5$.

## Case 43

Acute inferolateral myocardial infarction superimposed on a ventricular pacemaker pattern. Note the ST elevations in leads II, III, $aV_F$, $V_5$, and $V_6$, and the reciprocal ST depressions in leads $V_1$, $V_2$, and $V_3$.

## Case 44

B. Diffuse ST depressions (except in lead $aV_R$), most marked in the anterior leads. These findings are consistent with non–Q wave myocardial infarction.

## Case 45

A. Q waves and ST-T changes consistent with evolving inferoposterolateral myocardial infarction.

## Case 46

C. Q waves and persistent ST elevations consistent with anterior wall myocardial infarction and ventricular aneurysm.

## Case 47

D. Diffuse ST elevations and characteristic PR segment deviations, diagnostic of acute pericarditis.

## Case 48

Hypocalcemia. Calculate the $QT_C$, with $QT = 0.48$ sec and $RR = 0.85$ sec. Hence $QT_C = 0.48/\sqrt{0.85} = 0.52$. The prolonged $QT_C$ here is due to a long ST segment. The T wave is normal. Thus the most likely diagnosis is hypocalcemia. In contrast, hypokalemia generally flattens the T wave and prolongs the QT(U) interval.

## Case 49

Note the combination of the tall peaked T waves from *hyperkalemia* with the voltage criteria for left ventricular hypertrophy (LVH). (Left atrial abnormality is also present.) This combination strongly suggests *chronic renal failure,* the most common cause of hyperkalemia. Patients with hyperkalemia typically have hypertension as well, leading to LVH. QT prolongation may also be present in patients with chronic renal failure from concomitant hypocalcemia. The QT interval here is prolonged for the rate ($QT_c = .50$), which may be due to hypocalcemia, another common finding with chronic renal failure.

## Case 50

Cardiac arrest. The rhythm strip shows sinus rhythm with ST segment depressions that are consistent with *ischemia,* followed by the abrupt onset of *ventricular flutter* degenerating quickly into *ventricular fibrillation.* The treatment is defibrillation/resuscitation as described in Chapter 19.

# Answers to Chapter Questions

## Part 1 Basic Principles and Patterns

### Chapter 1
1. See Fig. 1-1.
2. An electrocardiogram (ECG) is a graph that records cardiac electrical activity by means of electrodes placed on the surface of the body.
3. True

### Chapter 2
1. **a.** 50 beats/min
   **b.** 150 beats/min
   **c.** Approximately 170 beats/min. Seventeen QRS cycles occur in 6 seconds. Notice the irregularity of the QRS complexes and the absence of P waves. This rhythm is *atrial fibrillation* (see Chapter 15).
2. **a.** Abnormally wide QRS complex (0.16 sec)
   **b.** Abnormally long PR interval (approximately 0.3 sec)
   **c.** Abnormally long QT interval (0.4 sec) for rate. The RR interval measures 0.6 sec; therefore the heart rate is 100 beats/min (see Table 2-1). The rate-corrected $(QT_c = QT/\sqrt{RR})$ is also prolonged, at 0.52 sec $(0.4/\sqrt{0.6})$. Normal is 0.44 sec or less.
3. **a.** Prolong the PR interval.
4. **b.** Prolong the QRS interval.
5. **a.** R wave
   **b.** qRS complex
   **c.** QS complex
   **d.** RSR' complex
   **e.** QR complex

6. Drugs (amiodarone, disopyramide, ibutilide, procainamide, quinidine, sotalol), electrolyte abnormalities (hypocalcemia, hypokalemia), systemic hypothermia, and myocardial infarction. See Chapter 24 for more extensive list.
7. **c.** Depolarization of the His bundle is not seen on the ECG. This physiologic event occurs during the isolectric part of the PR interval. His bundle activation, however, can be recorded using a special electrode system inside the heart during cardiac electrophysiologic (EP) procedures.

### Chapter 3
1. Lead II = lead I + lead III; therefore, according to Einthoven's equation, lead III = lead II - lead I, as shown below:

III

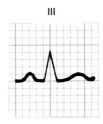

   Notice that the voltages of the P wave, QRS complex, and T wave in lead II are equal to the sum of the P, QRS, and T voltages in leads I and III.
2. The voltages in lead II do *not* equal those in leads I and III. The reason is that leads II and III

321

were mislabeled. When you reverse the labels, the voltage in lead II equals the voltages in leads I and III.

**3.** See Fig. 3-7C.

**4.** The positive poles of leads $aV_R$ and II point in opposite directions (see Fig. 3-7).

## Chapter 4

**1. a.** Yes. The P waves are positive (upright) in lead II and negative in lead $aV_R$, with a rate of about 75 beats/min.

  **b.** Electrically vertical. The R waves are most prominent in leads II, III, and $aV_F$.

  **c.** The transition zone is in lead $V_3$. Notice that the RS complexes have the R wave approximately equal to the S wave.

  **d.** The PR interval is about 0.16 sec. This is within normal range (0.12 to 0.2 sec).

  **e.** The QRS width is 0.08 sec. This is normal (less than or equal to 0.1 sec).

  **f.** Yes

**2.** No. Although a P wave appears before each QRS complex, it is negative in lead II. With sinus rhythm, the P should be positive (upright) in lead II. Thus, in this patient, the pacemaker must be outside the sinus node (ectopic), probably in a low atrial focus near the atrioventricular junction. Inverted P waves such as these are called *retrograde* because the atria are depolarized in the opposite direction from normal (i.e., from the bottom to the top rather than from the top [sinus node] to the bottom [atrioventricular junction]; see also Chapters 13 and 14).

## Chapter 5

**1.** The QRS axis is roughly +60°. Notice that the QRS complex in lead $aV_L$ is biphasic. Therefore the mean QRS axis must point at a right angle to -30°. In this case, the axis is obviously about +60° because leads II, III, and $aV_F$ are positive. Note that the R wave in lead III is slightly taller than the R wave in lead I. If the axis were exactly +60°, these waves would be equally tall. Thus the axis must be somewhat more positive than +60°, probably around +70°. Estimating the QRS axis to within 10° or 20° is usually quite adequate for clinical diagnosis.

**2.** *A*, lead II; *B*, lead I; *C*, lead III. *Explanation: If the mean QRS axis is –30°, the QRS axis is pointed*

toward lead I (which is at 0°) and away from lead III (which is at +120°). Obviously lead I must be B and lead III must be C. Lead II is A, which is biphasic. The positive pole of lead II is at +60° on the hexaxial diagram. If the mean QRS axis is -30°, lead II must show a biphasic complex because the mean QRS axis is at right angles to that lead.

**3. e.** Left anterior fascicular block (hemiblock)

## Chapter 6

**1. a.** About 75 beats/min

  **b.** The PR interval is prolonged (about 0.22 sec) indicating mild "first-degree AV block" (see Chapter 17). The P wave in lead II is also abnormally wide and notched (notice the two humps) as a result of left atrial abnormality (enlargement).

**2.** True

## Chapter 7

**1.** See Fig. 7-6.

**2. a.** 0.12 sec

  **b.** Right bundle branch block

  **c.** Secondary T wave inversions can be seen in the right chest leads with right bundle branch block (see text and answer to Question 4).

**3.** Left bundle branch block. The PR interval is also somewhat long (0.24 sec) due to prolonged AV conduction ("first-degree AV block").

**4.** *Primary* T wave abnormalities are due to actual changes in ventricular repolarization caused, for example, by drugs, ischemia, or electrolyte abnormalities. These abnormalities are independent of changes in the QRS complex. *Secondary* T wave changes, by contrast, are related entirely to alterations in the timing of ventricular depolarization and are seen in conditions in which the QRS complex is wide. For example, with bundle branch block, a change in the sequence of depolarization also alters the sequence of repolarization, causing the T wave to point in a direction opposite the last deflection of the QRS complex. Thus, with right bundle branch block, the T waves are secondarily inverted in leads with an rSR' configuration (e.g., $V_1$, $V_2$, and sometimes $V_3$) due to a delay in right ventricular repolarization. With left bundle branch block, the secondary T wave inversions are seen in leads with tall wide R waves ($V_5$ and

$V_6$) due to a delay in left ventricular repolarization. Secondary T wave inversions are also seen with ventricular paced beats (see Fig. 7-8) and the Wolff-Parkinson-White preexcitation pattern (Chapter 12). Sometimes, primary and secondary T wave changes are seen on the same ECG, as when ischemia develops in a patient with a bundle branch block (see Fig. 8-21).

5. True
6. True
7. True
8. False. It will produce a right bundle branch block pattern since the left ventricle will be stimulated before the right.

## Chapters 8 and 9

1. **a.** 100 beats/min
   **b.** Yes. In leads II, III, and $aV_F$, with reciprocal ST depressions in leads $V_2$ to $V_4$, I, and $aV_L$
   **c.** Yes. Best seen in leads III and $aV_f$
   **d.** Acute inferior wall infarction
2. **a.** About +90°. Between 80° and 90° is acceptable.
   **b.** No
   **c.** No. Notice the inverted T waves in leads $V_2$ to $V_6$, I, and $aV_1$.
   **d.** Anterior wall infarction, possibly recent or evolving
3. Reciprocally depressed
4. Ventricular aneurysm
5. **b.** Non–Q wave infarction
6. Marked ST segment depressions. This patient had severe ischemic chest pain with a non–Q wave infarct.
7. The ECG shows a right bundle branch block pattern with an evolving anterior Q wave infarct. With uncomplicated right bundle branch block, the right chest leads show an rSR′ pattern. Note that leads $V_1$, $V_2$, and $V_3$ show wide QR waves (0.12 sec) because of the anterior Q wave myocardial infarction and right bundle branch block. The ST elevations in leads $V_1$, $V_2$, and $V_3$ and the T wave inversions across the chest leads are consistent with recent or evolving myocardial infarction.
8. False. Thrombolytic therapy only has demonstrated benefit in acute ST segment elevation MI (STEMI), not with non–ST segment elevation MI.

## Chapter 10

1. **b.** Early repolarization pattern
   **d.** Ventricular aneurysm
   **g.** Pericarditis
2. **a.** Digitalis effect, B
   **b.** Hyperkalemia, A
   **c.** Hypokalemia, C
3. **b.** Hypokalemia

## Chapter 11

1. **a.** Pericardial effusion with cardiac tamponade
2. False

## Chapter 12

1. **d.** Wolff-Parkinson-White (WPW) pattern. Notice the diagnostic triad of a wide QRS complex, a short PR interval, and a delta wave (slurred initial portion of the QRS complex). Compare this with Figs. 12-3 and 12-4, which also show the WPW pattern. These patterns are sometimes mistaken for hypertrophy (tall R waves) or infarction (pseudoinfarction Q waves). The negative delta waves in lead aVL and positive waves in lead V1 are consistent with a left lateral bypass tract in this case.

### Part 2 Cardiac Rhythm Disturbances

## Chapter 13

1. Yes. The P waves are negative in lead $aV_R$ and positive in lead II. Do not be confused by the unusual QRS complexes (positive in lead $aV_R$ and negative in lead II) produced by the abnormal axis deviation. The diagnosis of normal sinus rhythm depends only on the P waves.
2. No. Each QRS complex is preceded by a P wave. Notice, however, that the P waves are negative in lead II. These retrograde P waves indicate an ectopic pacemaker, probably located in a low atrial site near the AV junction.
3. **d.** Isoproterenol
4. True

## Chapter 14

1. The palpitations could be due to occasional atrial premature beats. Notice that the fifth complex is an atrial premature beat (or possibly a junctional premature beat because the P wave is not seen).

2. Junctional escape beat. Notice that it comes after a pause in the normal rhythm and is not preceded by a P wave.
3. **a.** Approximately 210 beats/min. Count the number of QRS complexes in 6 sec and multiply by 10.
   **b. (2)** Paroxysmal supraventricular tachycardia (PSVT). A retrograde P wave may be seen just after the QRS complex, making atrioventricular nodal reentrant tachycardia (AVNRT) the most likely mechanism for the arrhythmia. A concealed bypass tract, however, cannot be excluded here.
4. False. PSVT is not a sinus rhythm variant, but is due to an ectopic rhythm originating in the atria (atrial tachycardia) or the AV node area (AV nodal reentrant tachycardia) or involving an atrioventricular bypass tract (AV reentrant tachycardia).

## Chapter 15

1. **a.** About 300 beats/min
   **b.** About 75 beats/min
   **c.** Atrial flutter with 4:1 atrioventricular (AV) conduction
2. **a.** About 70 beats/min. Count the number of QRS complexes in 6 sec and multiply by 10.
   **b.** Atrial fibrillation. This is a subtle example because the fibrillatory waves are of very low amplitude. The diagnosis of atrial fibrillation is suspected when an irregular ventricular response is found along with fine wavering of the baseline between QRS complexes.
3. Slower
4. Faster
5. False
6. False

## Chapter 16

1. Ventricular tachycardia (monomorphic)
2. Torsades de pointes. Notice the changing orientation and amplitude of the QRS complexes with this type of polymorphic ventricular tachycardia. Contrast this type of polymorphic ventricular tachycardia with the monomorphic ventricular tachycardia in Question 1, where all QRS complexes are the same.
3. Hypoxemia, digitalis or other drug toxicity, hypokalemia, hypomagnesemia (see text)
4. Sinus rhythm with ventricular bigeminy

## Chapter 17

1. **a.** Sinus rhythm with AV Wenckebach block. Notice the succession of P waves, with increasing PR intervals followed by a nonconducted (dropped) P wave. This pattern leads to "group beating." Blocked premature atrial complexes can also cause group beating, but the nonconducted P wave comes early (before the next sinus P wave is due). The P waves in this example come on time.
2. **a.** 100 beats/min
   **b.** 42 beats/min
   **c.** No
   **d.** Sinus rhythm with complete heart block. Notice that some of the P waves are hidden in QRS complexes or T waves.
3. True.

## Chapter 18

1. Hypokalemia, hypomagnesemia, hypoxemia, acute myocardial infarction, renal failure (Other answers can be found in the text of Chapter 18.)
2. True
3. False
4. False
5. True
6. False
7. True

## Chapter 19

1. No. By definition, patients with electromechanical dissociation have relatively normal electrical activity. The problem is that this electrical activity is not associated with adequate mechanical (pumping) action, due, for example, to diffuse myocardial injury, pericardial tamponade, or severe loss of intravascular volume. A pacemaker would not help in this situation because the patient's heart already has appropriate electrical stimulation.
2. **a.** Idioventricular escape rhythm
   **b.** External cardiac compression artifacts
3. Digitalis (digoxin), epinephrine, cocaine, flecainide (also quinidine, procainamide, disopyramide, ibutilide, dofetilide, and most other antiarrhythmic agents)

## Chapter 20

1. **a.** Irregular
   **b.** No. The baseline shows an irregular fibrillatory pattern.
   **c.** Atrial fibrillation

**2.** Ventricular tachycardia

**3.** Paroxysmal supraventricular tachycardia (probably atrioventricular nodal reentrant tachycardia; see Chapter 14)

**4.** Sinus rhythm with 2:1 AV block, indicated by a sinus rate of about 74 beats/min and a ventricular rate of about 37 beats/min

**5.** Digitalis toxicity, excess beta blocker, excess calcium channel blocker (e.g., verapamil or diltiazem), amiodarone, lithium carbonate, hyperkalemia, hypothyroidism

## Chapter 21

**1. b.** Symptomatic bradyarrhythmia

**2. b.** Failure to pace. In this example of intermittent failure to pace, the fourth pacemaker spike is not followed by a QRS complex. The two most common causes of failure to pace (with a pacemaker spike that does not capture) are dislodgment of the electrode wire and fibrosis around the pacing wire tip. In some cases of pacemaker failure, no pacing spikes are seen (see Fig. 21-9).

**3.** Atrial pacing. Notice the sharp pacemaker spike before each P wave, which is followed by a normal QRS complex (see Fig. 21-3).

**4. b.**

**5.** False.

## Chapter 23

**1.** Syncope can be caused by a variety of bradyarrhythmias or tachyarrhythmias, including marked sinus bradycardia, sinus arrest, atrioventricular (AV) junctional escape rhythms, second- or third-degree AV block, atrial fibrillation with an excessively slow ventricular response, sustained ventricular tachycardia, paroxysmal supraventricular tachycardias (PSVTs), and atrial fibrillation or flutter with a rapid ventricular response.

**2.** False

**3.** False. The sensitivity of a test is a measure of how well the test can detect a given abnormality. False-positive results (abnormal results in normal subjects) lower a test's specificity, not its sensitivity.

# Bibliography

## BASIC CONCEPTS

Berne RM, Levy MN: Cardiovascular Physiology, 8th ed. St. Louis, Mosby, 2001.

Fisch C: Centennial of the string galvanometer and the electrocardiogram. J Am Coll Cardiol 2000;26:1737–1745.

Mirvis DM: Electrocardiography: A Physiologic Approach. St. Louis, Mosby, 1993.

## NORMAL AND ABNORMAL ECG PATTERNS

Ashley EU, Raxwal VK, Froelicher VF: The prevalence and prognostic significance of electrocardiographic abnormalities. Curr Probl Cardiol 2000;25:1–72.

Goldberger AL: Myocardial Infarction: Electrocardiographic Differential Diagnosis, 4th ed. St. Louis, Mosby, 1991.

Mirvis DM, Goldberger AL: Electrocardiography. In Zipes D, Libby P, Bonow RO, Braunwald E: Braunwald's Heart Disease: A Textbook of Cardiovascular Medicine, 7th ed. Philadelphia, WB Saunders, 2004.

Park MK, Guntheroth WG: How to Read Pediatric ECGs, 3rd ed. St. Louis, Mosby, 1992.

Surawicz B, Knilans TK: Chou's Electrocardiography in Clinical Practice, 5th ed. Philadelphia, WB Saunders, 2001.

## ARRHYTHMIAS, PACEMAKERS, AND IMPLANTABLE CARDIOVERTER DEFIBRILLATORS

Josephson ME: Clinical Cardiac Electrophysiology, 3rd ed. Philadelphia, Lippincott Williams & Wilkins, 2002.

Saksena S, Camm AJ, Boyden PA, Dorian P, Goldschlager N: Electrophysiological Disorders of the Heart. Philadelphia, Churchill Livingstone, 2005.

Zipes D: Cardiac arrhythmias. In Zipes D, Libby P, Bonow RO, Braunwald E: Braunwald's Heart Disease: A Textbook of Cardiovascular Medicine, 7th ed. Philadelphia, WB Saunders, 2004.

Zipes D, Jalife J: Cardiac Electrophysiology: From Cell to Bedside, 3rd ed. Philadelphia, WB Saunders, 2004.

## FREE WEB-BASED ECG/ARRHYTHMIA RESOURCES

American College of Cardiology. ECG of the month: http://www.acc.org/education/online/

American Heart Association: www.americanheart.org

Heart Rhythm Society: www.hrsonline.org

Medical Multimedia Laboratories. SVT tutorial: www.blaufuss.org

Nathanson LA, McClennen S, Safran C, Goldberger AL: ECG Wave-Maven: Self-Assessment Program for Students and Clinicians: http://ecg.bidmc.harvard.edu

327

Note: Page numbers followed by f refer to figures; page numbers followed by t refer to tables.